Goldberger
on
Pellagra

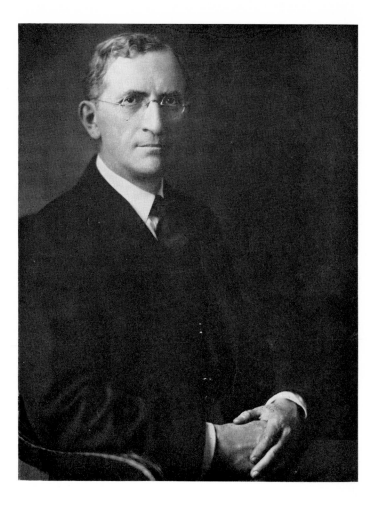

Joseph Goldberger

Goldberger
on
Pellagra

Edited, with an Introduction by

MILTON TERRIS

Professor of Preventive Medicine

New York Medical College

Louisiana State University Press : Baton Rouge

Editor's Preface

The seventeen papers included in this volume have been chosen to present the most significant publications on pellagra by Joseph Goldberger and his associates. The complete list of fifty-four publications appears in the appendix.

The papers are reproduced in their entirety with the exception of certain tables, figures, and appendices which were not considered essential. These deletions have been noted in the text. The tables have been renumbered and the references have been arranged in a uniform style in order to maintain the unity of the text.

The editor wishes to acknowledge the patient, discerning, and invaluable editorial assistance of Mrs. Dorothy C. Clair.

Contents

List of Tables

Goldberger
on
Pellagra

Introduction

It is a curious fact that American epidemiology reveres *Snow on Cholera*[1] as the classic demonstration of epidemiologic method and neglects its own masterpiece, the work of Joseph Goldberger on pellagra.

Snow on Cholera was published by the Commonwealth Fund in 1936. The first edition was exhausted in 1945, and a second printing was undertaken in 1949 to satisfy the urgent requests from schools of public health. It has since maintained an honored place in the epidemiology curriculum. The Broad Street pump which Snow immortalized has become a veritable symbol of the public health movement; it is not uncommon for those who deplore our backwardness in coping with new health problems to blame this on our "Broad Street pump fixation."

On the other hand, the "Rankin Farm" and the "Seven Cotton-Mill Villages of South Carolina," where Goldberger and Edgar Sydenstricker did much of their basic work, have no such place of honor. Goldberger's investigation of pellagra, the American classic of epidemiology, has remained buried on the back shelves of medical libraries, hidden in the massive red volumes of old *Public Health Reports*, gathering dust for more than three decades.

Perhaps one of the reasons for this contrast in appreciation is that Americans really do venerate antiquity and will accept a work as a classic only if published in a previous century. Another explanation might be that despite multiple signs of fierce independence, we still suffer feelings of inferiority and tend to place a greater value on British products than on our native articles.

It is evident that much of American public health derives directly from British theory and practice. Stephen Smith, the founder and first president of the American Public Health Association, tells us that when he wrote the initial draft of the Metropolitan Health Law of New York he "was guided chiefly in its details by the English sanitary laws."[2] The outstanding theoretician of the American public health movement for the past half century, C.-E. A. Winslow, states that "the impulse of the 'great sanitary awakening' actually came to

---

1 *Snow on Cholera* (New York: The Commonwealth Fund, 1936).
2 M. P. Ravenel (ed.), *A Half Century of Public Health* (New York: American Public Health Association, 1921).

us in this country from London" and that Lemuel Shattuck's *Report of the Massachusetts Sanitary Commission* "drew its inspiration directly from Chadwick and Simon."[3] Winslow himself, coming from a background of ten generations of New England stock, also looked to England for inspiration and example and urged us "to go forward step by step, in the tentative and experimental fashion which is characteristic of British and American social progress."[4]

Whether such general influences have played any role in the differential treatment accorded to the work of Snow and Goldberger, it is difficult to say. There was, however, a direct and immediate factor which was responsible for the emphasis placed on Snow's work by American epidemiologists. This was the influence of Wade Hampton Frost, Professor of Epidemiology at The Johns Hopkins School of Hygiene and Public Health. For almost twenty years, from 1919 until his death in 1938, Frost was the leading teacher of epidemiology in the United States. Since Johns Hopkins trained students from all parts of the globe, his influence was world-wide, and it has been continued and extended by his students, many of whom now hold the highest academic and official positions.

It was no accident that Frost wrote the introduction to *Snow on Cholera*, which he considered to be "a nearly perfect model."[5] As Kenneth Maxcy, his close collaborator and successor to the chair of epidemiology at Johns Hopkins wrote: "Frost profoundly admired Snow's achievement—his accurate and painstaking observations, his patient collection of facts and clear and exact statement, his coldly logical reasoning, his restraint, his confidence in his methods, and his courage in following through the implications of an analysis which brought him into direct conflict with the authoritative opinion of his day. In his admiration for Snow, Frost revealed himself. In Snow's work, he had found an example of the perfection for which he had been striving throughout his career."[6]

There is no question that Frost's admiration for Snow's "nearly perfect model" of epidemiologic study is eminently justified. Brilliant as it was, however, Snow's work on cholera remained necessarily at the level of observation. It could not achieve the additional certainty of experimental demonstration because the fatal character of the dis-

---

3 C.-E. A. Winslow, *The Evolution and Significance of the Modern Public Health Campaign* (New Haven: Yale University Press, 1923).
4 *Ibid.*
5 *Snow on Cholera.*
6 K. F. Maxcy (ed.), *Papers of Wade Hampton Frost, M.D.* (New York: The Commonwealth Fund, 1941).

ease precluded human experimentation. As a model of epidemiologic study, therefore, it must be considered incomplete.

Although Frost recognized the importance of experimental research, his own work was concerned entirely with observational studies of the distribution of diseases in communities and with the development of techniques and methods appropriate to such investigations. Goldberger, on the other hand, was a master of both observation and experiment. His investigation of Schamberg's disease in 1909 provides a brief but impressive illustration of the Goldberger style of investigation:

The cause of the peculiar affection which we are considering was until recently very obscure. During the months of May and June, 1909, an outbreak (20 cases) of this eruptive disease developed among the crew upon a private yacht docked in the Delaware River. At almost the same time 33 more cases appeared among the crews of 4 other boats. Besides these 53 cases we learned in the course of our investigation of about 70 other cases in 20 different private residences and boarding houses scattered about the city of Philadelphia and its vicinity. In practically every case we were able to determine that the patient had either recently slept upon a new straw mattress or had freely handled the same. The facts elicited by our inquiry enabled us to exclude from consideration the jute or cotton topping or the ticking of the mattresses and we satisfied ourselves that the essential causative factor was connected with the wheat straw. The mattresses were made by 4 of the leading manufacturers, all of whom received a large proportion if not quite all of their straw from the same source in New Jersey.

In order to establish the etiological role of the straw mattresses experimentally, one of us[7] exposed his (left) bare arm and shoulder for one hour between two straw mattresses. At the end of about 16 hours the characteristic itching eruption appeared. Later 3 volunteers slept upon a mattress during a night and each one developed the eruption at the end of about the same period.

We next took some of the straw and sifted such particles as would pass through the meshes of a fine flour sieve. The sifted particles were divided into two portions and placed in two clean glass Petri dishes. One of these was then applied for one hour to the left axilla of a volunteer. At the end of about 16 to 18 hours the characteristic eruption was present in the area of the left axilla to which the Petri dish of straw siftings had been applied.

Having therefore determined not only by deduction from the epidemiological facts but by experiment that the straw in the straw mattresses was in some way capable of producing the eruption we next sought in the straw for the responsible factor. First we exposed for an hour the second

7 This was Goldberger. R. P. Parsons, *Trail to Light, a Biography of Joseph Goldberger* (Indianapolis: Bobbs-Merrill, 1943).

portion of the siftings in a Petri dish to the vapour of chloroform under a bell jar with a view to killing any insect or acarine that might be present. These siftings were then applied to the right axilla of the volunteer to whose left axilla the untreated siftings were applied. While, as has been stated, the application of the untreated siftings was followed by the appearance of the characteristic eruption, the skin to which the chloroformized siftings were applied remained perfectly normal. We inferred, therefore, that the essential causative factor residing in the straw had been killed by the chloroform fumes. Careful scrutiny of some of the fresh siftings from the straw disclosed the presence of a small almost microscopic mite. Five of these mites were fished out, placed in a clean watch crystal and then applied to the axilla of another volunteer. At the end of about 16 hours following this application 5 of the characteristic lesions appeared on the area to which the mites had been applied.

We established, therefore, that the minute mite which we fished out of the straw siftings was the factor in the straw that was responsible for the production of the eruption. This mite was identified for us by Mr. Nathan Banks, expert in acarina of the United States Bureau of Entomology, as very close to, if not identical with, *Pediculoides ventricosus*.[8]

Goldberger's work on Schamberg's disease is an admirable example of the synthesis of observation and experiment to provide an incontrovertible answer to an epidemiologic problem. It is a little gem, a miniature classic which foreshadows his later achievement in pellagra.

That achievement did not occur by accident. It was the culmination of years of field and laboratory study during which Goldberger learned the tools of the epidemiologist's trade and sharpened the cutting edge of an incisive intellect.

Joseph Goldberger was an immigrant Jew who grew up in New York City's Lower East Side, studied engineering for two years at the City College of New York, and then switched careers to enter Bellevue Hospital Medical College. He graduated with honors in 1895, interned at Bellevue Hospital, practiced unsuccessfully in New York City and successfully in Wilkes-Barre, Pennsylvania, and then joined the United States Public Health Service in 1899.

For several years Goldberger served as a quarantine officer at various ports, including Tampico and Vera Cruz, Mexico. Here he studied yellow fever and its transmission by mosquitoes and assisted

8 J. Goldberger and J. F. Schamberg, "Epidemic of an Urticarioid Dermatitis Due to a Small Mite *(Pediculoides ventricosus)* in the Straw of Mattresses," *Public Health Rep.*, Vol. 24 (1909), 973–75.

Dr. Milton Rosenau, chief of the Hygienic Laboratory, in yellow fever and malaria studies. In 1905 he was one of a group of Public Health Service officers, including C. H. Lavinder and Wade Hampton Frost, assigned to control the yellow fever epidemic in New Orleans. It was at this point that he did his first experimental work—curiously enough, with humans—in a study with Rosenau on the hereditary transmission of the yellow fever virus in the mosquito. Rosenau and Goldberger allowed the progeny of heavily infected mosquitoes to feed on thirteen nonimmune men with negative results.

Goldberger conducted a sanitary survey of the drainage basin of the Potomac River, made other studies related to the investigation of typhoid fever in Washington, D.C., investigated dengue in Texas, and carried on painstaking research on parasitic worms in the Hygienic Laboratory's department of zoology. In 1909 he solved in very short order the epidemiology of Schamberg's disease and in that year began his important work on typhus fever with John F. Anderson, Director of the Hygienic Laboratory.

Anderson and Goldberger succeeded in producing typhus fever in monkeys by intraperitoneal inoculation of blood from human cases of tabardillo, the typhus fever of Mexico. They then attempted to demonstrate that typhus fever is louse-borne on the basis of epidemiological reasoning that provides some striking parallels to the logic which Goldberger used four years later in his remarkable first paper on pellagra:

The peculiarities of the epidemiology of tabardillo must strike even the most casual reader who is familiar with the advances in our knowledge of the role of insects in disease transmission as highly suggestive of the existence of an intermediary host. We were very early convinced that this disease is not contagious, using this word in its ordinary sense. We could cite a long series of facts, both from the literature and from our own observations, in support of this view. We shall, however, content ourselves with citing the following:

F. J., adult, American, nonimmune, lived at a hotel in Mexico City, but came in daily intimate contact with cases of tabardillo between November 22 and December 16, 1909. On the nights of January 5 and 6 he slept in a bed that had been occupied on January 2, 3, and 4 by a patient in the first three days of a well-marked attack of tabardillo. None of the bedding or bedclothes had been in any way disturbed in the interval prior to their use by this individual. At the end of three days the bedclothes were changed, but with this exception the bed and room remained as they had been when occupied by the patient. F. J. inhabited this room for three weeks longer. On careful search no insects other than fleas were found in the room. During a period of observation of 17 days this man continued in his usual health.[9]

The following data, for which we are indebted to Miss Ella Wilson, superintendent of the American Hospital in Mexico City, are significant in this connection. From January 9, 1908, to November 24, 1909, 30 cases of typhus fever had been treated in the typhus pavilion of that hospital. Each of these cases had had a special nurse who was an American non-immune. None of these nurses contracted the disease.

Having satisfied ourselves that neither contagion in the ordinary sense nor that fomites as usually understood played any role in the transmission of the disease, and with the impression strongly in our minds that some intermediary host was the probable transmitting agent of the infection, we took up a consideration of the insects which might be expected to play this role. The insects which immediately suggested themselves as worthy of serious attention in this connection were the flea, the bedbug, and the body louse.

The flea.—A review of certain facts enabled us very quickly to eliminate the flea from consideration. The ubiquity of the flea and the well-recognized limitation of the prevalence of the disease in the lowest social classes obviously do not harmonize with the idea that this insect is the transmitting agent. It is a well-recognized fact that in houses and families of the better classes secondary cases are rarely observed, though far from being free from infestation by fleas. Furthermore, it is a well-recognized fact that the striking distance of the infection is decidedly circumscribed, a fact with which the agility of the flea also does not harmonize.

The bedbug.—This insect is only a temporary parasite of man. As is well known, it lurks and hides in cracks and crevices and in the folds of bedding during the day, coming out at night to feed, retiring again toward morning. It is only rarely that it remains on the body of an individual. With this in mind, and assuming for the moment that the bedbug is the carrier, tabardillo should have the characteristics of a house disease, i.e., the infection should appear to be attached to houses and practically not at all to individuals, such as is the case in yellow fever. As a matter of fact, however, such is not the case. The distribution of the bedbug among the social classes is much more general than tabardillo, which, in a general way, is fairly limited to the poverty-stricken portion of the population. These facts appear to us to rule out this insect as the probable transmitter of tabardillo.

Finally, both the bedbug and the flea seem to us to be pretty definitely ruled out of consideration by the further fact that these insects are found

9 The "F. J." of this experiment was undoubtedly J. F. Anderson. We know from Parsons' biography of Goldberger (*Trail to Light*, pp. 209–17) that Anderson arrived at the Hotel Iturbide in Mexico City on November 22, saw cases of typhus daily with Goldberger, and had to return temporarily to Washington on December 16.

in the lowlands of Mexico, where the disease is unknown except as isolated imported cases.

The body louse.—Having eliminated the flea and the bedbug as the probable transmitters of the disease, there remains for consideration only the body louse (*Pediculus vestimenti*). This insect, as is well known, is parasitic on man, but may be said never to occur on persons or classes of people of cleanly habits. This fact may be seen very clearly in Mexico and is in entire harmony with the distribution of the disease among the social classes.

Students of the epidemiology of typhus fever have long observed that the disease, while apparently highly contagious, requires a fairly intimate contact for this contagiousness to manifest itself. Now, the body louse is a relatively sluggish insect. It practically makes only short excursions in the seams of the clothing of the individual and from these to the body of its host to feed. Its transfer from person to person takes place only when individuals are in close association with one another or with infested clothes or when the insect is accidentally dislodged from the body of its host and is subsequently picked up, as it were, by another person.

Impressed by these considerations we attempted to transmit the disease by means of the body louse, *Pediculus vestimenti,* from man to monkey.[10]

While engaged in these attempts, Anderson and Goldberger learned that C. Nicolle, C. Comte, and E. Conseil had just reported the successful transmission of typhus fever from monkey to monkey by means of the body louse. And in April, 1910, H. T. Ricketts and R. M. Wilder, working independently in Mexico, reported success in louse transmission of typhus from man to monkey and from monkey to monkey. Anderson and Goldberger completed their studies and confirmed these reports. They also demonstrated transmission by the head louse from man to monkey and carried out numerous experimental studies of the characteristics of the virus, immunity, and means of transmission. One of their most interesting contributions was the demonstration that so-called Brill's disease was actually typhus fever.

In addition to their work on typhus, Anderson and Goldberger were the first to demonstrate that measles could be transmitted to an experimental animal, the rhesus monkey. They studied the period of infectivity of the blood in measles, demonstrated the presence of measles virus in the mixed buccal and nasal secretions of patients, investigated the characteristics of the virus, and tested the infectivity of the desquamating scales of measles with negative results.

10 J. F. Anderson and J. Goldberger, "On the Infectivity of Tabardillo or Mexican Typhus for Monkeys and Studies on its Mode of Transmission," *Public Health Rep.,* Vol. 25 (1910), 177–85.

In 1913, Goldberger was assigned to investigate the high prevalence of diphtheria in Detroit. Here he carried out the first community-wide study of the prevalence of diphtheria carriers, using house-to-house visits in representative sections of the city and attempting to obtain cultures from a sample representative of the age and sex distribution of the general population. Goldberger completed his work in Detroit in March, 1914, in order to begin a new assignment in charge of the pellagra studies of the U.S. Public Health Service.

The Surgeon General's letter assigning Goldberger to the pellagra work starts with these words: "Within the past several weeks the importance of pellagra has been urged on me by members of Congress and other prominent people from sections in which the disease prevails. It is undoubtedly one of the knottiest and most urgent problems facing the Service at the present time."[11]

Pellagra was not recognized in the United States until the twentieth century although a few case reports had appeared as early as 1863. H. F. Harris of Atlanta, Georgia, reported a case in 1902, but nothing further was heard about the disease until 1907 when reports began to come in from state asylums and many communities of the South.[12] In 1912, C. H. Lavinder of the U.S. Public Health Service estimated that more than 25,000 cases had occurred in the United States in the previous five years, with a case fatality rate of 40 per cent.[13]

Lavinder also commented a year later that: "the literature of pellagra continues to increase in volume, but our actual knowledge of the nature of the disease still leaves much, very much, to be desired. The etiology of pellagra remains in obscurity. The Italian school continues to ring changes on the corn theory, while the American school seems largely inclined to regard pellagra as an infectious disease of some undetermined nature."[14]

The dominant thinking in the United States at the time Goldberger began his investigations was, as Lavinder indicates, clearly oriented to an infectious etiology. Thus the Pellagra Commission of the State of Illinois ended its investigations in 1911 with these

11   Parsons, *Trail to Light*, 277.
12   G. M. Niles, *Pellagra, An American Problem* (Philadelphia: Saunders, 1916).
13   C. H. Lavinder, "The Prevalence and Geographic Distribution of Pellagra in the United States," *Public Health Rep.*, Vol. 27 (1912), 2076–88.
14   C. H. Lavinder, "Pellagra, Brief Comments on our Present Knowledge of the Disease," *Public Health Rep.*, Vol. 28 (1913), 2461–63.

conclusions: "(1) According to the weight of evidence pellagra is a disease due to infection with a living micro-organism of unknown nature; (2) A possible location for this infection is the intestinal tract; and (3) Deficient animal protein in the diet may constitute a predisposing factor in the contraction of the disease."[15]

The Thompson-McFadden Pellagra Commission, in the first progress report of its studies in Spartanburg County, South Carolina, similarly concluded in 1913 that: "(1) The supposition that the ingestion of good or spoiled maize is the essential cause of pellagra is not supported by our study; and (2) Pellagra is in all probability a specific infectious disease communicable from person to person by means at present unknown."[16] In a paper presented at the Annual Session of the American Medical Association in June, 1914, the commission bolstered its original conclusions with these additional findings:

In the group of incident cases most thoroughly studied, evidence of close association with a preexisting case was disclosed in more than 80 per cent.

A house-to-house canvass of the homes of over 5,000 people living in six endemic foci of pellagra failed to disclose any definite relation of the disease to any element of the dietary.

In these six villages new cases of pellagra originated almost exclusively in a house in which a preexisting pellagrin was living, or next door to such a house, suggesting that the disease has spread from old cases as centers.

So far as we have observed, pellagra has spread most rapidly in districts where insanitary methods of sewage disposal have been in use.[17]

Despite this climate of opinion, Goldberger came in a very short period of time to diametrically opposite conclusions. In June, 1914, less than three months after beginning his investigations, Goldberger published his first paper on pellagra. This document of a little over three pages defines boldly and accurately the epidemiology of the disease: pellagra cannot be communicable; the cause is dietary; and prevention consists of a "reduction in cereals, vegetables, and canned foods that enter to so large an extent into the dietary of many of the

15 *Report of the Pellagra Commission of the State of Illinois, November, 1911* (Springfield, Ill.: Illinois State Journal Co., 1912).
16 J. F. Siler, P. E. Garrison, and W. J. MacNeal, "Pellagra, A Summary of the First Progress Report of the Thompson-McFadden Pellagra Commission," *J. Am. Med. Assn.*, Vol. 62 (1914), 8–12.
17 J. F. Siler, P. E. Garrison, and W. J. MacNeal, "Further Studies of the Thompson-McFadden Pellagra Commission. A Summary of the Second Progress Report," *J. Am. Med. Assn.*, Vol. 63 (1914), 1090–93.

people in the South and an increase in the fresh animal food component, such as fresh meats, eggs, and milk." The achievement is all
the more remarkable because it is based almost entirely on a chain
of reasoning from three epidemiological facts which were well known
to his contemporaries: (1) in institutions where pellagra was prevalent, no case had ever occurred in nurses or attendants; (2) the disease
was essentially rural; and (3) it was associated with poverty.

In a second short paper, published in September, 1914, Goldberger's hypothesis was buttressed by new observations: numerous
attempts to infect rhesus monkeys had proved futile, and the age
distribution of pellagra in a children's orphanage was found to correlate only with the dietary differences already noted. "A practical
test or demonstration" was needed.

In 1915, Goldberger and his colleagues demonstrated that pellagra
could be prevented in institutional patients by a diet which included
generous amounts of milk, eggs, meat, beans, and peas. Almost simultaneously, they reported success in producing pellagra by means of a
deficient diet in healthy volunteer convicts at the Rankin Farm of
the Mississippi State Penitentiary. The next year, in a series of
thorough and highly distasteful experiments on sixteen volunteers—
including Goldberger, Sydenstricker, W. F. Tanner, G. A. Wheeler,
D. G. Willets, and Goldberger's wife—they were unable to demonstrate any transmissibility of pellagra via blood, nasopharyngeal
secretions, epidermal scales from pellagrous lesions, urine, and feces.

In 1915, Sydenstricker used available economic and dietary data
to explain the prevalence of pellagra in southern wageworkers' families, particularly since 1907. The following year, intensive field
studies were carried out by Goldberger, Wheeler, and Sydenstricker
in seven cotton-mill villages of South Carolina. These studies differed
from previous field investigations in certain important methodologi-
cal features: (1) the diagnosis of pellagra was based on house-to-house
visits and inspection of all village households by a physician
(Wheeler) at two-week intervals from the middle of April to the
end of the year; (2) dietary and other pertinent data were obtained
for the season (April 16 to June 15) immediately preceding the period
of expected high incidence of the disease; and (3) the dietary data
were obtained by an objective method—that is, a special fifteen-day
recording of all household purchases by type and amount of foods in
the local stores—instead of relying solely on information obtained by
interview. The latter method was used only to obtain data on foods
obtained from sources other than the stores.

The results were clear-cut. Pellagrous households had, in comparison with nonpellagrous households, much more restricted supplies of animal protein foods, namely, lean meats, milk, butter, cheese, and eggs. No association was demonstrable, however, between the amount of the household corn meal supply and the incidence of pellagra. Independent sanitary ratings of the villages revealed no correlation of sanitary factors with pellagra incidence. There was a very marked correlation, on the other hand, between low income and pellagra incidence due to the association of the former with a restricted diet. An important factor in the occurrence of the disease in local communities was the availability of food supplies as determined by home ownership of cows, poultry, and gardens, the character of the local markets, the supply of produce from adjacent farm territory, and the marketing conditions.

Goldberger and Sydenstricker went considerably farther in their investigation of the epidemiology of pellagra. A careful analysis was made of the economic factors related to pellagra prevalence in the lower Mississippi River area, including the speculative character of cotton production, the sharecropping system which maintained the average tenant farmer "chronically on the verge of deprivation," and the one-crop type of agriculture with the consequent lack of diversification. From these studies there emerged a total epidemiologic picture of pellagra in the South.

Two problems remained: (1) to determine the pellagra-preventive action of various foods, and (2) to identify the specific deficiency responsible for the disease. At first, Goldberger and his colleagues had to rely entirely on experiments with humans; later they succeeded in demonstrating that blacktongue of dogs is identical with pellagra in man, and they were able therefore to develop their investigations through animal experiments. Most of these studies are not included in the present collection because of limitations of space, since the total writings of Goldberger and his colleagues on pellagra amount to almost a thousand pages (see Appendix). The three most important papers, however, are included; it is in these that we see the development of Goldberger's thinking—based on the experimental evidence—on the identity of the pellagra-preventive factor.

At first, Goldberger and Tanner considered amino-acid deficiency as probably the primary etiological factor in pellagra. This conclusion was based on the failure of diets containing a liberal supply of minerals and vitamins A, B, and C to prevent pellagra, on the marked pellagra-preventive value of animal protein foods, and on preliminary tests with cystine and tryptophan in three patients. It is of interest in this connection that G. A. Hundley states:

Apparently, tests with tryptophan alone were conducted but they were never reported. The author of this review is in possession of a copy of a progress report to Goldberger from Tanner, dated August 5, 1921, which has never been publicly reported. In it, Tanner relates the course of one pellagrous patient who was given "one-half dram" of tryptophan before each meal. There was no improvement in the diarrhea at the time of the report, but prompt and marked improvement in the patient's extensive dermatitis was noted. After describing the progress of the skin lesions, Tanner stated: "I might add that the improvement in this patient's skin condition has surpassed anything I have ever seen in a case of pellagra in an equal period of time." There is no record of the final result.[18]

Goldberger and Tanner soon shifted their position because of the results of additional human experiments. Soybean-supplemented diets, considered adequate in protein, failed to prevent pellagra; casein-supplemented diets, presumably rich in protein of good quality, did not completely prevent pellagra; but a dried-yeast–supplemented diet, relatively poor in protein, proved very efficient in preventing the disease. They came to the conclusion that the prevention of pellagra depended on "a heretofore unrecognized or unappreciated dietary factor which we designate as factor P-P. This may be effective with but little, possibly without any, cooperation from the protein factor."

Finally, Goldberger and his colleagues concluded on the basis of experiments with dogs and rats that "water soluble B" vitamin included at least two distinct factors: one a heat-sensitive antineuritic or beriberi preventive, and the other a heat-resistant, pellagra-preventive factor.

Goldberger did not succeed before his untimely death in 1929 in carrying any further the work of identifying the pellagra-preventive factor. In 1937, C. A. Elvehjem and his associates demonstrated that nicotinic acid cured blacktongue in dogs. This finding was immediately confirmed for human pellagra, and nicotinic acid was shown to be the pellagra-preventive factor which Goldberger had postulated. Furthermore, work since 1945 has demonstrated that the amino acid, tryptophan, is converted to nicotinic acid in man as well as in many species of animals; approximately 60 mg. of dietary tryptophan appears to be equivalent to 1 mg. of nicotinic acid.[19]

18 W. H. Sebrell and R. S. Harris, *The Vitamins: Chemistry, Physiology, Pathology* (New York: Academic Press, 1954), II, 553.

19 G. A. Goldsmith, "Niacin-Tryptophan Relationships in Man and Niacin Requirement," *Am. J. Clin. Nutrition,* Vol. 6 (1958), 479–86.

Goldberger's work on pellagra represents a major contribution of American medicine which is of general interest to physicians and of specific interest to workers in the field of nutrition. Above all, however, it is one of the great classics of epidemiology, deserving careful study by all those interested in the investigation of disease in human population groups.

The pellagra studies provide a brilliant example of the use of epidemiologic reasoning—that is, reasoning based on the behavior of a disease in the population—to develop an etiologic hypothesis. Even more remarkable is the complete and incontrovertible demonstration, step by step, of the truth of that hypothesis. Finally, the whole epidemiologic picture is presented; attention is focused not only on the dietary causes of pellagra but also on the underlying reasons for the dietary deficiencies. There emerges a thorough analysis of the economic and social basis of pellagra in the South, that is, of the total context in which pellagra took root and flourished.

This last achievement was undoubtedly due in large measure to the work of the economist Edgar Sydenstricker, whose investigations in the cotton-mill villages of South Carolina led in a direct line to his pioneer morbidity studies in Hagerstown; he was later to become one of the great figures in public health and the author of the first American textbook of social medicine.[20] Sydenstricker's contributions to the pellagra studies are notable for their realism, comprehensiveness, and methodologic rigor; they represent an outstanding example of the effective collaboration of medical and social scientists.

Students of epidemiology will discover in Goldberger's work on pellagra a rich sourcebook of epidemiologic methodology. Not only will they find rewarding a careful study of the specific methods used, but also the over-all approach will spur them to look beyond the borders of traditional epidemiology. Too often the latter is hampered by its one-sided concern with purely observational studies and its divorce from clinical medicine and the laboratory. Goldberger knew no such limitations; he not only observed pellagra as it occurred in the community but carried out human experiments in the field, utilized careful clinical observation, and did not hesitate to extend his investigations into the laboratory.

A vigorous epidemiology, capable of making significant contributions to the solution of the major disease problems of our day, must utilize both observational and experimental studies wherever this is possible—or rather, wherever human ingenuity can make this pos-

20   E. Sydenstricker, *Health and Environment* (New York: McGraw-Hill, 1933).

sible. It needs to operate, furthermore, in close collaboration with clinical and laboratory personnel and facilities. Finally, it should not hesitate to use all scientific methods, whether derived from the natural or the social sciences, which can be helpful in determining and explaining the behavior of specific diseases in the population. The effectiveness of such an approach is amply demonstrated in Goldberger's classic studies of pellagra.

PART ONE

Preliminary Observations and Hypothesis

1. The Etiology of Pellagra.
The Significance of Certain Epidemiological Observations with Respect Thereto[1]

JOSEPH GOLDBERGER

The writer desires to invite attention to certain observations recorded in the literature of pellagra the significance of which appears entirely to have escaped attention.

At the National Conference on Pellagra held in Columbia, S. C., November 3, 1909, Siler and Nichols in their paper on the "Aspects of the pellagra problem in Illinois" stated that certain facts "would seem to indicate that the exciting cause of the disease is present within the institution" (Peoria State Hospital), and add that "at the same time no nurses, attendants, or employees have shown the disease."

Manning, medical superintendent of the asylum at Bridgetown, Barbados, on the same occasion, in arguing against the identity of a disease that he called psilosis pigmentosa, with pellagra, but which undoubtedly is this disease, states that he had never seen it develop in an attendant.

At the same conference Mobley, from the Georgia State Sanitarium, in the course of his discussion of the relation of pellagra to insanity, presents data showing that at the Georgia State Sanitarium a considerable proportion of the cases of pellagra develop in inmates who have been residents therein for considerable periods, mentioning one case in an inmate after 10 years' residence. In this connection he remarks, what must have struck him, as it no doubt must have appealed to Siler and Nichols at the Illinois institution, as a curious fact, that "so far as can be ascertained there has never been a case of pellagra to develop among the nurses, white or colored, while employed as such in the Georgia State Sanitarium."

Sambon (1910) in his "Progress report" states that in Italy "no precautions are ever taken to avoid propagation of the malady in any of the pellagrosari, locande sanitarie, hospitals, insane asylums, and other institutions in which very numerous pellagrins are collected every year. Long experience has taught that there is no danger

1 *Public Health Rep.*, Vol. 29, No. 26 (June 26, 1914), 1683–86.

whatever of transmission from the sick to the healthy in any collective dwelling within urban precincts."

Sambon's statement is confirmed by Lavinder, who in a personal communication states that on careful inquiry while visiting a large pellagrosario near Venice, one in which some 300 to 500 pellagrins are constantly present and cared for by a large number of Sisters of Charity and other employees, he was assured that no employee had ever developed the disease while at the institution.

The results of personal inquiry at some of our State asylums in which pellagra occurs confirm the reported observations above cited. Thus at the South Carolina State Hospital for the Insane, where Babcock (1910 Ann. Rept.) states that cases of pellagra develop in patients who have been there for years, no case so far as the writer was able to ascertain has occurred in the nurses or attendants. It may be of interest to recall in this connection that in his annual report for 1913 Babcock states that a total of about 900 pellagrins had been admitted to his institution during the preceding six years.

At the State hospital for the insane at Jackson, Miss., there have been recorded 98 deaths from pellagra for the period between October 1, 1909, and July 1, 1913. At this institution cases of institutional origin have occurred in inmates. Dr. J. C. Herrington, assistant physician and pathologist, told me at the time of my visit of a case in an inmate after 15 and in another after 20 years' residence at the institution. No case, so far as I was able to learn, has developed in a nurse or attendant, although since January 1, 1909, there have been employed a total of 126 who have served for periods of from 1 to 5 years.

In considering the significance of the foregoing observations it is to be recalled that at all of these institutions the ward personnel, nurses, and attendants spend a considerable proportion of the 24 hours, on day or night duty, in close association with the inmates; indeed at many of these institutions, for lack of a separate building or special residence for the nurses, these live right in the ward with and of necessity under exactly the same conditions as the inmates.

It is striking therefore that although many inmates develop pellagra after varying periods of institutional residence, some even after 10 to 20 years of institutional life, and therefore it seems permissible to infer, as the result of the operation within the institution of the exciting cause or causes, yet nurses and attendants living under identical conditions appear uniformly to be immune. If pellagra be a communicable disease, why should there be this exemption of the nurses and attendants?

To the writer this peculiar exemption or immunity is inexplicable on the assumption that pellagra is communicable. Neither "contact" in any sense nor insect transmission is capable of explaining such a phenomenon, except on the assumption of an incubation or latent period extending over 10 to 20 years. In support of such an assumption there exists, so far as the writer is aware, no satisfactory evidence.

The explanation of the peculiar exemption under discussion will be found in the opinion of the writer in a difference in the diet of the two groups of residents. At some of the institutions there is a manifest difference in this regard; in others none is apparent.

The latter would seem to be a fatal objection to this explanation, but a moment's consideration will show that such is not necessarily the case. The writer from personal observation has found that although the nurses and attendants may apparently receive the same food, there is nevertheless a difference in that the nurses have the privilege—which they exercise—of selecting the best and the greatest variety for themselves. Moreover, it must not be overlooked that nurses and attendants have opportunities for supplementing their institutional dietary that the inmates as a rule have not.

In this connection brief reference must be made to two other epidemiological features of pellagra. It is universally agreed (1) that this disease is essentially rural, and (2) associated with poverty. Now there is plenty of poverty and all its concomitants in all cities, and the question naturally arises why its greater predilection for rural poverty? What important difference is there between the elements of poverty in our slums and those of poverty in rural dwellers? It is not the writer's intention to enter at this time into a detailed discussion of these questions; he wishes to point out one difference only. This difference relates to the dietary. Studies of urban and rural dietaries (Wait—Office of Experiment Stations, Bull. 221, 1909) have shown that on the whole the very poor of cities have a more varied diet, than the poor in rural sections. "Except in extreme cases, the city poor . . . appear to be better nourished than the mountaineers" of Tennessee.

With regard to the question of just what in the dietary is responsible, the writer has no opinion to express. From a study of certain institutional dietaries, however, he has gained the impression that vegetables and cereals form a much greater proportion in them than they do in the dietaries of well-to-do people; that is, people who are not, as a class, subject to pellagra.

The writer is satisfied that the consumption of corn or corn products is not essential to the production of pellagra, but this does not mean that corn, the best of corn, or corn products, however nutritious and however high in caloric value they may be, are not objectionable when forming of themselves or in combination with other cereals and with vegetables, a large part of the diet of the individual.

In view of the great uncertainty that exists as to the true cause of pellagra, it may not be amiss to suggest that pending the final solution of this problem it may be well to attempt to prevent the disease by improving the dietary of those among whom it seems most prevalent. In this direction I would urge the reduction in cereals, vegetables, and canned foods that enter to so large an extent into the dietary of many of the people in the South and an increase in the fresh animal food component, such as fresh meats, eggs, and milk.

It may be of interest to add that intensive studies along the lines so strongly suggested by the observations above considered are being prosecuted by several groups of workers of the United States Public Health Service.

2. *The Cause and Prevention of Pellagra*[1]

JOSEPH GOLDBERGER

Because of the prevalence of pellagra throughout a considerable part of the United States, and the fact that this disease has so far baffled all attempts to ascertain its cause and means of prevention, the following letter from Surg. Joseph Goldberger, in charge of the Government's pellagra investigations, is of interest.

Evidence seems to be accumulating to show that pellagra is due to the use of a dietary in which some essential element is reduced in amount or from which it is altogether absent, or to the use of a dietary in which some element is present in injurious amount.

UNITED STATES PUBLIC HEALTH SERVICE
Washington, September 4, 1914.

The SURGEON GENERAL,
Public Health Service.

SIR: As indicated in my progress report of June 5, 1914, the primary object of the pellagra studies that are being conducted under my general direction is the determination of the essential cause of the disease.

Although pellagra has been known and studied abroad for nearly two centuries, not only is its essential cause not known, but the broad question of whether it is to be classed either as a dietary or as a communicable (contagious or infectious) disease has never been satisfactorily determined.

Abroad, the spoiled-maize theory of Lombroso has for many years been the dominating one. Its adequacy, however, has on various grounds been repeatedly questioned.

In the United States, with the progressive and alarming increase in the prevalence of the disease, there has developed both in the lay and in the medical mind the opinion that pellagra is an infectious disease. This opinion has received important support, first, from the Illinois Pellagra Commission and, second, from the Thompson-McFadden Commission (Siler, Garrison, and MacNeal). In planning

1 *Public Health Rep.*, Vol. 29, No. 37, (September 11, 1914), 2354–57.

our investigations, therefore, due consideration was given to these two distinct possibilities, and the problem was attacked from both points of view.

From the point of view that we might be dealing with an infection, a comprehensive series of inoculations in the monkey was begun last fall by Drs. C. H. Lavinder and Edward Francis. Although every kind of tissue, secretion, and excretion from a considerable number of grave and fatal cases was obtained and inoculated in every conceivable way into over a hundred rhesus monkeys, the results have so far been negative.

At my suggestion Dr. Francis is making a culture study of the blood, secretions, and excretions of pellagrins by the newer anaerobic methods. This has been in progress about six weeks, but has so far given only negative results.

Epidemiologic studies were begun and have been in progress at the Georgia State Sanitarium in immediate charge of Dr. David G. Willets, and at an orphanage in Jackson, Miss., in immediate charge of Dr. C. H. Waring. These studies have brought out facts of the very greatest significance.

In a paper published in the Public Health Reports of June 26, 1914, I called attention to certain observations which appear inexplicable on any theory of communicability. These observations show that although in many asylums new cases of pellagra develop in inmates even after 10, 15, and 20 years' residence, clearly indicating thereby that the cause of the disease exists and is operative in such asylums, yet at none has any one of the employees contracted the disease, though living under identical environmental conditions as the inmates, and many in most intimate association with them.

In order to obtain precise data bearing on these observations, Dr. Willets is making a careful study of the records of the Georgia State Sanitarium. These show that of 996 patients admitted during 1910—excluding those that died, were discharged during their first year, or had pellagra on admission or within a year of admission—there remained at the institution after one year 418, and of this number 32, or 7.65 per cent, have developed pellagra since that time. Of the present employees of this asylum, 293 have been in more or less intimate association with pellagrins and have lived in substantially the same or in identical environment as the asylum inmates for at least one year. If pellagra had developed among these employees at the same rate as it has among the inmates, then 22 of them should have the disease. As a matter of fact not a single one has it.

The studies at the orphanage at Jackson show that on July 1, 1914, of 211 orphans 68, or 32 per cent, had pellagra.

The distribution of these cases with respect to age developed the remarkable fact that practically all of the cases were in children between the ages of 6 and 12 years, of whom in consequence over 52 per cent were afflicted. In the group of 25 children under 6 years of age there were 2 cases and in the group of 66 children over 12 years of age there was but 1 case. Inasmuch as all live under identical environmental conditions, the remarkable exemption of the group of younger and that of the older children is no more comprehensible on the basis of an infection than is the absolute immunity of the asylum employees.

A minute investigation has been made at both institutions of all conceivable factors that might possibly explain the striking exemption of the groups indicated. The only constant difference discoverable relates exclusively to the dietary. At both institutions those of the exempt group or groups were found to subsist on a better diet than those of the affected groups. In the diet of those developing pellagra there was noted a disproportionately small amount of meat or other animal protein food, and consequently the vegetable food component, in which corn and sirup were prominent and legumes relatively inconspicuous elements, forms a disproportionately large part of the ration. Although other than this gross defect no fault in the diet is appreciable, the evidence clearly incriminates it as the cause of the pellagra at these institutions. The inference may therefore be safely drawn that pellagra is not an infection, but that it is a disease essentially of dietary origin; that is, that it is caused in some way such as, for example, by the absence from the diet of essential vitamins, or possibly, as is suggested by Meyer and Voegtlin's work, by the presence in the vegetable-food component of excessive amounts of a poison such as soluble aluminum salts.

One-sided eccentric diets such as were consumed by the affected groups above referred to are in the main brought about by economic conditions. Poverty and the progressive rise in the cost of food oblige the individual, the family, and the institution to curtail the expensive elements—meat, milk, eggs, legumes—of the diet and to subsist more and more largely, especially in winter, on the cheaper cereal (corn), carbohydrate (sirup, molasses), and readily procurable vegetables and fats ("sow belly"). In the well-to-do, more or less well-recognizable eccentricities of taste may cause the individual, without himself realizing it, to subsist on a one-sided or eccentric diet. Somewhat similar eccentricities of taste are more or less common in the insane, some of whom, indeed (as the demented), because of apathy and indifference, will not eat at all. These, for the most part included in the "untidy" class, require special care in feeding. The poorer the institution, the fewer and of lower grade is likely to be its attendant personnel and therefore the greater the danger that these very trying and troublesome types of inmates will receive inadequate attention, and so be improperly (one-sidedly) fed. It has repeatedly been noted by observers that at insane asylums the "untidy" (the group in which my observations show scurvy and beriberi most likely to develop) were the most afflicted with pellagra. By some this supposed excessive susceptibility is explained as dependent on the untidiness which favors filth infection. The true explanation, however, is that both the untidiness and the supposed excessive susceptibility of these inmates are primarily dependent on the apathy and indifference typical of most of this group. The deteriorated mental condition causing apathy and indifference results not only in untidiness of person, but passively or actively in an eccentricity in the diet. I believe that in this, in conjunction with a diet admittedly low in the animal protein component we have the explanation of the excessive prevalence of the disease at the Peoria State Hospital, a hospital almost all of whose inmates in 1909 were of the "hopeless, untidy, incurable" class, drawn from the other Illinois institutions.

While confident of the accuracy of our observations and of the justice of our inferences, there is nevertheless grave doubt in my mind as to their general acceptance without some practical test or demonstration of the correctness of the corollary, namely, that no pellagra develops in those who consume a mixed, well-balanced, and varied diet, such, for example, as the Navy ration, the Army garrison ration, or the ration prescribed for the Philippine Scouts.

Respectfully,
Jos. GOLDBERGER,
Surgeon in Charge of Pellagra Investigations

PART TWO

Human Experiments

3. The Prevention of Pellagra. A Test of Diet Among Institutional Inmates[1]

JOSEPH GOLDBERGER
C. H. WARING
DAVID G. WILLETS

Introduction

In a paper published June 26, 1914, attention was called to certain epidemiological observations relating to pellagra which appeared inexplicable on any theory of communicability. These observations showed that, at certain institutions at which pellagra was either epidemic or had long been endemic among the inmates, the nurses and attendants, drawn from the class economically and socially identical with that most afflicted in the population at large, appeared uniformly to be immune, although living in the same environment and under the same conditions as did the inmates. Neither "contact" nor insect transmission seemed capable of explaining such a phenomenon. It was suggested that the explanation was to be found in a difference, which was believed to exist, in the diet of the two groups of residents.

From a study of the dietaries of certain institutions in which pellagra prevailed the impression has been gained that cereals and vegetables formed a much greater proportion in them than they did in the dietaries of well-to-do people; that is, people who as a class are practically exempt from pellagra. It was suggested, therefore, that it might be well to attempt to prevent the disease by reducing the cereals, vegetables, and canned foods and increasing the fresh animal foods, such as fresh meats, eggs, and milk; in other words, by providing those subject to pellagra with a diet such as that enjoyed by well-to-do people, who as a group are practically free from the disease.

In planning the field studies for 1914 it was proposed, with the approval of the bureau and the department, to put this suggestion to a practical test.

In accordance with the original plan to carry on the test for at least two years, the experiment is still in progress. The results so

1   *Public Health Rep.,* Vol. 30, No. 43 (October 22, 1915), 3117–31.

far recorded are so striking, however, and of such profound practical importance that they are reported at this time.

In planning the test of the preventive value of diet it was decided to take advantage of the universally recognized fact that "normally" pellagra tends to recur in the individual from year to year.

In order to obtain significant and perhaps decisive results, it was decided to submit to the test as large a number of individuals as possible at some institution where the disease was endemic. After some search an orphanage with a high incidence of pellagra among its residents was found at Jackson, Miss.

As a preliminary, a study was made of the epidemiology of the disease at this institution, and the singular fact was very quickly discovered that the disease was practically exclusively confined to those between 6 and 12 years of age. After a detailed inquiry the only explanation that could be found for the remarkable restriction of the disease to this group was a difference in the diet of the resident groups.

In the diet of the affected group, as contrasted with that of the exempt groups, there was noted a disproportionately small amount of lean meat or other animal protein food, so that the vegetable component, in which biscuits (wheat flour), grits, meal (corn), and sirup were prominent and legumes relatively inconspicuous, formed a disproportionately large part of the ration. Inquiry at other institutions developed analogous conditions, and as a whole the findings, in the light of the recent advances in our knowledge of beriberi, very strongly suggested the idea that the disease was dependent upon a diet that was for some reason faulty and that this fault was in some way either prevented or corrected by including in the diet larger proportions of the fresh animal protein foods. These findings not only confirmed the writer's previous tentative deductions but helped in defining these deductions more clearly, and moreover made it possible more definitely to formulate plans, which were temporarily broadened to include a test of diet in the treatment as well as in the prevention of the disease.

At the suggestion of the writer, Dr. W. F. Lorenz, special expert, United States Public Health Service, who was at that time studying the psychiatric manifestations of pellagra at the Georgia State Sanitarium, treated a series of 27 cases in the insane at that asylum exclusively by diet. Considering the class of cases with which he was dealing, his results, as well as those of Dr. D. G. Willets, who for a time continued the work begun by Lorenz, were notably favorable.

When the various recent methods of treatment, each warmly advocated by its author, are critically reviewed in the light of the test made by Lorenz and by Willets, one cannot fail to be struck by the fact that the one thing they all appear to have in common is the so-called "nutritious" diet, and it is difficult to escape the conclusion that it is to this single common factor that the marked success that is usually claimed for the "treatment" should properly be assigned.

It is of much interest to note that fully 50 years ago Roussel (Roussel 1866, pp. 529-530), on the basis of long experience and from a critical review of the literature of his day, came to precisely the same conclusion. This is so much to the point that it is quoted herewith: "Without dietetic measures *all remedies fail* [italics are Roussel's] . . . when drugs and good food are simultaneously employed it is to the latter that the curative action belongs, the former exercises simply an adjuvant action and is without proved efficacy except against secondary changes or accidental complications."

Important as the treatment of the individual case may be, it seemed to the writers of much more fundamental importance to apply their resources to the problem of prevention. Arrangements were therefore made to extend the preventive study to a second orphanage and later to two groups of insane at the Georgia State Sanitarium.

Orphanage Study

Both the orphanages at which the value of diet in the prevention of pellagra has been tested are located in Jackson, Miss.

The first of these to be considered will be spoken of as orphanage "M. J." Cases of pellagra have been recognized at this institution every spring for several years. During the spring and summer of 1914, up to September 15, 79 cases of the disease were observed in children at this orphanage. Although several of these were known to have had pellagra on admission or had developed it a short time after admission, a number appeared to have developed the disease for the first time after considerable periods of residence at this institution. The factor or factors causing pellagra and favoring its recurrence seemed, therefore, to be operative at this orphanage.

The second of the orphanages, which will be referred to as orphanage "B. J.," is located about half a mile east of orphanage "M. J." Here, as at "M. J.," cases of pellagra have been recognized every spring for several years. The writers are informed by the superintendent that a condition which he cannot distinguish from that now called pellagra has occurred every year among the children ever since his connection with the institution, a matter of some 12 to 13 years.

From his description it is believed that there can be but little doubt that pellagra has prevailed at this institution almost, if not quite, since its foundation in 1897.

During the spring and summer of 1914, up to September 15, there were observed among the children at this institution 130 cases of pellagra. As at "M. J.," some of these were in recent admissions; a large proportion, however, occurred in long-time residents.

There appears to be little if any reason to doubt that the factor or factors causing the disease and favoring its recurrence have been operative at this institution for many years.

At both institutions the hygienic and sanitary conditions found left much to be desired. Both were much overcrowded.

The drinking water at each is drawn from the public supply.

One is equipped with a water carriage sewerage system connected with that of the city; the other has the unscreened surface privy type of sewage disposal and, incidentally, we found here a great deal of soil pollution.

At the very outset it was requested that no change be made in hygienic and sanitary conditions, and it is believed that these have remained as they were found and as they have been for several years.

Since about the middle of September, 1914, the diet at both orphanages has in certain respects been supplemented by the Public Health Service. At both institutions a very decided increase was made in the proportion of the fresh animal and of the leguminous protein foods.

The milk supply was greatly increased. Provision was made to give every child under 12 years a cup of about 7 ounces of milk at least twice a day. Those under 6 years had it three times a day. Until the spring of 1915 the milk used was all fresh sweet milk. In April of this year buttermilk was added to the diet. This was served at first only on alternate days to those over 12 years of age; later, when a sufficient supply became available, it was served daily at the midday meal to all.

Eggs, except in cooking or for the sick, had previously not entered into the regular diet of these children. The writers prescribed at least one egg at the morning meal for every child under 12 years of age. It had been the custom to serve the children with fresh meat but once a week; under the writers' direction it was increased to three or four times a week.

Beans and peas, which had been conspicuous in the diet only during the summer and fall, were made an important part of nearly every midday meal at all seasons.

The carbohydrate component of the institution diets was also modified. The breakfast cereal was changed from grits to oatmeal, partly because it was believed to be an advantage to reduce the corn element and in part because it was believed that the oatmeal would favor the increased consumption of milk. The corn element, though much reduced, was not wholly excluded. Corn bread was allowed all children once a week and grits to those over 12 years of age once or twice a week. Cane sirup or molasses, which it had been customary to serve freely at two or three meals each day, was for some weeks entirely excluded, and later allowed in small amounts at only three or four evening meals a week. The object in this was to reduce the proportion of the carbohydrate element. A more detailed idea of the character of the diet furnished may be obtained by reference to the menus herewith submitted. (See pp. 34–35.)

Results

Orphanage "M. J."—Of the 79 cases of pellagra observed at "M. J." during the spring and summer of 1914, not less than 67 completed at least the anniversary date of their attacks under the observation of the writers. Of these not less than 9 have had at least 2 annual attacks. In none of the 67, following the change in diet, has there been observed so far this year any recognizable evidence of a recurrence, nor have the writers been able to detect any evidence justifying a diagnosis of pellagra in any of the nonpellagrin residents, numbering 99 children and adults, who have been continuously under observation for at least one year. In other words, barring recent admissions, there has been no pellagra at this institution this year.

Orphanage "B. J."—Of the 130 cases of pellagra observed in the children at "B. J." during the summer of 1914, not less than 105 have completed at least the anniversary date of last year's attack under the writers' observation. Not less than 14 of these have histories of at least 2 successive annual attacks. In only 1 of these 105 pellagrins, following the above change in diet, has there, so far this year, been recognized evidence justifying the diagnosis of a recurrence.

Of the residents of this orphanage that did not present any definite evidence of pellagra in 1914, 69 have remained continuously under observation for at least a year; none has thus far developed recognizable evidence of the disease this year. Recent admissions aside, there has been but one case of pellagra at this institution this year.

Orphanage, M. J.—January 1 to 7, 1915.

BREAKFAST

All ages:

Oatmeal, with sugar and milk, biscuit with butter, daily. Frankfurters (boiled), one morning, in place of fried bacon or eggs.

Matrons and "big" boys:

Fried bacon on six mornings.

All under 12 years:

Milk (about 7 ounces) as a beverage, daily; one egg (scrambled, fried, or boiled), six mornings.

DINNER

January 1:
  All—
    Vegetable soup (tomatoes, Irish potatoes, corn, onions, rice).
    Baked sweet potatoes.
    Corn bread.
    Light bread.
  Matrons—
    Biscuit.

January 2:
  All—
    Navy beans (boiled).
    Baked sweet potatoes.
    Light bread.
    Pie (blackberry, peach).
  Matrons—
    Hot biscuit.
    Corn muffins.

January 3:
  All—
    Roast beef.
    Lima beans (boiled).
    Layer cake.
  Matrons—
    Baked sweet potatoes.
    Boiled rice custard.
    Blackberry preserves.

January 4:
  All—
    Vegetable soup (tomatoes, rice, onions, navy beans).
    Hash for three tables.
    Baked sweet potatoes.
    Boiled navy beans.
    Light bread.

January 4—Continued.
  Matrons—
    Corn bread.
    Hot biscuit.

January 5:
  All—
    Vegetable soup (tomatoes, rice, onions).
    Roast beef.
    Baked sweet potatoes.
    Boiled lima beans.
    Light bread.
  Matrons—
    Biscuits, corn bread.

January 6:
  All—
    Roast beef.
    Boiled navy beans.
    Baked sweet potatoes.
    Blackberry pie (five tables).
    Stewed pears (three tables).
    Light bread.
  Matrons—
    Biscuit.
    Corn muffins.

January 7:
  All—
    Vegetable soup (tomatoes, rice, onions).
    Boiled frankfurters
    Boiled lima beans.
    Baked sweet potatoes.
    Light bread.
  Matrons—
    Biscuit.
    Corn muffins.

N. B.—Children under 6 years of age received about 7 ounces of mik each daily in addition to the above.

SUPPER

January 1:
  All—
      Stewed prunes or pumpkin.
      Light bread.
  Over 12—
      Boiled grits.

January 2:
  All—
      Sirup.
      Light bread.
  Over 12—
      Boiled rice.
      Fried bacon.

January 3:
  All—
      Cakes.
      Light bread.
      Milk.

January 4:
  All—
      Stewed apples.
      Light bread.
  Over 12—
      Fried bacon.
      Boiled rice.

January 5:
  All—
      Light bread.
      Sirup.
  Over 12—
      Boiled grits.
      Fried fresh pork.

January 6:
  All—
      Light bread.
      Stewed apples.
  Over 12—
      Beef hash.
      Boiled rice.

January 7:
  All—
      Light bread.
      Sirup.
      Milk.
  Over 12—
      Fried bacon.
      Boiled rice.

N. B.—All under 12 years received about 7 ounces of milk daily in addition to the bread and stewed fruit or sirup. The matrons and teachers were served with hot biscuits daily in addition to the other articles noted.

Asylum Study

Through the courtesy and with the very helpful cooperation of the board of trustees, superintendent, clinical director, and staff of the Georgia State Sanitarium, two wards were turned over to the writers for a test of the value of diet in the prevention of pellagra. To this asylum, the largest in the South, there are admitted annually a considerable number of cases of pellagra. Besides this, cases of institutional origin are of frequent occurrence. This asylum must, therefore, be regarded as an endemic focus of the disease.

Of the two wards placed at our disposal one is in the colored and the other in the white female service; the former was organized in October, the latter in December, 1914.

Each ward has a capacity of about 50 beds. To each there were admitted about 40 adult pellagrins who had had attacks at one time or another during 1914. In organizing the wards and selecting our patients the list of female pellagrins that at that time were known to have had attacks in 1914 was practically exhausted. In selecting the

patients only one condition was observed, namely, that the patient
should, if possible, be of such a mental type as would give the highest
degree of probability of remaining under observation for at least a
year. In consequence a very considerable proportion of them were
of a much deteriorated, untidy class. There were, nevertheless, unavoidably included several in whom the mental condition improved
to such a degree that we felt obliged to permit them to go when a
request for their discharge was made. Not all, therefore, of our original patients remained under observation long enough to be included
in the present discussion.

Very few of the patients presented active symptoms on admission
to the writers' wards, the object so far as this test was concerned
being not a study of the treatment of active symptoms but the prevention of recurrences. A very considerable number of the patients,
however, presented marked residuals of a recent attack. Many of the
colored patients had been dieted by either Dr. Lorenz or Dr. Willets
during the acute stage of their attacks in the same ward prior to its
organization for the purpose under consideration. A number of the
white females had been dieted during the acute stage by Dr. Y. A.
Lyttle, of the asylum staff, and formed part of a series reported on by
him at the meeting of the Southern Medical Association in November, 1914. The writers are especially indebted to Dr. Lyttle for his
courtesy in subordinating his own study and turning these patients
over to them.

The diet furnished the inmates of these two wards was prescribed
by the writers, and instructions were given to the nurses to give more
than ordinary care in supervising the feeding. As at the orphanages,
a decided increase was made in the animal and leguminous protein
foods. A cup of sweet milk, about 7 ounces, is furnished each patient
for breakfast and one of buttermilk at both dinner and supper.
About half a pound of fresh beef and 2 to 2½ ounces of dried field
peas or dried beans enter into the daily ration. Oatmeal has almost
entirely replaced grits as the breakfast cereal; sirup has been entirely
excluded. Corn products, though greatly reduced, have not been
entirely eliminated.

The menu that follows will serve to give a more detailed idea of
the character of the diet furnished. (See p. 37.)

Aside from the change in diet and the increased watchfulness over
the individual feeding enjoined on the nurses and attendants, no
change in the habitual routine of the corresponding services was
made. The patients were permitted and encouraged to visit the yard

Weekly menu for Ward 23.

MONDAY

Breakfast: Grits, sweet milk, sugar, broiled steak, hot rolls, biscuits, coffee.
Dinner: Roast beef, gravy, peas, potatoes, rice, biscuits, buttermilk.
Supper: Stewed apples, light bread, coffee, buttermilk, sugar.

TUESDAY

Breakfast: Oatmeal, sweet milk, sugar, Hamburg steak, biscuits, hot rolls, coffee.
Dinner: Beef stew, potatoes, rice, bread, buttermilk.
Supper: Baked beans, light bread, coffee, sugar, buttermilk.

WEDNESDAY

Breakfast: Oatmeal, sweet milk, sugar, beef hash, hot rolls, biscuits, coffee.
Dinner: Pea soup, corn bread, gravy, potatoes, rice, bread, buttermilk.
Supper: Stewed prunes, light bread, coffee, sugar, buttermilk.

THURSDAY

Breakfast: Oatmeal, sweet milk, sugar, fried steak, hot rolls, biscuits, coffee.
Dinner: Beef stew, peas, potatoes, rice, bread, buttermilk.
Supper: Baked beans, bread, coffee, sugar, buttermilk.

FRIDAY

Breakfast: Oatmeal, sweet milk, sugar, broiled beefsteak, hot rolls, biscuits, coffee.
Dinner: Pea soup (purée), roast beef, potatoes, rice, bread, buttermilk.
Supper: Light bread, coffee, sugar, buttermilk, apples, baked beans.

SATURDAY

Breakfast: Oatmeal, sweet milk, sugar, Hamburg steak, hot rolls, biscuits, coffee.
Dinner: Beef stew, potatoes, rice, bread, buttermilk.
Supper: Bread, baked beans, buttermilk, coffee, sugar.

SUNDAY

Breakfast: Oatmeal, sweet milk, sugar, mackerel, bread, coffee.
Dinner: Loaf beef and gravy, peas, potatoes, rice, bread, buttermilk, pudding.
Supper: Beef hash, bread, sugar, coffee, buttermilk.

NOTE.—Green vegetables in season at irregular intervals. Milk and eggs, as a special diet, are furnished those patients who may require them.

and take the air as frequently as their physical condition and the weather permitted.

Results.—Of the pellagrins admitted to the writers' wards at the time of their organization, or shortly thereafter—that is, not later than December 31, 1914—72 (36 colored and 36 white), have remained continuously under observation up to October 1, 1915, or remained at least until after the anniversary date of their last year's attack. Of the 36 colored patients, 8 have histories of at least 2 annual attacks; of the 36 white patients, 10 have histories of at least 2 attacks. None of this group of 72 patients has presented recognizable evidence of a recurrence of pellagra.

Significance

The significance of the results set forth naturally depends upon the rate of recurrence that may properly have been expected to occur in the groups studied under "normal" conditions; that is, without interference of any kind.

The ideal form of the experiment would have been, of course, to retain for purpose of comparison a control group at each of the institutions. This was impracticable at the orphanages. In estimating the significance of the results of the orphanage study, the writers are therefore obliged to depend on general observations and on experience at other similar institutions. Satisfactory observations on the rate of recurrence either in children or adults are, so far as the writers are aware, not available in the accessible literature. There are to be found for the most part simply general statements that the disease tends as a rule to recur from year to year. Fortunately, Dr. H. W. Rice, of Columbia, S. C., has very kindly given a copy of his records of the cases of pellagra observed by him in children at an orphanage to which he has been attending physician. These records show that of 31 children who had pellagra in 1912, 18, or 58 per cent, had recurrences in 1913; of the 21 who had it in 1913, 16, or 76 per cent, had it in 1914; and of 75 who had the disease in 1914, 56, or 75 per cent, had it again in 1915. The rate of recurrence in children at this institution seems to have varied, therefore, between 58 per cent and 76 per cent. These very valuable data enable one to form a definite conception of the frequency of recurrence that one might expect from year to year in children at such institutions as those at which the writers have worked.

Taking 50 per cent, a rate somewhat lower than the lowest of the above rates, as being fairly and conservatively representative and applying it to the orphanages at Jackson, it is found that 33 recurrences at "M. J." and 52 at "B. J." might reasonably have been expected this year, whereas, as already stated, there actually was none observed at the former and only one at the latter institution.

Although not specifically so planned, conditions at the Georgia State Sanitarium have been such as to give a control group of pellagrins in both the colored and the white female service. This permits the making of a direct comparison of the results observed in the writers' wards with those in other wards of the corresponding services at this institution.

The control group of colored female pellagrins of 1914 consists of 17 who have remained under observation for a period comparable to that of the group on the special diet. Of these, 9, or 53 per cent, have already presented recurrences.

The control group of white female pellagrins of 1914 consists of 15 individuals. Of these, 6, or 40 per cent, have had recurrences this year. Combined, the two control groups have thus far presented an average of 47 per cent of recurrences. Besides the recurrence rates in these control groups, the rates of recurrence in previous years in these services have been determined from a study of the records. It is found that in the colored female service the average rate for the four years 1911, 1912, 1913, and 1914 has been 52.5 per cent, the rate in different years having varied from 40 to 70 per cent. In the white female service the average recurrence rate for the same period has been 37.5 per cent, the rate having varied between 22 and 48 per cent.

It must be quite evident, therefore, that on the basis of any of the foregoing rates a considerable number of recurrences in the groups of insane pellagrins subsisting on the modified diet might reasonably have been expected. On the basis of the average recurrence rate, 47 per cent, observed this year in the control groups, we might have expected some 34 recurrences, or on the basis of the average rate, 37.5 per cent, for four years, for the white female service, a rate lower than the average for the colored female service, we might have expected some 20 to 27 recurrences. As already stated, however, none has actually been observed.

Viewing the foregoing results as a whole, bearing in mind that three different institutions in two widely separated localities are involved, each institution being an endemic focus of the disease, and bearing in mind, also, that the number of individuals considered is fairly large, it seems to the writers that the conclusion is justified that pellagra recurrences may be prevented and, in view of the conditions of the test, that they may be prevented without the intervention of any other factor than diet.

In this connection the question arises whether the conclusion is justified that the development of pellagra, apart from its recurrence, may be prevented by diet. The character of the answer to the question will depend on the view held as to the nature of the pellagra recurrence.

Among the epidemiologic features of pellagra none is more striking than the tendency for the disease not only to develop in the spring or early summer, but to recur year after year at about the same season. Various explanations of this singular phenomenon have been advanced. According to Sambon (1910, p. 49), "this peculiar peri-

odicity of symptoms can be explained only by the agency of a parasitic organism presenting definite alternating periods of latency and
activity." A somewhat similar conception appears to be held by the
workers of the Thompson-McFadden Commission (Siler, Garrison,
and MacNeal, Oct. 15, 1914), who distinguish between conditions
favorable for the development of the disease, in the first place, and
those that permit its subsequent recurrence. Why Sambon and many
other observers should consider this periodicity of symptoms as
explicable only by the agency of a parasitic organism or of a virus
or a toxin presenting definite alternating periods of latency and
activity is rather hard to understand when it is recalled that in
endemic scurvy (Lind, 1772, pp. 33, 84, 130, 306) and particularly in
endemic beriberi, diseases of well-known dietary origin, a strikingly
similar periodicity is present. The following description of the clinical course of beriberi taken from Scheube (1903, pp. 199–200) well
illustrates this point: "After developing the disease" [beriberi], says
Scheube, "the condition of the patient may remain the same for
months. Then, especially on the appearance of the cold season, improvement sets in and recovery ensues. The predisposition is not
extinguished by recovery from the disease; on the other hand, he
who has once had beriberi is apt to be attacked again. The relapses
are sometimes milder, sometimes more severe than the initial attack,
and are repeated every year for shorter or longer periods, sometimes,
10, 20, or even 30 years. Sometimes the disease remains absent for
one or several years, and then appears anew. Occasionally two or
even three attacks occur during the course of one year."

In the light of this striking analogy, it would seem entirely permissible to invoke as an explanation of the periodic recurrence in
pellagra, what undoubtedly is the explanation of the same phenomenon in beriberi, namely, a modification or change in diet brought
about by or incidental to the recurring seasons (Vedder, 1913, p. 29).
In accordance with this explanation the recurrence in pellagra is to
be considered as in beriberi, etiologically, at least, essentially identical with the initial attack; it would seem permissible to conclude,
therefore, that the means found effective in the prevention of recurrences will be found effective in the prevention of the initial attack.

From the foregoing it will be observed that the writers' results are
at variance with those of some other recent workers in this field,
notably, the Thompson-McFadden Pellagra Commission. In a summary of their second progress report (Siler, Garrison, and MacNeal,
Sept. 26, 1914, p. 1093) this commission concludes that its efforts to
discover the essential pellagra-producing food or the essential

pellagra-preventing food have not been crowned with success, and that their evidence suggests that neither exists in the population studied by them.

In the opinion of the writers this conclusion is due to the way in which they analyzed what is undoubtedly a very valuable mass of data. They assume that the relation of a particular food to pellagra can be determined by comparing the incidence of the disease in groups of families using this particular food with different degrees of frequency. This assumption, however, fails to take into account the possibility that more than one food having a relation to the disease may have been present in the dietaries of the families studied.

Thus it seemed to them, and at first thought it no doubt would seem to others, that if meat, for instance, had any relation to pellagra, this would be revealed by a comparison of the incidence of the disease in a group of families using this food daily with the incidence in a group using it rarely. As a matter of fact, however, although a comparison of the incidence of pellagra in different families grouped on the basis of the frequency of the use of fresh meat might result, let us say, in finding a greater relative incidence in families using it daily than in those using it rarely, it would not on that account be permissible to conclude that meat had no preventive value, for it may very well be that the families using meat rarely were protected by some other food or foods, such as milk, eggs, or peas, of which they may have been abundant consumers.

In fact, it is believed by the writers that an analysis of the commission's data from this point of view will show, for instance, that there does exist, or may exist, in a group of cotton-mill villages an inverse proportional relation between degree of pellagra morbidity and the percentage of families using fresh meat and milk "daily" and "habitually." In other words, the disagreement in our results from those of the commission is more apparent than real.

It is beside the present purpose to enter into a discussion of the etiology of pellagra. In order that the position of the writers may be clear, however, it is pointed out that they are not to be understood as meaning that pellagra is necessarily due to a lack or deficiency of fresh animal or leguminous protein food. All that they wish to say at present is that the dietary "fault" upon which in their judgment the development of pellagra essentially depends is capable of being corrected or prevented by including in the diet a suitable proportion of these foods. Nor are they to be understood as meaning that the pellagra-causing "fault" is capable of correction or prevention in this way only. The possibility is not excluded that there may be other foods capable of serving the same purpose. Indeed, there is some reason to justify at least a suspicion that barley, rye, and millet may have this power in some degree.

Moreover, it may be, if Funk's suggestion that pellagra is a vitamin deficiency, brought about by the consumption of overmilled corn, is proven to be correct, that the use of undermilled corn will of itself correct the "fault" in a diet in which this cereal is the staple. For the present at least the point of chief, of fundamental, practical importance is the recognition of the fact that the pellagra-producing dietary "fault," whatever its essential nature or however brought about, is capable of correction or prevention, as the results above presented seem to clearly indicate, by including in the diet suitable proportions of the fresh animal and leguminous foods.

Summary and Conclusion

1. The diet at two orphanages, "M. J." and "B. J.," for several years endemic foci of pellagra, was modified in accordance with the directions of the writers in September, 1914. Hygienic and sanitary conditions have remained unchanged.

2. The modification in the diet consisted principally of a marked increase in the fresh animal and the leguminous protein foods.

3. Since the change in diet at orphanage "M. J." there has not been observed any recognizable evidence of a recurrence in any of the pellagrins of 1914, 67 of whom remained under observation until they had completed at least the anniversary date of their attacks. Nor have any new cases been observed among the nonpellagrin residents of 1914, 99 of whom have been under observation for not less than a year.

4. Since the change in diet at orphanage "B. J." there has been observed this year but a single individual with recognizable evidence of a recurrence among the pellagrins of 1914, 105 of whom remained under observation until they had completed at least the anniversary date of their attacks. Nor has any new case been observed among the nonpellagrin residents, 69 of whom have been under observation not less than a year.

5. At the Georgia State Sanitarium, an endemic focus of pellagra, a ward of pellagrins in the colored female service and one in the white female service was organized in October and December, 1914, respectively, for a test of diet in the prevention of pellagra.

6. The diet in these wards was modified on the same principle as that at the orphanages. The institution routine and the hygienic and sanitary conditions have remained unchanged.

7. Since the change of diet and up to October 1, 1915, there has not been observed this year any recognizable evidence of a recurrence in any of the pellagrins in these wards, 72 of whom (36 colored and 36 white females) have remained continuously under observation throughout this period or at least until the completion of the anniversary date of their 1914 attacks.

8. During the corresponding period of observation not less than 15 (47 per cent) of 32 control female pellagrins have presented recurrences.

9. The conclusion is drawn that pellagra may be prevented by an appropriate diet without any alteration in the environment, hygienic or sanitary.

Application

The practical application of the foregoing to the problem of the prevention and eradication of pellagra seems so obvious that extended discussion is not called for in the present communication, particularly as a somewhat detailed outline of treatment and prevention has already been published (Goldberger, Willets, and Waring, 1914). At this time it is desired simply to submit for consideration some general recommendations that appear to be pertinent to the problem.

In order that a suitable modification in the diet of the population chiefly affected may be brought about, the writer would recommend:

1. An increase in the diet of fresh animal and leguminous foods, particularly during the late winter and spring.
    a. Ownership of a milk cow and increase in milk production for home consumption.
    b. Poultry and egg raising for home consumption.
    c. Stock raising.
    d. Diversification and the cultivation of food crops (including an adequate pea patch) in order to minimize the disastrous economic effects of a crop failure and to make food cheaper and more readily available.
    e. Making these foods as accessible as possible in the more or less isolated industrial communities by providing markets, particularly butcher shops, throughout the year.
2. A reduction in the diet of the carbohydrate (starchy) foods.
    a. Improve economic conditions; increase wages, reduce unemployment.
    b. Make the other class of foods cheap and readily accessible.

References

Funk, C. *Die Vitamine* (Wiesbaden, 1914).

―――. "Prophylaxie und Therapie der Pellagra ins Lichte der Vitamin-lehre," *Münch. Med. Wchnschr.* (1914), pp. 698–99.

Goldberger, J. "The Etiology of Pellagra; the significance of certain epi-demiological observations with respect thereto," *Public Health Rep.* (Washington, D.C.), June 26, 1914, pp. 1683–86.

―――. "The Cause and Prevention of Pellagra," *ibid.* (September 11, 1914).

―――. "Beans for Prevention of Pellagra," *J. Am. Med. Assn.* Vol. 63 (October 10, 1914), p. 1314.

Goldberger, J., Waring, C. H., and Willets, D. G. "The Treatment and Prevention of Pellagra," *Public Health Rep.* (Washington, D.C.), Octo-ber 23, 1914, pp. 2821–25.

―――. Reprint No. 228 from *Public Health Rep.* (Washington, D.C.), October 23, 1914.

―――. Reprint No. 228 from *Public Health Rep.* (Washington, D.C.), October 23, 1914; revised edition (January 15, 1915).

Lind, J. *A Treatise on the Scurvy* (3d ed.; London, 1772).

Lorenz, W. F. "The Treatment of Pellagra," *Public Health Rep.* (Wash-ington, D.C.), September 11, 1914.

Lyttle, Y. A. "The Dietetic Treatment of Pellagra. With report of eleven cases," *Southern Med. J.* Vol. 8 (August, 1915), pp. 659–62.

Roussel, T. *Traité de la Pellagra et des Pseudo-Pellagres* (Paris, 1866).

Sambon, L. W. "Progress Report on the Investigation of Pellagra," Reprint from the *J. Trop. Med. and Hyg.* (London, 1910).

Scheube, B. *The Diseases of Warm Countries* (London, 1903).

Siler, J. F., Garrison, P. E., and MacNeal, W. J. "A Statistical Study of the Relation of Pellagra to Use of Certain Foods, etc." *Arch. Int. Med.* (Chicago), Vol. 14 (September 15, 1914), pp. 292–373.

―――. "Further Studies of the Thompson-McFadden Pellagra Commis-sion. A summary of the second progress report," *J. Am. Med. Assn.* (Chicago), Vol. 63 (September 26, 1914), pp. 1090–93.

―――. "The Relation of Methods of Disposal of Sewage to the Spread of Pellagra," *Arch. Int. Med.,* Vol. 14 (October 15, 1914), pp. 453-74.

Vedder, E. B. *Beriberi* (New York, 1913).

4. Pellagra Prevention by Diet Among Institutional Inmates[1]

JOSEPH GOLDBERGER
C. H. WARING
W. F. TANNER[2]

In 1914, when the study herein reported was begun, American opinion as to the etiology and prophylaxis of pellagra may be said to have been very unsettled, if not chaotic. The spoiled-maize theory of the cause and as the basis for prevention, though stoutly held in some important quarters, was declining in favor; and the belief that the disease was an infection of some kind, supported as it was by such important studies as those of the Illinois and of the Thompson-McFadden pellagra commissions (Report of the Pellagra Commission, 1912; Siler, Garrison, and MacNeal, 1914), was gaining a ready and rapidly widening acceptance. The state of mind, both lay and professional, is well indicated by the following from Lavinder (1909, pp. 1617-24) even though written five years earlier:

There are several very good reasons just now why this question of communicability should have arisen to much importance in this country. . . . In the first place, the disease has arisen and grown to large proportions, apparently like the proverbial mushroom, almost in a single night. It is something new, a malady with which we are not familiar, and in some of its manifestations is repulsive, if not actually loathsome; indeed, some of the older writers, evidently struck with this fact, applied to it the name "leprosy," a term which, since the days of Moses, has been a synonym to mankind of all that is repulsive and loathsome in human disease. Then, too, it has been associated in our minds very frequently with mental alienation, a state naturally abhorrent to all; and its reported death rate has been very large indeed. Furthermore, the indefinite and pervasive character of its etiology, with the lack, not only of any specific treatment, but the apparent inefficacy of all treatment, has added further color to an already vivid picture.

---

1 *Public Health Rep.*, Vol. 38, No. 41 (October 12, 1923), 2361-68.
2 During the first two years of the study at the Georgia State Sanitarium, Dr. David G. Willets, late assistant epidemiologist, United States Public Health Service, was associated with us. His premature separation was unhappily made necessary by the development in December, 1916, of what proved to be a fatal illness.

All these features have given to the disease an air of strangeness, not to say of actual mystery, which has made a strong appeal to the public mind and which has probably, to a certain extent, reacted upon the professional mind. The result in certain communities has been to produce a very uneasy state of feeling, almost an hysterical condition, at times actually bordering on panic.

The fear that the disease was communicable led here and there to the adoption of such drastic measures of control as isolation and quarantine.

The situation called urgently for renewed investigation with a view of testing these conflicting views and, if possible, establishing a sound basis for the prevention of the disease. Considering this problem, one of the present writers was struck by the possible significance of the long recognized exemption from the disease enjoyed by well-to-do people. In reflecting on this striking phenomenon and in considering the elements differentiating affluence from poverty, diet, in view of the conspicuous place it had always had in discussions of the disease, naturally arrested attention. It seemed possible that the well-to-do owed their exemption to their superior diet. Coupled with certain other epidemiological observations, this led him (Goldberger, 1914) to suggest that it might be well to attempt to prevent the disease by providing those persons subject to pellagra with a diet such as that enjoyed by the class practically free from it. Accordingly, in the fall of 1914, the Public Health Service undertook to put this hypothesis to the test. A report covering the work and results of the first year was published in 1915 (Goldberger, Waring, and Willets, 1915). It was originally intended to make a detailed presentation of the study on its completion; but the confirmation of the published results of the first year by White (1919), among Armenian refugees at Port Said, and by Stannus (1920) among the inmates of Central Prison, Nyasaland, before this could be done, has rendered a detailed account superfluous. And this all the more as the later results, as will presently be seen, were in close harmony with and in complete confirmation of those of the first year. We therefore present now but a general summary of this study with brief mention of only the more important and significant details.

Since the study was carried on throughout along the lines adopted at its beginning, and since, as stated, later results were in close harmony with those of the first year, it will be helpful to review at the outset the methods and results of the first year.

First year.—The test of the preventive value of diet was begun at two orphanages at Jackson, Miss., in September, 1914, and in two wards of the Georgia State Sanitarium later that same year. These institutions had been endemic foci of the disease for some years. During the spring and summer of 1914, 79 cases of pellagra had been observed among the children of one orphanage and 130 among those of the other. Besides a variable number of cases of pellagra annually admitted as such (see below), cases of intramural origin were of frequent occurrence at the sanitarium.

At the orphanages the diet of all the residents, and at the sanitarium that of a group of selected inmates of two wards set aside for the purpose, was modified in several respects, among others in that oatmeal almost entirely replaced grits as the breakfast cereal and the allowance of fresh animal protein foods (milk, meat, and, at the orphanages, eggs) and legumes was greatly increased. The allowance of maize was thus reduced but not abolished. Aside from these modifications in diet and increased watchfulness over the individual eating, all administrative routine and hygienic and sanitary conditions remained unchanged. Furthermore, in order, at the same time, to test the hypothesis of infection, no restrictions were imposed on new admissions by reason of any manifestations of pellagra or of a history of an attack of the disease, and thus association and contact with newly admitted active cases were permitted without hindrance and, from time to time, actually took place, particularly at the sanitarium, the opportunities there being better.

At about the end of the first year following the inauguration of the modified diet, it was found that, at the orphanages, of an aggregate of 172 pellagrins who had completed at least the anniversary date of the 1914 attack under observation, only 1 had showed any evidence of a recurrence, and not a single case developed among an aggregate of 168 nonpellagrins who had been continuously under observation at least one year; and at the sanitarium of an aggregate of 72 pellagrins who had either remained continuously under observation up to October 1, 1915, or, at least, until after the anniversary date of the 1914 attack, not one presented recognizable evidence of a recurrence, although at the same time 47 per cent of a comparable group of 32 pellagrins not receiving the modified diet had recurrent attacks of the disease.

Second year.—The results of the first year afforded no support for the idea that pellagra was communicable, but very clearly indicated that the disease could be prevented by an appropriate diet. Nevertheless, by reason of the importance of the question involved, and in order to make the test and demonstration of preventability as convincing as possible, it seemed desirable to continue the investigation, as originally planned, for at least another year and, if possible, on a larger scale.

The study at the orphanages and at the asylum was accordingly continued and, in addition, was extended to include an orphanage at Columbia, S. C., and a third ward of insane pellagrins, with recent attacks, at the State Sanitarium.

It was extended to the Columbia institution on September 1, 1915. At this orphanage the disease, after its recognition there in 1907 or 1908, had prevailed from year to year in spite of various efforts to control it. With this purpose in view, a water carriage sewerage system had been installed in 1914 in place of the surface privies theretofore used, but without appreciable effect, for in 1915 the number attacked and the rate of recurrence were higher than ever, upward of 100 cases being recognized among the children by the orphanage physician (Rice, 1916). At the time of taking charge there were present 235 residents at this orphanage, of whom 106 had been reported to us as having had pellagra that year; and of these 15 still presented recognizable evidence of the attack.

At the sanitarium the additional ward of pellagrins was taken under observation and provided with the modified and supplemented diet about November 1, 1915.

The result of this more extensive test of the preventability of pellagra by dietary means was in the closest harmony with that of the first year. In not a single one of the individuals receiving the modified diet at the three orphanages and at the hospital for insane did pellagra develop either as an initial or a recurrent attack. So impressive was this outcome that it seemed unnecessary longer to continue the demonstration on so large a scale. Accordingly, the study at the orphanages was discontinued on September 1, 1916; but because of the much greater significance likely to attach to results of tests in the insane, that at the state Sanitarium was continued through a third year; that is, until December 31, 1917.

Third year.—The third year's study at the sanitarium was continued with three wards under observation, one in the white and two in the colored service, as during the second year. The modifications of and supplements to the institution diet, the hygienic conditions, the administrative routine, the mingling with other inmates (including those with active pellagra) in the wards and in the recreation yards were continued as during the first and second year.

The result of the third year's study was exactly like that of the second year: no recurrence and no new case among those inmates taking the modified diet.

Result as a whole.—The result of the investigation considered as a whole may be summed up as follows: The individuals under observation, disregarding those who were present for periods too brief to be significant, numbered 702, of whom 414 were pellagrins and 288 nonpellagrins.

Two hundred and fifty of the pellagrins and 268 of the nonpellagrins were included in the study at the orphanages and were under continuous observation for at least one year. Of this group, 107 of the pellagrins and 85 of the nonpellagrins were under observation for a period of at least two years (Table 1).

Of the 414 pellagrins included in the study, 164 were observed at the sanitarium and were under observation until at least the first anniversary date of the attack, during which or shortly after which they entered the study. Of these 164, 109 were under observation until at least the second anniversary date, and, of the latter group, 57 until at least the third anniversary date. Resident on the same wards and receiving the same diet as these pellagrins, were nonpellagrins, 20 of whom (not including nurses and attendants) were under observation for at least one year, 16 of these for not less than two years, and, of the latter, 10 for not less than three years.

As has already been stated, but a single case of pellagra occurred among all these pellagrins and nonpellagrins. This one case, a recurrence in a boy at one of the Jackson orphanages, developed during the first year of the study. The boy continued under observation during the second year without again developing any evidence of the disease.

At this point mention may be made of the history of pellagra at one of the institutions subsequent to the discontinuance of the foregoing study. Immediately following our withdrawal, there was a return to the unmodified and unsupplemented institution diet.

TABLE 1—*Number of specified classes of individuals observed for pellagra during specified periods, according to orphanage of residence.*

Class.	Period of observation.										
	At least one year.				One year but less than two years.				At least two years.		
	Total	MJ.[*]	BJ.[*]	EC.[+]	Total	MJ.[*]	BJ.[*]	EC.[+]	Total	MJ.[*]	BJ.[*]
Pellagrins.....	250	59	99	92	143	22	29	92	107	37	70
Nonpellagrins..	268	100	69	99	183	58	26	99	85	42	43

[*] Two orphanages at Jackson, Miss., indicated by "MJ" and "BJ."
[+] Orphanage at Columbia, S. C., indicated by "EC."

During the period of from 3½ to 9½ months following this, approximately 40 per cent of those who were affected by the change in diet developed pellagra. Thereupon there were added to the institution diet, again under our direction, 4 ounces of fresh beef, about 7 ounces of sweet milk, and about 14 ounces of buttermilk per adult per day; and during an observation period of 14 months immediately succeeding the adoption of these supplements no evidence of pellagra developed in any of the group.

Discussion

It appears, then, that at each institution at which the test was made, barring cases admitted as such during the progress of the test, pellagra promptly disappeared. And it is perhaps important to note that this was not merely a marked reduction in prevalence, but in each instance a complete disappearance of the disease. It may be noted also that the disease disappeared from the institutions at a time when it was highly prevalent at large in the corresponding states. Thus, judging by mortality reports, we find that in Mississippi there were 1,192 deaths from pellagra in 1914, 1,535 in 1915, 840 in 1916, and 1,086 in 1917; that in South Carolina there were 1,649 in 1915, 729 in 1916, and 714 in 1917. For Georgia no reports are available for this period, but admissions to the Georgia State Sanitarium will serve as a good index of the yearly prevalence in that state. In 1914, of 1,427 patients admitted, 194, or 13.59 per cent, were active cases of pellagra; in 1915, of 1,683 admissions, 272, or 16.16 per cent, were cases of pellagra; in 1916, of 1,331 admissions, 111, or 8.34 per cent, were pellagra; and in 1917, of 1,219 admissions, 121, or 9.93 per cent, were active cases.

Clearly, therefore, the disappearance of pellagra from the institutions under consideration must have been due to something not operative at large or operative only to an inappreciable degree. Recalling the conditions of the test—namely, that hygienic and sanitary conditions (excepting diet) continued unaltered, that admission of active cases and association of these with persons in the test continued without hindrance (and was particularly frequent and free at the sanitarium), that considerable groups of persons in four separate endemic foci in three widely separated localities were involved— the something that operated to bring this disappearance about must have been the one factor, diet, close upon the modification of which disappearance of the disease followed. Since both pellagrins and exposed nonpellagrins were carried for as long as two and three years without manifesting recognizable evidence of a return or of the development of an initial attack of the disease, and since in one group of these the disease reappeared on departing from and again disappeared on returning to what, for this purpose, is considered to have been an appropriate diet, the inference seems clearly warranted that not only may pellagra be completely prevented by diet, but that it may be prevented indefinitely as long as a proper diet is maintained and without the intervention of any other factor, hygienic or sanitary.

What food or foods, food factor or factors, in the diet are to be credited with the result under discussion, this experiment in itself does not definitely reveal. In planning the test diet we were guided by general observation of the character of the dietary of well-to-do people and the results of certain epidemiologic observations (Goldberger, Waring, and Willets, 1915) which suggested that the disease was dependent upon a diet that was faulty and that this fault was, in some way, either prevented or corrected by including in the diet larger proportions of the fresh animal protein foods. The experiment may be therefore considered as, at most, suggesting that the fresh meat and milk of the diet were concerned in bringing about the protective effect, or, in other words, that fresh meat and milk supplied some factor or factors which operated to prevent the development of pellagra.

Since the results here reported are but a confirmation, on a more extended and more convincing scale, of those previously reported for the first year of this study, which alone and in connection with the results of certain other phases of the general investigation of which they are parts, have already been sufficiently considered,[3] both in their implications and in their relation to the results of the studies of other investigators, further discussion at this time seems uncalled for.

Summary and Conclusions

A report of a three years' study of the preventability of pellagra by means of diet, the result of the first year of which was reported eight years ago, is briefly presented.

The study was carried on for a year at one and for two years at two of three orphanages, and for three years in a section of the Georgia State Sanitarium, each of the institutions being recognized as an endemic focus of the disease.

The institution diet was in each instance modified by reducing

3 Goldberger, Waring, and Willets, 1915; Goldberger, 1916; Goldberger and Wheeler, February, 1920; Goldberger and Wheeler, May, 1920; Goldberger, Wheeler, and Sydenstricker, 1920; Goldberger, 1922.

the maize element and increasing the fresh animal protein foods—meat, milk (and at the orphanages, eggs), and legumes.

All other conditions, hygienic and sanitary, including association with active cases which from time to time were admitted, remained unchanged.

The individuals under observation, not counting those who were present for periods too brief to be significant, numbered 702 in all, of whom 414 were pellagrins and 288 nonpellagrins.

Among the pellagrins a single recurrent case was noted during the first year following the inauguration of the modified diet; none in the second nor in the third year. Among the nonpellagrins there was not a single case.

A return to the institution diet immediately after the discontinuance of the formal study at one of the institutions was shortly followed by an incidence of pellagra of approximately 40 per cent among the affected group. Resumption of the modified diet was again followed during a period of observation of 14 months by complete disappearance of the disease.

During the study the disease disappeared from the institutions, although a considerable prevalence at large in the corresponding states continued.

The idea that pellagra is a communicable disease receives no support from this study.

Pellagra may be completely prevented by diet.

References

Goldberger, J. *Public Health Rep.* (Washington, D.C.), Vol. 29 (June 26, 1914), pp. 1683–86.

————. *J. Am. Med. Assn.*, Vol. 66 (February 12, 1916), pp. 471–76.

————. *J. Am. Med. Assn.*, Vol. 78 (June 3, 1922), pp. 1676-80.

————, Waring, C. H., and Willets, D. G. *Public Health Rep.* (Washington, D.C.), Vol. 30 (October 22, 1915), pp. 3117–31.

Goldberger, J., and Wheeler, G. A. *Hyg. Lab. Bull.* (Washington, D.C.), No. 120 (February, 1920).

————. *Arch. Int. Med.*, Vol. 25 (May, 1920), pp. 451–71.

————, and Sydenstricker, E. *Public Health Rep.*, Vol. 35 (March, 1920), pp. 648–713.

Lavinder, C. H. *Public Health Rep.* (Washington, D.C.), Vol. 24 (October 29, 1909), pp. 1617–24.

Report of the Pellagra Commission of the State of Illinois (Springfield, Ill., 1912).

Rice, H. W. *Southern Med. J.*, Vol. 9 (September, 1916), pp. 778–85.

Siler, J. F., Garrison, P. E., and MacNeal, W. J. *J. Am. Med. Assn.*, Vol. 62 (January 3, 1914), pp. 8–12.

Stannus, H. S. *Trans. Roy. Soc. Trop. Med. & Hyg.* (London), Vol. 14 (1920), p. 16.

White, R. G. *Report on an Outbreak of Pellagra Amongst Armenian Refugees at Port Said. 1916–17* (Cairo, Egypt, 1919).

5. The Experimental Production of Pellagra in Human Subjects by Means of Diet[1]

JOSEPH GOLDBERGER
G. A. WHEELER

Introduction

The experiment presented in this report is part of an investigation of pellagra begun in the spring of 1914 and still in progress. Brief reports, in part preliminary, of some of the more important phases of this investigation have already been published.[2]

In the course of some preliminary surveys relating to the prevalence of pellagra, especially at such institutions as asylums for insane and orphanages, a very high incidence of pellagra in certain groups of inmates was found associated with a diet which differed from the diet of the exempt groups, so far as was then apparent, only in that it included but minimal quantities of the animal protein foods. In the light of certain broad, previously well-recognized, epidemiological features of the disease and with the then recent advances in our knowledge of beriberi in mind it was tentatively inferred that this very striking association had etiologic significance. At the beginning of 1915 an opportunity presented itself to put this inference to the test of experiment in the human subject. Through the kind offices of Dr. E. H. Galloway, then secretary of the Mississippi State Board of Health, the interest of Gov. Earl Brewer was enlisted, who, on the offer of a pardon, secured 12 convicts for this purpose. Advantage was immediately taken of this opportunity and the experiment carried out between February 4 and October 31, 1915, a preliminary report of which was published November 12, 1915 (Goldberger and Wheeler, 1915).

In the following pages we give the details of this experiment, presentation of which has been unavoidably delayed by the pressure of continuing field investigations.

1   *Hygienic Laboratory Bulletin*, No. 120 (February, 1920), 7–116.
2   Goldberger, 1914; Goldberger, 1916; Goldberger, Waring, and Willets, 1915; Goldberger, Wheeler, and Sydenstricker, 1918; Sydenstricker, 1915.

Purpose

The purpose of the experiment was to test the possibility of producing pellagra in previously healthy men by feeding a one-sided, monotonous, principally cereal diet of the type found in previous studies to be associated with a high incidence of pellagra.

Plan of Experiment

The experiment was carried out at the Rankin farm of the Mississippi State Penitentiary. The subjects were white male convicts who volunteered in consideration of a pardon which was to be and was granted them by the governor on completion of the study. In order to make the test as rigorous as possible white male adults were chosen, for, judging by the available data with respect to incidence, this race, sex, and age group would seem to be least susceptible to the disease.

The volunteers were segregated and kept under special guard primarily for the purpose of preventing access to food other than the prescribed diet. Incidentally, this served also to minimize access of any hypothetical infection. As a check on the latter, we had under observation as controls the remaining population of the farm, both convict and free.

In planning the experiment it was believed that its value and significance would be enhanced if, in the event of success in producing pellagra, the attack or attacks developed at a season when the incidence and the prevalence of the disease were normally on the decline, say in August or September. Accordingly, having estimated that it would take some three or four months to develop the disease, it was proposed to begin with the experimental diet early in May. As the organization of the volunteer squad was completed on February 4 this plan provided a period of three months for preliminary observation. The growing impatience of the volunteers to begin and to get through with their ordeal obliged us, however, to begin the feeding experiment about two weeks earlier than planned, that is, on April 19, 1915.

During the first or preliminary period the men were kept under observation with no change in the regular prison fare. This period afforded a desirable opportunity for a close scrutiny of the men for any evidence of pellagra that might conceivably already have existed. It also afforded time for the men to become habituated to the routine of work and discipline. One or two of the squad had previously been "trusties," doing clerical work; for these this period served as a period of training, accustoming them to work in the field.

As a condition of their volunteering it was agreed that the men would not be kept on the experimental diet for a period longer than six months, at the end of which time they were to be pardoned and freed. It was agreed also that in the event that symptoms of pellagra were late in appearing that this period might be extended somewhat. Events proved this stipulation to have been wise, but, unfortunately, we were permitted an extension of but two weeks, the men being freed on November 1, 1915. The second period of the study, the feeding experiment strictly speaking, extended therefore from April 19 to and including October 31, 1915, a period of approximately six and a half months.

Controls and Subjects

The population of the prison farm consists ordinarily of the prison officials, a warden, two assistant wardens, and a night watchman, and their families, and a fluctuating number of white male convicts. All of the work of the farm was done by the latter under the supervision of the officials.

About one-half of the prisoners serve as clerks, cooks, guards, teamsters, etc. These are the "trusties"; they are selected from among the more dependable prisoners and have the freedom of the farm, and, on occasion, even beyond. The others are at all times under armed guard and are therefore spoken of as "under the gun," or "gunmen." Dereliction of duty on the part of a "trusty" may be punished by return "under the gun." Depending on the needs of the prison and good conduct, such convict may again be detailed to special work and again become a trusty. A prisoner may, therefore, alternate as gunman and trusty. The gunmen when not at work in the field were confined within the limits of a stockade, later to be described.

Controls.—All persons other than the volunteers resident on the farm during the study were under observation as controls. At the beginning of the study this included 65 prisoners; before the end a number of these were transferred, released, or escaped, while others, 43 in all, were admitted and remained for varying periods. There were therefore under observation for varying periods as controls a total of 108 convicts. Of these 108 convict controls 30 were present at the beginning and remained under observation to the end of the study. The other 78 were under observation for periods which varied between two or three weeks and eight to nine months. [Tabulation of this material deleted. ED.]

Of the 8 men who were under observation between eight and nine months, 4 were present at the beginning of the study and continued under observation to October 5, 12, 14, and 26, respectively, while 4 were admitted in February, early during the preliminary observation period, and remained to the end. Of the former group, 1, at least, may be considered to have been under observation practically to the end, while all 4 of the latter group were clearly under observation throughout the most significant period, both with respect to the pellagra season in general and the experimental feeding period in particular. For practical purposes, then, it may be stated that we had under observation a group of, in all, 35 convicts for a period comparable to the period of observation of the subjects of the experiment; these are our full-time convict controls.[3]

While all of the controls were under satisfactory observation, it was not practicable to examine all of them as regularly and systematically as was done with the volunteers. In this respect only 20 are fully comparable to the volunteers and will be referred to as our special full time convict controls.

In age the convict controls varied between 19 and 64 years, the full-time convict controls varying between 19 and 61 years, and the special group between 19 and 51 years (See Table 2).

The convict controls all denied having had pellagra, but 6 gave histories of the disease in members of the family or near relatives. Of these 6, 1 was under observation through the entire period of study, 1 from May to the end, 1 from April 19 to August 24, 1 from February 4 to June 12, and the remaining 2 for the briefer, less significant periods of 1 and 3 months, respectively.

In addition to the convict population there were resident at the farm a varying number of free individuals (officers and their families) of whom 12 were present throughout the study, our full-time free controls. These, though not regularly or systematically examined, were nevertheless under such observation as would have permitted us to detect the occurrence of pellagra, and, therefore, may properly be considered as controls. Included in this group were

3 The official pellagra morbidity reports for Mississippi show that in 1915 approximately 80 per cent of the cases were incident between Apr. 1 and Oct. 1. It is of interest therefore to note that of the control group under observation for less than the whole period of study 9 were under observation from not later than Apr. 1 to at least Oct. 1. Taken with the 30 who were under observation throughout the entire period of study we have in all a control group of 39 men who were under observation throughout that season when 80 per cent of the pellagra in the state developed.

6 adult males, 4 adult females, and 2 children, 1 a boy of 12 and the other a girl of 2 years (See Table 2). This group is of special interest because of the supposedly greater susceptibility of women and children. In this connection it may be of interest to note that this group was increased by one, a young married woman, who took up her residence at the home of the warden on May 7 and who remained under observation throughout the remainder of the period of study.

None of this group of "free controls" gave a history of pellagra.

TABLE 2—*Age distribution of volunteer subjects and full-time controls.*

Age periods.	2	12	19	20 to 24	25 to 29	30 to 34	35 to 39	40 to 44	45 to 49	50	51	52	54	57	61	78	Total
Volunteers..........	0	0	0	1*	1	0	4+	0	5	1	0	0	0	0	0	0	12
Full-time controls:																	
Convict--																	
All...........	0	0	2	8	5	5	3	4	4	0	2	0	1	0	1	0	35
Special......	0	0	1	8	3	2	2	2	1	0	1	0	0	0	0	0	20
Free--																	
Male.........	0	1	0	0	0	3	0	0	0	0	1	1	0	1	0	0	7
Female.......	1	0	0	0	0	1	0	0	1	0	0	0	0	1	0	1	5

*This man was 24 years old.   +One of these dropped out July 1.

Subjects.—The squad of 12 volunteers, or "Pellagra Squad" as it came to be called, was organized between February 1 and February 4, segregated and placed under a special guard of men employed for that purpose and under our control. On April 9, while still under preliminary observation, one of these men attempted to escape. He was promptly recaptured and turned back to the general (or control) group of prisoners, his place in the squad being taken by another volunteer (G. R.) until then under observation among the general group (controls).

The age distribution of the men in the squad thus constituted is shown in Table 2. As may be noted, the ages varied between 24 and 50 years.

As may be seen by reference to the individual records none gave a history of ever having had pellagra or of the occurrence of this disease in any member of the family or a near relative.

On July 1 one of this group of men was released because of the development of a condition that later was thought to be a prostatitis. This left 11 men, who remained in the test to its termination.

General Environment

Farm.—Rankin farm is located in Rankin County, about 8 miles east of the city of Jackson, Miss., on the Alabama & Vicksburg Railway. It is roughly a square of about 3,200 acres. The country surrounding the farm is sparsely settled, the nearest hamlets, hardly villages, being Greenfield, about 1½ miles to the east, and Pearson, about 3½ miles to the west (See map below).

Camp.—A little to the north of the center of the farm is located the group of prison, official residence, and farm buildings, locally designated as the "camp" (See map p. 60).

Near the center of the camp is a quadrangular area inclosed by a board fence, at each corner of which is a small guardhouse. Within this stockade are four frame structures, namely, the "cage," "old hospital," dining hall, and church. In the cage and old hospital are the dormitories in which the general convict population is lodged. All were quartered in these buildings during the period of the study, with the exception of the volunteers. The latter were lodged in the "new hospital," a small, one-story cottage, of recent construction, about 500 feet southeast of the cage and outside the

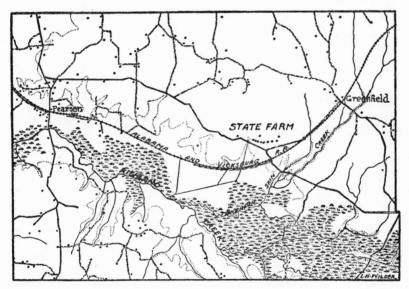

Location of Rankin State Prison Farm and sparsely settled surrounding country. (Modified from U.S. Geological Survey quadrants.)

stockade. Originally intended for use as the camp hospital, this cottage had served instead as a tailor shop and as quarters for one of the trusties and one of the assistant wardens. By reason of these facts, this cottage was, by comparison with the quarters of the other convicts, exceptionally clean. It was given a general overhauling and thorough cleaning before the volunteers were lodged therein. One of the rooms continued to be used by the assistant warden, but the trusty convict was moved April 18, the day before the beginning of the second period of the study.

A little to the north of the cage was a one-story cottage which served as the residence of the warden and his family. Another cottage about 300 yards northeast of the cage designed for use by one of the assistant wardens served, during the study, to lodge the special

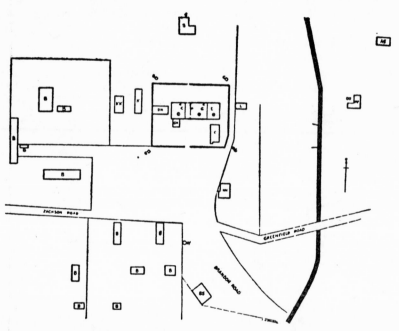

Location of buildings constituting the camp at the Rankin Prison Farm. (Diagrammatic.) AS, assistant warden's cottage; B, farm buildings; BS, blacksmith shop; C, church; DH, dining hall for gunmen; G, convict guard; K, convict kitchen; KK, commissary; L, laundry; MP, sawmill and water pump; NH, new hospital, volunteers' quarters; OH, old hospital adjoining cage, convicts' dormitories; S, warden's cottage; W, water tank; II, surface privy.

guard of the volunteers. The second assistant warden and his family resided in a cottage about a quarter of a mile to the west of the cage.

Other buildings included in the group were the general kitchen, including the dining room for the trusties, commissary, blacksmith shop, mill and pump house, and barns.

Screening.—All of the residence buildings and quarters were more or less completely screened against flies.

The screening of the cage and old hospital was incomplete and defective, so that flies and mosquitoes had easy access to these quarters, the quarters of the convict controls.

The cottage occupied by the volunteers was carefully screened at all doors and windows. This screening was carefully scrutinized before the beginning of the study and all defects repaired and kept so throughout the study. Its efficiency, while not perfect, was superior to that of any in the camp and notably so to that of the quarters occupied by the other convicts.

In this connection it may be noted that the cage and old hospital were infested with fleas and bedbugs, whereas the cottage lodging the volunteers was kept entirely free of this vermin throughout the study.

Water supply.—The water supply of the camp was from two shallow wells, located close to the mill and pump house. The water was pumped to an elevated tank from which it was piped to various points in the camp.

Sewerage.—One water-carriage sewer served the cage, old hospital, and warden's cottage, and a second the new hospital. Both discharged into an open ditch, which traversed the camp and emptied into a creek. In addition, there were four surface privies. One of these was back of the warden's cottage, one at each assistant warden's cottage, and the fourth was over a drainage ditch near the mill.

Disease prevalence.—Information with respect to disease prevalence for any period prior to 1909 was not available. Since that year Dr. A. G. McLaurin, of Brandon, has been prison physician, and to him we are indebted for the information that some cases of typhoid and a considerable number of cases of malaria have occurred, and that measles, pneumonia, "influenza," and colds have been observed. But although pellagra is fairly prevalent in the county, no case of this disease had been observed on the farm.

External communication.—Although an isolated community the camp was not without communication with the outside world. Visitors to the families of the officials were not infrequent, and from time to time friends or relatives visited the prisoners other than the volunteers. The officers and members of their families not infrequently visited the city of Jackson or more distant points, and the needs of the camp made it necessary for a trusty to call at the post office at Greenfield practically every day; occasionally also some teamsters (trusties) would drive to Jackson for supplies.

While no pellagrin is known to have visited the camp during the study, some of the free individuals or trusties may have come into direct contact with pellagra on the occasion of their visits to points beyond the farm. It was quite different, however, with the volunteers. From the beginning, as already stated, these were segregated and under special guard. No communication was permitted them with the outside except through one of us (G. A. W.) who resided at the camp throughout the study. While, therefore, some of the controls may have come into direct contact with pellagra, such contact was, we believe, absolutely excluded for the volunteers. In other words, while direct exposure of some of the controls to a hypothetical infection was possible and may have occurred, we believe that this possibility was excluded and did not occur in the case of the subjects of the experiment.

Hygiene.—The quarters of the convict controls were inadequately looked after and were for the most part dirty and vermin infested. The practice of personal cleanliness was left to the individual and therefore varied within wide limits. In contrast, the quarters of the volunteers were regularly and thoroughly cleaned. Once each week beds and bedding, personal effects, and furniture were taken out, aired, and sunned, and the dormitory well scrubbed. Each volunteer was required to wash hands and face before each meal and to take a full bath at least three times a week. Fresh clean underclothing and bedding were supplied each week and each man was required to make a change regularly.

Work.—The volunteers were required to do a share of the work of the farm. The character and amount of labor performed by them may be judged by the sample periods on the top of page 63.

The character and amount of work of the convict controls is indicated by the periods on the bottom of page 63.

For a proper estimate of the relative amount of work performed by the two groups, certain facts in addition to the foregoing must also be considered. The hours of the volunteers at first were those of the other prisoners, but after beginning the experimental diet they were shortened. After June 3 the volunteers were allowed to sleep 1 hour later in the morning than were the other prisoners, and when in the field were allowed a rest period of 10 minutes in every hour.

Week ended July 11, 1915:   Days
     Hoeing corn   2.0
     Shelling peas   2.5
     Rest   2.5

Week ended Aug. 8, 1915:
     Whitewashing fences and buildings   2.5
     Sawing lumber (ram sawmill)   2.0
     Rest   2.5

Week ended Sept. 12, 1915:
     Cutting weeds and grass   0.5
     Chopping cordwood   5.0
     Rest   1.5

Week ended Oct. 10, 1915:
     Baling hay   4.75
     Resting   2.25

Week ended Oct. 31, 1915:
     Walking   3.5
     Resting   3.5

During the last 6 weeks of the study, although maintaining this routine, the amount of work performed was very little, and during the final week no work at all was done, walking being their only exercise. In brief, when compared with the convict controls the volunteers were at no time pushed, had shorter hours of work, had

Week ended July 11, 1915:   Days
     Plowing   0.5
     Cutting and hauling wood   1.0
     Thrashing oats   3.0
     Resting   2.5

Week ended Aug. 8, 1915:
     Cutting and hauling wood   3.0
     Cutting grass and weeds   1.5
     Resting   2.5

Week ended Sept. 12, 1915:
     Squad of 15 men—
         Cutting and hauling wood   2.5
         Harvesting hay   3.0
         Resting   1.5
     Others—
         Working road   5.5
         Resting   1.5

Week ended Oct. 10, 1915:
     Working road   1.75
     Harvesting corn   4.0
     Resting   1.25

Week ended Oct. 31, 1915:
     Plowing   6.0
     Resting   1.0

regular rest periods when in the field, did less actual work, and toward the close of the study did practically no work at all. The work of the convict controls is rated by us as requiring moderate to hard, that of the volunteers as requiring moderate to light muscular exertion.

Diet of Controls

The diet of the controls varied somewhat with the different groups in respect, principally, to liberality of supply of certain foods. As might be anticipated, the diet of the free controls (officials) included a more generous supply of milk, butter, lean meat, and eggs than that of the convict groups. As there were no notable differences in availability in other respects, we shall confine ourselves to a consideration of the character of the more restricted diet provided the convict controls. During the first period of the study this was also the diet of the volunteers. A general idea of the character of this diet may be formed by reference to Table 3, which shows how frequently the articles enumerated appeared at meals during the 74⅓ days (223 meals) of the first period of the study. It was evidently quite a restricted diet, although it included a fairly liberal amount of meat. Table 4 shows in a similar way the general diet of the convict controls during the second period of the study. This was somewhat more varied than that during the first period. The influence of season is clearly indicated; there is noticeable a marked

TABLE 3—*Food* served convict controls and volunteers during period February 4 to April 19, 1915.*
(Days, 74⅓; meals, 223)

Food.	Times served.[+]	Food.	Times served.[+]
Biscuit........	195	Pork, cured["]	201
Corn bread.....	74	Brown gravy.........	109
Rice...........	78	Potatoes, Irish.....	8
Oatmeal........	4	Rutabagas..........	7
Butter.........	1	Tomatoes, canned....	2
Buttermilk.....	5	Tomato gravy........	8
Eggs[#]...........	23	Navy beans..........	37
Beef, fresh....	14	Cowpeas, dried......	14
Kid, fresh.....	3	Sugar..............	166
Pork, fresh....	14	Sirup, cane.........	223

*Not including coffee and condiments.
[+]Maximum possible 223.
[#]Served to volunteers.
["]Includes salt pork, "backs" and "sides."

reduction in lean meat, an increase in milk and in fresh vegetables, particularly greens. An idea of the more intimate make-up of this diet is afforded by Table 5, which shows the approximate composition and energy value of the convicts' diet for a period of one week. [Tabulation of three other sample weeks deleted. ED.] This table was computed with the aid of the Atwater and Bryant tables (U. S. Dept. Agr. Bull. 28); chemical analyses on the ground being impracticable, and as in the case of some of the cooked dishes we were unavoidably obliged to content ourselves with an estimate of the quantity in lieu of an actual weighing of the individual ingredients, the composition shown is an approximation and is not to be interpreted too closely.

TABLE 4—*Food* served convict controls during period April 19 to October 31, 1915.*

(Meals, 586)

Food.	Times served.[+]	Food.	Times served.[+]
Bakers' bread........	3	Ice cream................	1
Biscuit..............	559	Vegetable soup...........	21
Biscuit pudding......	21	Beets....................	1
Cake................	1	Cucumbers................	35
Crackers, sweet......	4	Potatoes, Irish..........	83
Fritters.............	2	Potato soup..............	1
Corn, fresh..........	6	Sweet potatoes...........	11
Corn bread...........	190	Sweet potatoes, canned...	5
Grits, hominy........	25	Cabbage..................	35
Oatmeal..............	14	Lettuce..................	14
Rice.................	114	Mustard greens...........	2
Rice pudding.........	2	Okra....................	25
Rice with tomatoes...	3	Peppers, green...........	79
Butter...............	58	Tomatoes, fresh..........	33
Buttermilk...........	36	Tomatoes, canned.........	4
Skimmed milk.........	122	Tomato soup..............	12
Cheese, cream........	2	Tomato gravy.............	1
Eggs.................	4	Turnips..................	4
Beef, fresh..........	40	Turnip greens............	27
Beef hash............	6	Onions...................	50
Beef liver...........	2	Apples, stewed...........	16
Beef soup............	9	Apple pie................	9
Beef gravy...........	13	Bananas..................	1
Beef dressing........	1	String beans.............	34
Kid, fresh...........	5	Navy beans...............	86
Kid soup.............	1	Bean soup................	1
Pork, fresh..........	5	Peas, English, fresh.....	2
Salt pork............	547	Cowpeas, fresh...........	19
Salt pork dumpling...	3	Cowpeas, dried...........	11
Brown gravy..........	15	Sugar....................	390
Fish, fresh..........	1	Sirup, cane..............	585
Sardines, French.....	2	Pickle, mixed............	5

*Not including coffee and condiments.   [+]Maximum possible 586.

TABLE 5—*Approximate composition of diet of convict controls (33 men) during week ended June 6, 1915.*

Food.	Quantity con-sumed.	Protein.	Fat.	Carbo-hydrate.
	Pounds.	Pounds.	Pounds.	Pounds.
Biscuit............	234.12	20.36	6.09	129.47
Corn bread........	76.13	3.92	2.44	31.44
Oatmeal...........	55.13	1.20	.28	6.34
Rice..............	23.12	.41	.02	5.64
Butter............	3.05	.03	2.99	.00
Buttermilk........	206.10	6.18	.62	10.51
Eggs, fried.......	6.06	.79	.55	.00
Beef gravy........	2.07	.09	.01	.02
Beef roast........	19.15	4.27	5.48	.00
Beef soup.........	4.05	.18	.02	.04
Salmon, canned....	1.14	.16	.09	.00
Salt pork.........	42.03	3.47	30.56	.00
Vegetable soup....	34.12	.99	.07	.17
Beets.............	18.00	.41	.02	1.33
Potatoes, Irish...	58.60	1.45	.06	12.25
Cabbage...........	12.10	.12	.04	.68
Onions, raw.......	13.90	.20	.04	1.38
Tomatoes, fresh...	6.09	.10	.02	.24
Turnips...........	16.10	.13	.14	.92
Turnip greens.....	19.00	.17	.04	.78
Sugar.............	33.50	.00	.00	33.50
Sirup, cane.......	72.00	.34	.00	54.42
Total.............		44.97	49.58	289.13

Grams per man per day were: Protein, 88; fat, 97; carbohydrate, 568.
Calories per man per day were 3,500.
Protein from animal food was 29 grams per man per day.
Per cent of total calories derived from protein, 10.

TABLE 6—*Summary of approximate average composition of the diet of convict controls for the specified sample periods per man, per day.*

Sample period, week ended--	Protein.			Fat (grams).	Carbohy-drate (grams).	Total calories.	Per cent of total calories derived from pro-tein.
	Total grams.	From animal food.					
		Grams.	Per cent of total.				
June 6.........	88	29	33	97	568	3,590	10
June 29........	97	35.	35	117	539	3,695	11
July 26........	110	32	29	134	566	4,020	11
October 21.....	92	18	20	96	579	3,645	10

Judging by the indications afforded by the four sample-week periods summarized in Table 6, the diet of the controls, although tending to be rather high in fat, conformed fairly well to recognized standards. The energy value varied between about 3,500 and 4,000 calories of which 10 to 11 per cent was derived from protein. The protein intake varied between approximately 90 and 110 grams, fat between 95 and 135 grams, and carbohydrate between 540 and 580 grams. Most of the protein was derived from cereals and peas and beans; about 20 to 35 per cent was from animal food.

Experimental Diet

The volunteers began the experimental diet with the midday meal of April 19, 1915, and continued it up to and including the midday meal of October 31, 1915. This is the second period of our study.

In planning the diet to be tested we followed, as closely as we could, the rather crude indications afforded by the institutional surveys previously referred to, and by other miscellaneous observations.

The ingredients of the diet were white wheat flour, corn (maize) meal, hominy grits, cornstarch, white rice, granulated cane sugar, cane sirup, sweet potatoes, pork fat, cabbage, collards, turnips, turnip greens, and coffee. In the preparation of biscuits and corn bread Royal baking powder was used. Table salt and pepper were freely allowed for seasoning. Up to July 28 buttermilk was used in making the wheat biscuit, this being the same biscuit as that provided the controls. During the week ending June 27, 3 pounds of beefsteak were served at one of the meals, thus giving each man approximately 4 ounces of lean beef on this occasion.

No fats other than those occurring naturally in the foods specified were used; the pork fat was extracted from salt pork by frying or boiling. The pork crackling or connective tissue remaining was not served. The sirup was home produced, made from "ribbon" sugar cane raised on the farm.

All ingredients appeared to be of excellent quality and, with one or two exceptions, part of the general camp supply. The principal exception was the maize meal. That of the camp was home ground from corn raised on the farm and was unbolted. As it was desired to keep the antineuritic vitamin content of the diet low, and as it was believed that the milling was a factor of importance in this and possibly other respects, we preferred to use a bolted meal and accordingly provided the volunteers with such.

Having in mind the great etiologic importance that had for so long attached to the quality of the corn, we provided the best quality of both meal and hominy grits obtainable on the local market. In order that we might have a biological check on the quality of these products we arranged to secure our supply from part of that being used at one of the orphanages (M. J.) at which a study of the preventability of pellagra by diet was being made at the time. (No pellagra occurred at this institution during 1915. See Goldberger, Waring, and Willets, 1915.) For purposes of additional check, we arranged also that the controls should share with the volunteers the hominy grits thus provided.

The diet was not absolutely uniform throughout the experimental period. Thus, as already mentioned, the biscuit included buttermilk up to July 28, after which date the milk was entirely excluded. Having the idea that corn bread was the cause of pellagra, the volunteers tended to minimize its consumption with a corresponding increase in the consumption of biscuit and vegetables. In order to counteract this tendency, the biscuit was sophisticated in the manner mentioned below and the quantity of vegetables provided gradually reduced.

Beginning about August 1, corn meal replaced part of the flour in the biscuit. The meal was objected to so that after August 14 it was replaced by cornstarch which was added in the proportion of 1 of cornstarch to 8 of flour. On August 29 an increase was made in the proportion of starch entering the biscuit so that after this date the biscuit included 1 of starch to 5 of flour. A further increase was made on September 29, the proportion becoming 1 of starch to 4 of flour.

In order to further counteract the tendency of the volunteers to minimize the consumption of maize, corn meal was added to the flour in making the gravy.

Besides these variations in the diet as served there were also individual variations in the diet consumed resulting from individual variations in preference for different dishes. Some would eat freely of one dish and some of another with, in addition, occasional trading of favorite dishes, a moderate amount of which was permitted.

The menu was varied so far as circumstances permitted, but this was very little. A typical weekly specimen is on page 69.

Our field studies (Goldberger, Wheeler, and Sydenstricker, 1918) of the past three years show that this diet differs most notably from the average diet associated with pellagra, at least in cotton-mill villages in South Carolina, in that it is very much more restricted, includes practically no animal protein, no dried legumes, and does include relatively considerable quantities of green vegetables. So far

Bill of Fare, Week Ended August 8, 1915.

AUGUST 2

Breakfast: Biscuits, fried mush, grits and brown gravy, sirup, coffee with sugar.
Dinner: Corn bread, cabbage, sweet potatoes, grits, sirup.
Supper: Fried mush, biscuits, rice, gravy, cane sirup, coffee, sugar.

AUGUST 3

Breakfast: Biscuits, mush, rice, gravy, sirup, coffee, sugar.
Dinner: Corn bread, collards, sweet potatoes, grits, sirup.
Supper: Biscuits, mush, grits, gravy, sirup, coffee, sugar.

AUGUST 4

Breakfast: Biscuits, mush, grits, gravy, sirup, coffee, sugar.
Dinner: Corn bread, collards, sweet potatoes, rice, sirup.
Supper: Biscuits, mush, grits, gravy, sirup, coffee, sugar.

AUGUST 5

Breakfast: Biscuits, mush, grits, gravy, sirup, coffee, sugar.
Dinner: Corn bread, collards, sweet potatoes, grits, sirup.
Supper: Biscuits, mush, rice, gravy, sirup, coffee, sugar.

AUGUST 6

Breakfast: Biscuits, mush, rice, sirup, coffee, sugar.
Dinner: Corn bread, collards, sweet potatoes, grits, sirup.
Supper: Biscuits, mush, grits, gravy, sirup, coffee, sugar.

AUGUST 7

Breakfast: Biscuits, mush, grits, gravy, sirup, coffee, sugar.
Dinner: Corn bread, collards, sweet potatoes, rice, sirup.
Supper: Biscuits, mush, grits, gravy, sirup, coffee, sugar.

AUGUST 8

Breakfast: Biscuits, mush, grits, gravy, sirup, coffee, sugar.
Dinner: Corn bread, collards, sweet potatoes, grits, sirup.
Supper: Biscuits, mush, rice, gravy, sirup, coffee, sugar.

as may be judged by such (surface) indications, our experimental diet was probably not altogether a typical or average one.

Weighings of food consumed were made for eight periods of a week each; the results for the first-week period, in terms of cooked food and raw ingredients, are shown in Table 7, having been computed by means of ratios previously determined. [Tabulations of quantities consumed in seven other weekly periods deleted. ED.] A chemical analysis of the diet on the ground was not practicable. (See, however, Sullivan and Jones, *Hyg. Lab. Bull.*, Feb., 1920.) The composition of the diet of these sample-week periods has been computed and the results are summarized in Tables 9 and 10. (Table 8 shows the composition of the diet for the first-week period.) Reference to these tables shows a variation in energy intake of between about 2,500 and 3,500 calories, or a variation of between about 40 and 54

TABLE 7—*Quantities, in pounds, of different articles of food consumed by twelve volunteers during the week ended May 27, 1915.*

	Cooked food.				Raw ingredients.								
Article.	Quan-tity.	But-ter-milk.	Cab-bage.	Corn meal.	Flour.	Grits.	Pork fat.	Rice.	Sugar.	Sweet pota-toes.	Sirup.	Tur-nips.	Tur-nip greens.
Biscuit........	37.75	8.30*	.....	.....	24.54*	.....	2.34*	.....	.....	.....	.....	.....	.....
Cabbage........	27.63	.....	17.13	.....	.....	.....	.83*	.....	.....	.....	.....	.....	.....
Corn bread.....	33.19	.....	.....	19.25	.....	.....	.....	.....	.....	.....	.....	.....	.....
Fried mush.....	62.63	.....	.....	26.93	.....	.....	8.77	.....	.....	.....	.....	.....	.....
Grits..........	39.37	.....	.....	.....	.....	8.66	.....	.....	.....	.....	.....	.....	.....
Gravy..........	38.00	.....	.....	.....	1.10	.....	5.32	.....	.....	.....	.....	.....	.....
Rice...........	19.25	.....	.....	.....	.....	.....	.....	4.04	.....	.....	.....	.....	.....
Sugar..........	10.12	.....	.....	.....	.....	.....	.....	.....	10.12	.....	.....	.....	.....
Sweet potatoes.	26.12	.....	.....	.....	.....	.....	4.96	.....	3.92	30.56	.....	.....	.....
Sirup..........	7.81	.....	.....	.....	.....	.....	.....	.....	.....	.....	7.81	.....	.....
Turnips........	11.56	.....	.....	.....	.....	.....	.35*	.....	.....	.....	.....	7.17	.....
Turnip greens..	30.63	.....	.....	.....	.....	.....	.92	.....	.....	.....	.....	.....	12.86
Total.....	344.06	8.30	17.13	46.18	25.64	8.66	23.49	4.04	14.04	30.56	7.81	7.17	12.86

*Estimated.

calories per kilogram of the average weight of the volunteers. This it will be recognized compares favorably with the requirement by the organism of "35 calories per kilogram of body weight in the average man doing light work on a mixed diet" (Lusk, 1917, p. 345). About 6 per cent of the calories were contributed by the protein.

The average protein intake varied between 41 and 54 grams, the fat between 91 and 134 grams, and the carbohydrate between 387 and 513 grams. The protein was predominantly (between 80 and 97 per cent of the total) from cereal sources (wheat flour, maize, and rice).

Comparison shows the experimental diet and the diet of the controls during the corresponding period to be much alike with respect to intake of fat and carbohydrate and, when due allowance is made for the difference in the amount of work done by the two groups, also with respect to energy.

In relation to protein, however, there are some rather outstanding differences between the two. The intake of protein by the convict controls was approximately twice that of the volunteers and while at least 20 to 35 per cent of the protein in the diet of the former group was from animal sources practically none at all of the protein in the diet of the latter was derived from this class of foods.

With respect to the mineral constituents and vitamins differences can be indicated in very general terms only. The inclusion of milk, butter, peas, and beans in the diet of the controls and their complete

TABLE 8—*Approximate average composition* of the diet of the volunteers during the week ended May 27, 1915.†

(Average per man per day.)

Article.	Quantity (gm.).	Protein (gm.).	Fat (gm.).	Carbohydrate (gm.).	Minerals (in grams).								Calories.
					Ca.	Mg.	K.	Na.	P.	Cl.	S.	Fe.	
Buttermilk......	44.8	1.34	0.22	2.15	0.047	0.007	0.068	0.029	0.043	0.044	0.012	0.0001	....
Cornmeal........	249.4	22.94	4.74	188.05	.045	.209	.531	.097	.474	.364	.277	.0022	....
Grits...........	46.8	4.40	.33	36.78	.005	.027	.081	.009	.067	.022	.064	.0004	....
Wheat flour.....	138.5	14.96	1.52	103.60	.028	.025	.159	.083	.127	.102	.245	.0014	....
Rice...........	21.8	1.74	.07	17.22	.002	.007	.015	.005	.021	.012	.026	.0002	....
Cane sirup.....	42.1	.20	....	31.82	....	....	....	....	....	....	....	....	....
Cane sugar.....	75.8	....	....	75.80	....	....	....	....	....	....	....	....	....
Sweet potatoes..	165.0	2.97	.12	45.21	.031	.046	.655	.064	.074	.155	.040	.0008	....
Turnips........	38.7	.50	.08	3.13	.025	.007	.131	.022	.018	.016	.025	.0002	....
Turnip greens..	69.4	2.91	.42	4.37	.241	.019	.213	.057	.034	.117	.048	.0012	....
Cabbage........	92.5	1.48	.28	5.18	.042	.014	.228	.025	.027	.022	.061	.0010	....
Pork fat.......	126.8	.11	126.50	......	....	....	....	....	....	....	....	.....	....
Total........	1,112.0	54.00	134.00	513.00	.470	.360	2.080	.390	.890	.850	.800	.0075	3,570

*Not including table salt or baking powder.
†Tabulation of average composition of the diet of volunteers for seven other weekly periods deleted. ED.

TABLE 9—*Summary of average composition of diet of the volunteers during specified sample periods.*

Sample period, week ended--	Protein (grams).	Fat (grams).	Carbohydrate (grams).	Total calories.	Calories per kilo.	Per cent of total calories derived from protein.
May 27.........	54	134	513	3,570	54	6
June 21........	41	99	426	2,835	45	6
July 12........	41	91	387	2,600	40	6
August 9.......	46	113	457	3,115	49	6
August 29.....	46	117	479	3,240	51	6
September 13..	47	119	481	3,265	52	6
September 20..	44	114	459	3,125	50	6
October 6.....	44	105	479	3,120	51	6

absence (milk, after July 28) from the diet of the volunteers would suggest that the former had a more satisfactory mineral composition because of the milk, at least, and was richer in both the fat soluble and the antineuritic vitamin.

Results

During the period of study various minor ailments and a number of rather sharp attacks of malaria were observed among the controls, but in none was there observed any evidence justifying even a suspicion of pellagra. On the other hand, of the 11 volunteers who remained in the test to the end, not less than 6 developed evidence

TABLE 10—*Sources of protein in diet of the volunteers during specified sample periods.*

Sample period, week ended--	Total grams.	From animal.		From cereal.		From other foods.	
		Grams.	Per cent of total.	Grams.	Per cent of total.	Grams.	Per cent of total.
May 27..........	54	1.5	3.0	44.0	81.0	8.0	16
June 21.........	41	1.4	3.4	33.0	80.5	6.6	16
July 12.........	41	.9	2.0	37.0	90.0	3.0	8
August 9........	46	.1	.3	40.0	87.0	5.8	13
August 29.......	46	.1	.3	42.5	92.0	3.4	8
September 13....	47	.1	.3	43.8	93.0	3.3	7
September 20....	44	.1	.3	40.5	92.0	3.0	7
October 6.......	44	.1	.3	40.0	91.0	3.8	9

which experienced observers joined with us in recognizing as that
of pellagra.

The volunteers were seen with us on three occasions, and a
diagnosis of pellagra concurred in, in 6 of the men, by Dr. E. H.
Galloway, then secretary of the Mississippi State Board of Health,
and by Dr. Nolan Stewart, one time superintendent of the Mississippi Asylum for the Insane, at Jackson, and among the first to
recognize pellagra in Mississippi. In excluding the known dermatoses
other than pellagra the special knowledge of Dr. Marcus Haase,
professor of dermatology in the Medical College of the University
of Tennessee, Memphis, Tenn., and that of Dr. Martin F. Engman,
professor of dermatology in the Washington University Medical
School, St. Louis, Mo., was utilized in consultation. Dr. Haase saw
these men on October 27, and Prof. Engman on October 29. In addition to the foregoing who were formally called into consultation,
the subjects were also seen by Drs. C. R. Stingily and F. L. Watkins,
of the state board of health, and by Dr. C. H. Waring, assistant
surgeon, United States Public Health Service, all of whom concurred in the diagnosis.[4]

4 So far as we are aware the diagnosis of pellagra in these cases has not been
   questioned by any of our fellow workers except MacNeal (1916). By reason of
   the tone and personal character of MacNeal's criticism we have not felt that it
   required any special notice, preferring to let the record of our work speak for
   itself. Some reference seems, however, to be called for by reason of the fact
   that McCollum, in a paper appearing (*J. Biol. Chem.*, May, 1919) after this
   manuscript had been submitted for publication, seems to have been led to
   attach importance to MacNeal's criticism. McCollum states that "Goldberger
   seems to have safeguarded his experimental men against infection and it is
   unfortunate that a sufficient number of undisputed authorities were not
   called into consultation to forestall the possibility of a question arising concerning the accuracy of the diagnosis of pellagra, such as MacNeal has raised."
   The question as raised by MacNeal is as follows: "The National Association
   for the Study of Pellagra held its third triennial meeting at Columbia, S. C.,
   October 21 and 22, 1915, or approximately one month after the appearance
   of the dermatitis in these cases. Dr. Goldberger attended this meeting. It may
   be pertinent to inquire why no mention of this alleged important discovery
   was made at this meeting and why recognized authorities on the diagnosis of
   pellagra, such, for example, as Dr. C. H. Lavinder, surgeon, Public Health
   Service, then president of the National Association for the Study of Pellagra,
   or Dr. J. F. Siler, captain, Medical Corps, United States Army, then vice
   president and now president of this association, were not invited to see such
   alleged important cases."

   The following comments are submitted for the information of those who,
   like Professor McCollum, may be led to attach to MacNeal's criticism an importance which, when rightly considered, it totally lacks.

   The announcement of the results of our experiment at the meeting of the

Discussion.—In formulating the diagnosis, we followed the conventional rule of not considering any case pellagra in the absence of definite skin lesions having the characters usually considered distinctive of the pellagrous dermatitis, namely bilateral symmetry, sharpness of delimitation, and, when sufficiently advanced, pigmentation, keratosis, and desquamation. As already stated, our consultants and ourselves agreed in a diagnosis of pellagra in six of the

---

National Association for the Study of Pellagra would have been premature, even though this meeting took place, as MacNeal states, "approximately one month after the appearance of the dermatitis in these cases," by reason of the fact that the dermatitis in these cases did not appear full-blown, as MacNeal seems to have assumed, but developed gradually and was not recognized by us as significant until after the date of this meeting.

It would have given us great satisfaction, had it been practicable, to have had Dr. Lavinder, Capt. Siler, and, indeed, Dr. MacNeal see our cases. As already stated, however, the evolution of the eruption on the genitalia was slow and that on the hands and neck very late in appearing, so that the evidence justifying a diagnosis of pellagra was not regarded by us as present until within a very few days of the close of the experimental period, which, as elsewhere stated, was abruptly terminated on November 1. We were obliged to limit our invitation, therefore, to such authorities on the diagnosis of pellagra as were quickly accessible. Fortunately Drs. E. H. Galloway and Nolan Stewart, to cite only those formally invited as clinical consultants, are well known to the medical profession of the state of Mississippi as careful clinical observers with large experience with pellagra. As for Profs. Haase and Engman, it would seem unnecessary to point out that their standing is in the front rank of American dermatologists with a large experience in pellagra; indeed, there are few, if any, larger pellagra clinics in the United States than that of Prof. Haase at the Memphis City Hospital. In this connection it may be stated that in response to a recent inquiry (August, 1918) addressed to these gentlemen as to whether they were still of the opinion that the known dermatoses other than pellagra could be excluded in our experimental cases Prof. Engman writes (Sept. 4, 1918): "Will say that I am at present even more confirmed in the opinion I gave you three years ago as to the nature of the eruption on the convicts in the experimental squad than I was at that time"; and Prof. Haase, under date of August 20, 1918, writes: "I have not changed my opinion in regard to cases seen with you and Wheeler at the prison farm near Jackson, Miss. As stated to you then, I knew of no dermatological condition except pellagra that would produce the lesions seen, and on my return home looked for early lesions occurring on scrotum and observed two such cases." It would seem to be unnecessary to comment further, particularly as the clinical notes of our cases are submitted as part of the present report. We may add that in the nearly four years since the close of the experiment we have seen many hundreds of cases of pellagra (over 1,000 cases were seen by us in the cotton-mill village study in South Carolina in 1917 alone), but have not only seen nothing that raises the slightest doubt as to the correctness of the diagnosis of pellagra in the convict volunteers but, indeed, our exceptionally large experience has throughout confirmed that diagnosis.

subjects. We believe, however, that a definite diagnosis of pellagra was justified in at least one other of the men (A–E. S.), but in deference to the opinion of our consultants who, in this case, did not regard the skin manifestations (a mild erythema of the scrotum) as sufficiently marked, this case was not included as such in our preliminary report.

It is a not infrequent observation that, in a family of several members, although only one may show the distinctive cutaneous lesions, some, if not all, of the others may present subjective and other manifestations which leave little room for doubt that they also are suffering from the same disease. Now it seems to us that our squad of volunteers is strictly comparable to a family group or unit; the members of this squad lived together, worked together, ate at the same table, and, within much narrower limits than obtained in any family, ate the same diet. It would appear to follow that, having recognized the six or seven cases presenting the skin lesions as pellagra, this diagnosis may properly be extended to apply to the four or five without the cutaneous lesions but presenting the other manifestations. In other words, we are of the opinion that every one of the volunteers developed pellagra, six or seven with skin lesions and four or five without ("pellagra sine pellagra").

In all the cases with distinctive skin lesions the eruption was first detected on the genitalia (scrotum). Although there was considerable individual variation with respect to the extent of the involved scrotal area and also with respect to the degree of involvement of the penis, nevertheless the genital lesions in these cases very clearly represent a single type, and by comparing our photographs with that of Deiaco's case and with the diagram from the report by Stannus of pellagra in Nyasaland it will at once be recognized that the genital lesion observed by us in our experimental cases is essentially identical with the lesion as observed in Europe and in Africa. [See *Hyg. Lab. Bull.*, Feb. 1920, pp. 32 ff., for photographic material which has been deleted. ED.]

The first appearance of the skin lesion on the scrotum in all our cases with definite eruption suggested to us that the scrotal lesion might be a much more common early skin manifestation than had theretofore been believed. The literature on this point at the time of the publication of our preliminary report was, and still is, extremely meager. There existed, as far as we are aware, only two first-hand reports of this lesion, a paper by Deiaco (1907), whose case was also seen by Merk (1909) who speaks of it in his monograph, and a report by Stannus (1913). In the one case reported by

Deiaco the scrotal eruption was not the initial one, but was preceded
by lesions in other locations. Although Merk by implication clearly
suggests (1909, p. 20) that the scrotal lesion may be the first to appear, Stannus seems to be the first to actually record such cases. In
his report of pellagra in Nyasaland, Stannus records 19 (out of 100
with eruption) that presented the scrotal lesion, and of these 19 four
presented the scrotal lesion alone; whether the scrotal lesion was the
first to appear in any other of his cases is not clear from his report.
Since the publication of our note a case of pellagra with the initial
lesion on the scrotum has been reported by Crosby (1917) from
South Carolina, and by Wood (1917) from North Carolina.

In the course of our study of pellagra in cotton-mill villages in
South Carolina in 1916 notes were made (by G. A. W.) of 23 male
cases examined for lesions on the genitals and of finding four with
lesions on these parts as the initial site. Of these four cases one was
a first and three were recurrent attacks. Of the 23 cases examined
8 were claimed to be first and 15 recurrent attacks, so that we had
one of 8 first-attack cases with the initial site of the dermatitis on
the genitals and three of 15 recurrent-attack cases with this lesion.

This experience would seem to bear out our suggestion that the
pellagrous eruption occurs on the male genitalia as an initial lesion
much more commonly than the literature might lead one to judge.
It remains a fact, however, that the genital lesion, whether early or
late, is a somewhat infrequent one. Its appearance in all our cases
with skin lesions as the initial lesion is therefore of exceptional interest. It is difficult to accept this as merely a chance phenomenon
or as an individual peculiarity. We are inclined to interpret it as a
specific reaction, direct or indirect, to some special factor or combination of factors in the diet, and it suggests to us further that the
site of at least the initial lesion in pellagra is bound up with a specific
quality of the diet. Thus, we are inclined to believe that the dietary
fault related to a case of pellagra with the initial lesion on the backs
of the hands differs in some essential detail from that associated with
a case in which the initial lesion appears on the backs of the feet, etc.

In this connection reference may be made to the opinion elsewhere expressed by us (Goldberger, Wheeler, and Sydenstricker,
1918) that pellagra, as conventionally defined, is probably not a
single entity but probably includes at least two syndromes which are
commonly associated but etiologically essentially distinct though
closely related. One of these is the complex comprehended by the
phrase "pellagra sine pellagra" and the other the dermal complex or
pellagra without or with only slight other manifestations. These two

complexes were in a measure represented in our volunteers. Thus volunteer "A–W" lost markedly in weight, falling from 124 to 99.5 pounds, and showed other marked manifestations but without the slightest appreciable eruption; on the other hand, volunteer "J–G. R." lost but little weight, which fell from 126 to 118 pounds, but developed the most marked and most extensive eruption of any of the men. It might be objected that these were but individual variations, particularly as all the volunteers had the same diet. While the possibility of the differences referred to being but individual variations in reaction cannot be definitely excluded, it is perhaps worth pointing out that although it is true that the same diet was served to all individuals of the volunteer group there were nevertheless distinct differences in the relative proportion of the individual foods actually eaten. Some ate their meals as served, others traded dishes so that some had more than the average allowance, say, of greens and less, of sweet potatoes, or vice versa. The possibility that there were essential differences in diet corresponding to differences in some of the reactions observed is therefore distinctly present.

We incline to the view that seems to us the more probable one, namely, that there were such differences, as we do also to the opinion that there exist essential differences in the intimate make-up of the diet corresponding to observed differences in some, at least, of the clinical types of the disease. We may have in this the explanation of some at least of the reported differences in the manifestations of pellagra in different localities and in the same locality in different years.

We now turn to the question as to what factor or factors in the diet are to be charged with bringing about the pellagra syndrome or syndromes. It has already been pointed out that with respect to the quantitative intake of energy, fat, carbohydrate, and protein the experimental diet differed from the diet of the controls significantly only in that the intake of protein was low though within the limits of recognized standards. These features of the diet do not, therefore, come up for consideration in this connection. With respect to the more intimate make-up of the diet, it has previously been noted that the protein was almost exclusively from products of highly milled cereals (wheat, maize, rice). In the light of recent studies, notably those of Osborne and Mendel and of McCollum and associates, this would suggest the probability of a deficiency in intake of some one or more of the amino acids, a probability that would be increased by the relatively low protein intake. This interpretation is strengthened by the indications afforded by the results of some feed-

ing experiments in rats carried out by Sullivan at the United States
Pellagra Hospital at Spartanburg, S. C., pointing to the protein as
one of the limiting factors of the diet, at least for this species (See
M. X. Sullivan, *Hyg. Lab. Bull.*, Feb., 1920).

The antineuritic vitamin content of the diet was planned to be
low, and feeding experiments by Sullivan show that it was actually
deficient in this factor for the common fowl and the pigeon. It is
of great interest to note, however, that none of the subjects developed
any distinctive clinical manifestations of beriberi; whether they
would have done so eventually had they continued on the diet is an
interesting speculation.

Judging by the fact that none of the men showed the slightest
recognizable indications of scurvy, the content of the diet in the
antiscorbutic factor would seem to have been adequate for the period
of the experiment at least.

With regard to the adequacy of supply of the fat soluble vitamin,
it is difficult to judge by reason of the meagerness of the available
fundamental data; none of the men developed the eye symptoms
currently considered indicative of a deficiency in this dietary
essential.

Compared to the average intake afforded by various American
dietaries as compiled by Sherman (1918, p. 271) the intake of
some, at least, of the mineral ingredients in the diet of our volunteers would seem to have been decidedly low (See Table 8). Thus,
for example, Sherman (1918, p. 264) considers that 0.45 gram of
calcium approximates the minimum of actual daily need, while
the average intake of the volunteers varied between about 0.13 and
0.20 gram during the period, after the buttermilk was excluded from
the diet. With respect to phosphorus, the average daily requirement,
according to Sherman (1918, p. 255) is 0.96 gram; the average intake
by the volunteers varied between about 0.89 and 0.67 gram. As to the
adequacy of sodium and chlorine little can be said, inasmuch as
the quantities shown in the tables do not include the salt used in
seasoning, which was freely allowed but not weighed; one is tempted
to assume that the intake of these elements was sufficient. Whether
the mineral intake as a whole was actually inadequate or improperly
balanced for normal nutrition, it is perhaps impossible to state at
the present time; that such may have been the case is rather strongly
suggested, however.

It would seem from the foregoing considerations that our test
diet was probably faulty in some degree with respect to the protein
(amino acid or acids), antineuritic vitamin and mineral constitu-

ents. Judging by the results of our field observations with reference particularly to the inclusion of dried legumes in the diet of pellagrous families and individuals, it seems to us well-nigh certain, however, that a deficiency in the antineuritic vitamin is not an essential element in the pellagra-producing dietary fault. Consequently, of the now generally recognized essential dietary factors, there remain for consideration in this regard only the protein (amino acids) and the inorganic factor, and possibly also the fat-soluble vitamin, although our experiment affords no satisfactory basis for an opinion as to the latter. McCollum, in the light of his extensive studies in rats, believes that our diet is faulty in all three of these respects. Whether this interpretation can be directly applied to man is uncertain and must await further study for determination.

As to which or what combination (or combinations) of these, if any, or whether some deficiency in an as yet unknown dietary factor (vitamin?) alone or in combination with some one or more of the known factors constitutes the specific pellagra-producing dietary defect or (more probably) defects cannot be stated.

By reason of the etiological importance that has attached to corn (maize), particularly spoiled corn, it is worth noting that the quality of the maize included in the diet seemed to be excellent, judging (1) by appearance and taste, and (2) by the fact that none of the controls at the penitentiary or the large number using the same maize meal and grits at one of the orphanages under our observation, developed any evidence of pellagra. Spoiled maize would, therefore, not seem to be an essential factor in the production of the disease.

Conclusions

Having due regard for the conditions of the experiment, the conclusion would seem to us to be warranted that pellagra developed in at least 6 of our 11 volunteers as the result of the restricted diet on which they subsisted.

Discussion.—The significance of our experiment has been questioned on the ground that it was carried out in an "infected" state. It seems to us that those who advance this criticism have failed to take account of the controlled conditions under which it was performed and especially of the large number of the controls—over four times the number of the subjects of experiment.

In considering its significance in relation to the etiology of the disease the experiment should be regarded as evidence not apart from but in conjunction with other evidence bearing on this problem. The most immediately pertinent part of this other evidence may be summarized as follows:

1. In institutions for the treatment of pellagra ("pellagrosario" or hospital) employees (nurses and attendants) in constant contact with the disease practically never contract it while so employed. (Lavinder, 1911; Goldberger, 1914.)

2. It has been found that employees (nurses, attendants, etc.) resident in institutions in which pellagra is and has for long periods been endemic (occasionally also epidemic), and many of them in frequent or constant contact with cases of the disease, practically never contract it while so employed. This exemption has been found associated with a decided difference in diet and in no other significant respect. (Goldberger, 1914.)

3. Active cases of pellagra respond promptly and strikingly to an appropriate dietary. Exceptions are relatively rare and no more than might be expected when the experience in beriberi and scurvy are kept in mind. The natural tendency to recovery from the attack without change of environment and without therapeutic interference is associated with a significant seasonal change in diet. (Goldberger, 1916; Goldberger, Wheeler, Sydenstricker, and King, unpublished data.)

4. Pellagra may be prevented completely by a suitable diet without intervention of any other known factor, hygienic or sanitary. There is no sound evidence that the disease is controllable in any other way. (Goldberger, Waring, and Willets, 1915; Nesbitt, 1916; Goldberger and Tanner, unpublished data; Goldberger, Wheeler, and Sydenstricker, unpublished data.)

5. Attempts to transmit the disease to the human subject by inoculations of blood and of nasopharyngeal secretions and by feeding with dermal scales, urine and feces from cases of pellagra in various stages and of varying degrees of severity were without result. (Goldberger, 1916.) The report by Harris (1913) of a successful inoculation of a monkey with a filtrate from pellagrous lesions remains unconfirmed, although extensive attempts have been made to do so, notably by Lavinder and Francis (1914) and by Harris[5] himself.

6. Chittenden and Underhill (1917) have by feeding succeeded in producing pellagra-like symptoms in dogs.

When now we add to all this the results of our experiment and

5 Communicated at a meeting of Louisiana health officers, New Orleans, July, 1915.

consider this evidence as a whole, it is our judgment that it clearly and consistently points to diet as the controlling factor in the causation as well as in the prevention of the disease.

The possibility of the existence of an essential infective etiological factor must next be considered. When the evidence that has been advanced in support of the conception of pellagra as a communicable disease is critically analyzed, it is found that much of it is susceptible of an interpretation in harmony with, or at least as not inconsistent with, the view that pellagra is primarily of dietary origin. Further consideration of this portion of the evidence need not, therefore, detain us, but we may proceed at once to examine what is perhaps generally regarded as the most weighty part of the remainder of the evidence in favor of infection.

Much significance has been attached to the observation by some of our fellow students that there is to be found in a very large percentage of cases of pellagra, a previous association with other cases. In estimating the importance of such observations it has been overlooked, however, that they were admittedly made in endemic areas of high prevalence. In such localities contact with pellagra is so difficult to avoid that we doubt if many residents or visitors escape some degree of such association for more than a short period. Evidently, then, such a study is without the significance which has been attached to it, a view which has already been expressed by Vedder. (Vedder, 1916, p. 148.) In this connection reference may be made to the "domiciliary" study of the Thompson-McFadden Commission (Siler, Garrison, and MacNeal, 1914 and Aug., 1917).

This commission believes that this "domiciliary" study of theirs revealed relationships of such significance as seemed to them conclusive evidence of the correctness of their view that pellagra is an infectious disease (Siler, Garrison, and MacNeal, 1914, p. 370). In this study the population was divided into three domiciliary zones on the basis of proximity to the residence of a pellagrin or pellagrins, and the results seemed to indicate an incidence which was higher as proximity to a resident pellagrin increased. It must suffice for the present to point out that whether such relationship actually does or does not exist, this study is devoid of significance, because, among other reasons, the "arbitrary rules" adopted with regard to the exposed population were such that in practical effect the question was begged. Thus, as between their "Zone 1" and "Zone 2" on the one hand, and "Zone 3" on the other, the rules adopted required a minimum of two weeks' residence for the former zones, but of three months for the latter, the effect of which would be to credit incident cases to "Zone 1" or "Zone 2" rather than to "Zone 3." Furthermore, under these rules, an incident case is not assigned to "Zone 2" if *"on account of previous residence in a house with a pellagrin (Zone 1) within a period of three months in summer or six months in winter, it has been possible to credit the case to Zone 1"* [italics ours].

In other words, under their "rules" if an incident case had resided 14 days in "Zone 1" and then, let us say, for as long as 2 months and 29 days in "Zone 2" before developing the disease, such case would be assigned to "Zone 1"; obviously the effect of the operation of such a rule is to favor "Zone 1" over "Zone 2" or, as we have said, it is begging the question. (See also Vedder, 1916, p. 150.)

Brief reference may also be made to another of the interesting studies of this commission. Having conceived that the methods of disposal of human wastes might prove to be a determining factor in the spread of pellagra,[6] the commission carried out an experiment, designed to test this hypothesis, at Spartan Mills, Spartanburg, S. C. (Siler, Garrison, and MacNeal, May, 1917). In this community, an endemic focus of pellagra, a water carriage system of sewage disposal was installed in 1913–14, replacing an insanitary system of surface privies. The commission reports (May, 1917) that subsequent to this change "the community has been transformed from a pellagra focus to a community in which pellagra no longer spreads." It so happens that in a study of factors influencing pellagra prevalence in cotton-mill communities in South Carolina during 1917 and 1918, Spartan Mill Village was one of the villages studied by us. We are, therefore, in a position to state that this commission seems again to have fallen into error, for we (Goldberger, Wheeler, and Sydenstricker, unpublished data) found pellagra quite as prevalent in this village as in a near-by village with sanitary conditions of the vilest character. Thus, in 1917 we recorded in Spartan Mill Village 37 first-attack cases, a rate of 26.2 per 1,000, while in the village without sewers and filthy in the extreme we recorded, on precisely the same basis, 17 first-attack cases, an incidence rate of 23.4 per 1,000, for the same year. Clearly, Spartan Mill Village has not only not ceased to be a pellagra focus, but the

---

6 This conception seems to have been developed, at least in part, as the result of the failure of their studies "to disclose any definite relation of the disease to any element of the dietary." This failure on their part seems to have been due to faulty and inadequate methods of study, as has elsewhere already been suggested by us (Goldberger, Waring, and Willets, 1915; Goldberger, Wheeler, and Sydenstricker, 1918) and by Vedder (1916).

disease was found by us during 1917 and 1918 at least as prevalent in this village as in some other near-by villages with but the crudest, most insanitary methods of sewage disposal.

This striking discrepancy between our results and those of the commission is probably due to a number of factors. At the outset the important question arises whether their data for newly incident cases occurring after the experiment was instituted are properly comparable to those for cases recorded before the beginning of the experiment. Doubt as to this point arises because of the fact that the field work of the commission is known to have been greatly restricted after October, 1914, so that, as they elsewhere implicitly suggest (Arch. Int. Med. 1916, vol. 18, p. 176) their data for 1915 and 1916 are probably not as complete as those for 1912, 1913, and 1914 when they were in the field for a large part of each year. The significance of this point would at first thought seem to be minimized by the apparently different course taken by pellagra in a control district immediately adjacent to Spartan Mill Village. In this district, with a population of approximately 300 or about one-sixth that of the mill village, pellagra, the commission states, continued to spread after 1913 (the year in which the installation of sewerage in Spartan village was begun) at about the same rate as it did before. In 1914, three new cases are reported to have appeared in the control district. "In 1915, after the general enforcement of the sanitary ordinance in regard to privies in Spartanburg City, *only* [italics ours] two new cases of pellagra appeared in this district." (Spartan village and the control district are included in the city of Spartanburg.) In 1916 four new cases are said to have occurred. A moment's consideration of these facts seems to us quite clearly to indicate, however, that this district cannot properly be considered a suitable control. Its population was actually and relatively so small, with so few cases of pellagra occurring from year to year, that it might readily be affected by circumstances of little or no general significance; these might manifest themselves in just such fluctuations as are indicated which, while relatively very great, are actually of no importance.

In the newly sewered village, the commission states, "the number of new cases each year has shown a progressive diminution since 1913, being 18 in 1914, 8 in 1915, and 2 in 1916." This result the commission considers to be due to the installation of the sewerage. Disregarding the question already raised of the comparability of these figures with those for the period preceding the beginning of the experiment, and granting that some reduction in numbers actually occurred, it seems to have escaped their notice that their own data show that in the year (1912) before the installation of sewerage was begun the number of new cases (8) was as low as in the year (1915) after the installation was completed (the number of new cases having fallen, according to the commission's figures, from 23 in 1911 to 8 in 1912). Clearly, before crediting the decline of pellagra after 1913 to the effect of improved sanitation, the factor or factors responsible for the marked drop in pellagra in 1912, whatever they may have been, should have been considered. This was not done, nor, what is still more important, has the commission presented any evidence to show that the behavior of pellagra in Spartan village during 1914, 1915, and 1916 differed essentially from that in other mill villages in South Carolina. Our own observations very clearly indicate that there was no such difference in 1917 and 1918, at all events.

It is but fair to say that these workers believe they have shown that certain factors of a general character, such as improved economic conditions were inadequate to explain the diminution in the number of newly incident cases. Thus, in discussing the possible influence of improved financial conditions, they say: "Granting, for the moment, that increased prosperity has caused a reduction in recurrent cases from 40 in 1914 and 40 in 1915 to 21 in 1916, it is evidently quite impossible to ascribe to it the decrease in newly incident cases from 30 in 1913 to 18 in 1914, when the recurrent cases increased from 26 to 40, or the further decrease to 8 incident cases in 1915, while the recurrent cases still remained at 40." This argument appears a weighty one until it is noted that numbers alone are stated without any indication of rates. Now, while such omission is of no significance with respect to newly incident cases in circumstances such as the present, where the population is reported as practically stationary, it is quite different when recurrences are considered, for where a distinction, such as the commission assumes, is drawn between the two classes of cases, the recurrence rate, unlike that for newly incident cases, must be based, not on the population but on the number of pellagrins included in that population. This basic point seems to have altogether escaped the commission. Fortunately, they publish the data (Arch. Int. Med. 1917, vol. 19, p. 688, Table 2) which enable one to compute the rate per cent of recurrences, and we find that the recurrence *rate* for 1913 and 1914, instead of increasing as the commission seems to have been led to believe by taking account of the number of cases alone, actually fell from 65 per cent to 61 per cent, and instead of being stationary for 1914 and 1915, as is suggested by a consideration of mere numbers, fell from 61 per cent to 49 per cent. Thus it is evident that the recurrence rate fell as the newly incident cases fell, and, even though not to the same degree, it nevertheless clearly suggests the possibility of the operation of the same cause in both classes of cases, which in turn suggests what we believe to be a fact, namely, the essential etiological identity of newly incident and recurrent attacks.

Other sources of error might be suggested, but enough have been pointed out to show that the significance which the commission has been inclined to attribute to this experiment is entirely unwarranted.

In connection with the foregoing, consideration may be given to the findings of Jobling and Petersen (1916) which appear to show a relationship similar to that which the Thompson-McFadden commission believed they had observed between increased pellagra prevalence and insanitation. In comparing the incidence of pellagra in two sections of the city of Nashville, Tenn., Jobling and Petersen assumed that, because these included approximately equal numerical groups of Negroes in their population, this indicated approximately equal economic "standards" in the two divisions. They state that "apart from the evidence afforded by the apparently equal distribution of the Negroes, the two divisions are representative of equal economic and social conditions in other respects," but submit no evidence in support of the assertion. The Negro may conceivably serve as an index of economic conditions sufficiently well for some, perhaps many, purposes, but where equality of economic condition is, as here, a vital consideration, some evidence would seem to be called for to show that this really was a valid index in the circumstances under consideration. Furthermore, these gentlemen have evidently assumed that there exists no difference worth considering in economic condition among the Negroes themselves, and, as a considerable proportion of the pellagra in Nashville occurred in the Negro population, it is evident that these workers failed to give due consideration to the possible influence on diet of factors of an economic character, and, therefore, they have failed to show that the relationship, which they claim to have found, is anything other than a spurious correlation.

The results of our (Goldberger, Wheeler, and Sydenstricker, unpublished data) own extensive field studies in which this phase has been carefully considered have failed to reveal any necessary relation between sanitary conditions and pellagra prevalence, and we venture to suggest that in those instances where a relation appears to have been found inadequate or faulty methods of study have been applied or some point has been overlooked, or its importance not sufficiently considered. This is well illustrated by the following: Jobling and Petersen (1917, pp. 122–123) in discussing the possible reasons for a rise in pellagra in 1915 and a decline in 1916 state that though "wages have either not advanced at all, or only in a limited measure during the fall of 1916," the cost of food products "increased at a most disproportionate rate" (in the fall of 1916), a fact which seemed to them inconsistent with the reduction of pellagra in 1916. Now, evidently what happened in the fall of 1916 could not much influence the pellagra incidence of that year, since the vast proportion of cases developed in the spring and early summer. If it had any effect this might be expected to show itself in 1917. As a matter of fact, this is just what did happen; there were more cases of pellagra in Nashville in 1917 than in 1916.[7] With respect to conditions in 1914–15 they say that "while unemployment was increased to some extent in 1914, the larger industries did not alter their forces, *nor did the applications for charity increase to our knowledge*" [italics ours]. Now, in discussing this phase of the subject in their first report (Jobling and Petersen, 1916, p. 528) they stated: "It appears then that there was a period of economic depression beginning about September, 1914, and lasting into the early summer of 1915. *This depression was made evident by the increase in the number of applicants for assistance at the charitable institutions*" [italics ours]. It would seem to us that this self-contradiction on a question of fundamental fact speaks for itself and renders further comment superfluous.

Finally, we desire very briefly to consider the views of McCollum (1917), whose brilliant studies in nutrition very justly give great weight to any opinions he may express. He states (1917, p. 110) that since "there seems to be good evidence that there sometimes occur cases of pellagra in individuals whose diets have included a certain amount of such articles as McCollum and his coworkers have designated as protective foods, viz., milk, eggs, and the leafy vegetables, the theory of infection is supported." No doubt pellagra does occur in individuals whose diets have included "a certain amount" of milk, eggs, and the leafy vegetables. Indeed, by reference to the account (p. 67 *et seq.*) of the diet of our convict volunteers it will be seen that this also included a "certain amount" of milk and leafy vegetables, but this, McCollum tells us (1917, p. 109), was not sufficient to make good the dietary deficiencies of the seed

7 Jobling (James W.): Personal communication. There was an increase also in other localities.

products which it included. And we would add that, so far as we are aware, there exists no good evidence of pellagra occurring in one whose diet was known (not simply assumed) to have included *enough* of the "protective foods." To be sure, pellagra in the nursing infant (an undoubted instance of a case in one exclusively breast fed we ourselves have never seen) might be cited as such an occurrence, but, when we recall reports of scurvy in nursing infants, such cases of pellagra may, with at least equal propriety, be interpreted as indicating that rarely the mother's milk may be faulty and pellagra-producing.

Continuing, McCollum states that "the prevalence of the disease in badly sewered districts supports this view" of an infection. We have already considered what may be regarded as the most important evidence on this point and have pointed out that there really exists no good reason for believing that this relation, when it occurs, is other than a spurious one.

Continuing further, this investigator says that the existence of a bacteriological factor in pellagra "is further supported in some degree by the fact that McCollum, Simonds, and Parsons observed only malnutrition without diarrhea or sore mouth in rats fed diets which, in the experience of Chittenden and Underhill, produce in dogs the gastrointestinal symptoms seen in pellagra in man. The sloughing of the mucous membrane of the mouth and the presence of ulcers in the intestine affords conclusive evidence of an infection in their dogs." These interpretations do not seem to us well founded. To us it seems quite as logical, if not more so, to interpret the difference in reactions observed in the rats on the Chittenden-Underhill diet as dependent on the difference in the species of the experimental animals as to attribute it, as McCollum does, to a chance infection in the dog. This view is strengthened by the fact that rats react to certain diets very differently from guinea pigs, for instance; the latter will develop scurvy on diets apparently entirely adequate for the former. Furthermore, to us the occurrence of the sloughing of the buccal mucous membranes and the intestinal ulcers affords no more conclusive evidence of an infection in the dogs so affected than the occurrence of inflammation of the eyes ("xerophthalmia") in rats on a diet too low in the fat soluble vitamin affords conclusive evidence that this is the result of an infection of the eye in the rat; or that the bleeding swollen gums, loosened teeth, painful, swollen muscles (calves) in man on a diet deficient in the antiscorbutic factor is conclusive evidence that scurvy is due to an infection.

He states, finally, that "it seems logical in the light of all the data available, to conclude that poor nutrition predisposes to infection and that there is an infectious agent involved in the production of pellagra." In this connection, a related argument not infrequently advanced in favor of pellagra as an infection is of interest chiefly, perhaps, because it seems directly to contradict the basic assumption just cited as favored by McCollum. The argument we have in mind most frequently takes the following form: "Inasmuch as bread lines and poor nutrition are of common occurrence in such large cities as New York, Chicago, etc., and as pellagra is of rare occurrence in these places, diet and poor nutrition can have nothing to do with pellagra." More recently this argument has at times been stated as follows: "Inasmuch as the people of Europe, particularly of the Central Powers, have been on starvation diets and necessarily badly nourished and we hear of no pellagra among them, diet and poor nutrition can have nothing to do with pellagra." Assuming the facts to be as stated by the advocates of this view, the fallacy in the argument at once becomes apparent when it is pointed out that beriberi, a disease well known to be dependent on a faulty diet, seems to have been no more prevalent than pellagra under the circumstances mentioned. Evidently, then, it does not necessarily follow that, because a disease is the result of a faulty diet, any faulty diet will bring it about. What this argument does suggest—and strongly— is that if poor nutrition favors infection as McCollum and others suggest, then (1) "poor nutrition" does not predispose to invasion with the hypothetical "infection" of pellagra, or (2) no such "infection" exists, or finally (3) that a specific kind of poor nutrition is necessary to permit the pellagrous "infection" to establish itself. In considering these possibilities it may be argued that "poor nutrition" does favor invasion with the specific pellagrous "infection" in localities where this "infection" is present in the environment. This would imply that in New York and Chicago and, incidentally, in our North as a whole the pellagrous infection is absent or held in restraint by some unknown factor. As a matter of fact, cases of pellagra, though relatively rare, are by no means of infrequent occurrence in our Northern states and in such cities as New York, Chicago, etc. The hypothetical infection of pellagra is present, therefore, and, it may be added, has been present in this environment at least since the notable epidemic of 1909 at the Peoria (Ill.) State Asylum. Consequently the important question presents itself, Why is the disease not more prevalent in these cities and in the North generally if poor nutrition favors its invasion? The restraint imposed by the cooler northern climate, the only explanation which suggests itself and one frequently advanced as the explanation of the relative rarity of the disease in the North, fails as the explanation when it is recalled that in Italy pellagra has for generations been chiefly, if not entirely, prevalent in the colder northern mountainous section and that the disease has long been highly endemic in such relatively rigorous climates as those of Bukowina, Rumania, and Bessarabia. In view of this consideration and, still more, when the available evidence bearing on the question is considered as a whole, one must conclude that the view that "poor nutrition" of a general character favors invasion with the "infection" of pellagra, and that this is the explanation of the rôle of diet in pellagra, is untenable. This does not, however, in strict logic exclude the third of the above-stated possibilities, namely, that a poor nutrition of a specific kind is essential to enable this "infection" to establish itself. It will at once be recognized that this is identical with the view still held by some with reference to the etiology of such diseases as beriberi and scurvy, namely, that each is due to a specific infection which can arise only in one subsisting on a deficient diet of a specific character; in other words, an etiological conception calling for the concurrence of two specific factors for each of these diseases.

In pellagra, as in beriberi and scurvy, however, no unequivocal evidence in support of the existence of an essential infective factor has yet been adduced. Nevertheless, if in spite of this fact and in spite of the evidence demonstrating the vital relation of diet to these diseases, one still considers it logical to hold that there is also a second essential factor, an infection, in beriberi and likewise one in scurvy, we recognize that it is equally logical to hold a like view with respect to pellagra. It is clear, however, that even in this event diet is necessarily recognized as the primary controlling etiological factor. This is of considerable practical importance, for, whichever view may happen to appeal to the minds of those charged with the duty of preventing or controlling the disease, the fundamental guiding principle will not be affected.

Summary

1. An experiment was carried out to test the possibility of producing pellagra in previously healthy men by feeding a monotonous, principally cereal diet of the type found in other previous studies to be associated with a high incidence of pellagra.

2. The experiment was carried out at the Rankin farm of the Mississippi State Penitentiary, about 8 miles east of Jackson.

3. The subjects of the experiment were white adult male convicts

who volunteered for the purpose. They were segregated and kept under special guard. Of 12 volunteers who entered the experiment, 11 remained throughout, 1 had to be released because of the development of a physical infirmity. None of these men gave a history of having had pellagra or of the occurrence of this disease in any member of the family or a near relative.

4. All persons other than the volunteers resident on the farm were under observation as controls. This included 108 convicts, of whom 35 were under observation for a period comparable to the period of observation of the subjects of the experiment. In addition, there were 12 free persons who were present throughout the study; included in these were 4 adult females and 2 children.

5. The general sanitary environment was the same for subjects and controls. With respect to personal cleanliness, cleanliness of quarters, and freedom from insects and vermin, the volunteers were decidedly better off than the convict controls.

6. No direct communication with the outside was permitted the volunteers. There was no special restriction imposed on the controls, convicts or free. Direct exposure of some of the controls to a hypothetical infection was possible and may have occurred when beyond the limits of the farm; this possibility is believed to have been excluded in the case of the subjects of the experiment. There is no history of the previous occurrence of pellagra on this farm.

7. The volunteers were required to do a share of the work of the farm, but, when compared with the convict controls, they were at no time pushed, had shorter hours of work, had regular rest periods when in the field, and did less actual work. The work of the convict controls is rated as requiring moderate to hard, that of the volunteers as moderate to light muscular exertion.

8. The study falls into two periods, one extending from February 4 to April 19, during which the volunteers were kept under observation without any change in the regular prison fare. This afforded an opportunity for a close scrutiny of the men for evidence of any existing pellagra and also permitted them to become accustomed to the desired routine of work and discipline. The second period extended from April 19 to and including October 31, during which the volunteers subsisted on the experimental diet.

9. The diet of the convict controls provided an average of approximately 3,500 to 4,500 calories, about 90 to 110 grams of protein, 95 to 135 grams of fat, and 540 to 580 grams of carbohydrate. Approximately 20 to 35 grams or 20 to 35 per cent of the protein was from animal food. The diet was superior to the experimental diet with

respect to the protein, mineral constituents, and antineuritic and fat soluble vitamins.

10. The ingredients of the experimental diet were highly milled wheat flour, maize meal and grits, cornstarch, white rice, cane sugar, cane sirup, sweet potatoes, pork fat, cabbage, collards, turnips, turnip greens, coffee, "Royal" baking powder, salt, and pepper. During the first three months some buttermilk was used in making wheat biscuits. All ingredients were believed to be of excellent quality and, with one or two exceptions, part of the general camp supply.

11. The average energy intake by the volunteers, as shown by eight periods of a week each during the experimental period, varied between approximately 2,500 and 3,500 calories. The average intake of protein varied between approximately 41 and 54 grams, of fat between approximately 91 and 134 grams, and of carbohydrate between approximately 387 and 513 grams. Eighty to ninety per cent of the total protein was from cereal sources (wheat, maize, rice). The antineuritic vitamin content was planned to be low, but in the absence of any distinctive clinical manifestations of beriberi in our volunteers it would seem to have been sufficient, at least not appreciably deficient, for their needs during the period of study. Similarly in the absence of recognizable indications of scurvy, the diet would seem to have included an adequate supply of the antiscorbutic factor. With regard to the adequacy of supply of the fat soluble vitamin, it is difficult to judge by reason of the meagerness of the available fundamental data; none of these men developed the eye symptoms currently considered indicative of a deficiency in this food element. The intake of some, at least, of the mineral ingredients of the diet was decidedly low. Whether the mineral intake was actually inadequate or improperly balanced for normal nutrition over a long period in man is uncertain.

12. The test diet was probably faulty in some degree with respect to the protein (amino acid deficiency), antineuritic vitamin, mineral constituents, and possibly also with respect to the fat soluble vitamin. In relation to the production of pellagra, this study suggests that the dietary factors to be considered as possibly essential are (1) an amino acid deficiency, (2) a deficient or faulty constitution of the mineral supply, possibly, but doubtfully, (3) a deficiency in the fat soluble vitamin intake and perhaps (4) an as yet unknown (vitamin?) factor. As to which or what combination (or combinations) of these constitutes the specific pellagra-producing dietary defect or defects remains to be determined.

13. Although both classes of controls (convict and free) were ex-

posed to the chance of direct contact with pellagra and although, as compared with the volunteers, the convict controls were at a disadvantage hygienically, and were required to work harder and further, although various minor ailments and a number of rather sharp attacks of malaria were observed among them, none of the convict (or other) controls developed any evidence of pellagra. On the other hand, although segregated and under special guard with the possibility of direct contact with pellagra excluded, and although under much more favorable hygienic conditions, not less than 6 of the 11 volunteers who remained in the test to the end developed evidence which experienced observers joined with us in recognizing as those of pellagra.

14. Having due regard for the conditions of the experiment, the conclusion seems warranted that pellagra developed in at least 6 of our 11 volunteers as the result of the diet on which they subsisted.

15. Significant subjective symptoms made their first appearance during the second month after beginning the test diet. These included weakness, abdominal discomfort or pain, and headache. All subjects lost weight, the loss becoming particularly marked during the last four weeks of the experiment. At least 6 of the 11 men developed a well-marked eruption. The earliest date of the beginning of this was September 12, or at about the end of the fifth month of the diet. The initial site in all of the cases was the scrotum; later classical lesions also developed on hands or neck of some of these. The knee jerk became exaggerated in five of the men, the earliest date being October 17, or at the close of the sixth month of the experiment.

16. The scrotal lesion is a much more common early skin manifestation of pellagra than has heretofore been realized, but is nevertheless a somewhat infrequent one.

17. It is suggested that the site of at least the initial dermatitis is bound up with a specific quality of the diet.

18. In its essential make-up the experimental diet was probably not entirely typical of the average pellagra-producing diet.

19. The view is advanced that there exist essential differences in the intimate make-up of the diet corresponding to observed differences in some at least of the clinical types of the disease. Pellagra, as conventionally defined, probably includes at least two commonly associated but etiologically essentially distinct syndromes.

20. Diet is at least the primary controlling etiological factor.

[Appendices deleted: A. Clinical record of volunteers; B. Analysis of symptoms; C. Tables of factors used in computing composition of

experimental diet; D. Clinical record of full-time convict controls.
ED.]

References

Chittenden, R. H., and Underhill, F. P. *Am. J. Physiol.*, Vol. 44 (1917), p. 13.

Crosby, C. E. "Pellagra with Erythema of Scrotum as Initial Skin Manifestation," *J. Am. Med. Assn.*, Vol. 68 (May 12, 1917), p. 1403.

Deiaco, P. "Über Lokalisation und Natur der Pellagrösen Hautsymptome," *Wien. Klin. Wchnschrft.*, Vol. 20 (1907), pp. 967–74.

Goldberger, J. "The Etiology of Pellagra; The Significance of Certain Epidemiological Observations with Respect Thereto," *Public Health Rep.* (Washington, D.C.), Vol. 29 (June 26, 1914), pp. 1683–86.

———. "Pellagra, Causation and a Method of Prevention," *J. Am. Med. Assn.*, Vol. 66 (February 12, 1916), pp. 471–76.

———. "The Transmissibility of Pellagra; Experimental Attempts at Transmission to the Human Subject," *Public Health Rep.* (Washington, D.C.), Vol. 31 (November 17, 1916), pp. 3159–73.

———, Waring, C. H., and Willets, D. G. "The Prevention of Pellagra, etc.," *Public Health Rep.* (Washington, D.C.), Vol. 30 (October 22, 1915), p. 3117.

Goldberger, J., and Wheeler, G. A. "Experimental Pellagra in the Human Subject, etc.," *Public Health Rep.* (November 12, 1915), p. 3336.

———, and Sydenstricker, E. "A Study of the Diet of Nonpellagrous and of Pellagrous Households, etc.," *J. Am. Med. Assn.*, Vol. 71 (September 21, 1918), pp. 944–49.

Harris, W. A. "The Experimental Production of Pellagra in the Monkey," *J. Am. Med. Assn.*, Vol. 63 (September 26, 1914), pp. 1093–94.

Jobling, J. W., and Petersen, W. "A Preliminary Report upon the Epidemiology of Pellagra in Nashville, Tenn.," *J. Infec. Dis.*, Vol. 18 (January, 1916), pp. 501–67.

———. "The Epidemiology of Pellagra in Nashville," *J. Infec. Dis.*, Vol. 21 (August, 1917), pp. 109–31.

Lavinder, C. H., and Francis, E. "Attempts to Transmit Pellagra to Monkeys," *J. Am. Med. Assn.*, Vol. 63 (September 26, 1914), pp. 1093–94.

McCollum, E. V. *The Newer Knowledge of Nutrition* (New York, 1917).

Merk, L. *Die Hauterscheinungen der Pellagra* (Innsbruck, 1909).

Nesbitt, C. T. "Sanitation and the Control of Pellagra," *J. Am. Med. Assn.*, Vol. 66 (February 26, 1916), pp. 647–48.

Sherman, H. C. *Chemistry of Food and Nutrition* (New York, 1918).

Siler, J. F., Garrison, P. E., and MacNeal, W. J. "A Statistical Study of the Relation of Pellagra to Use of Certain Foods and to Location of Domicile, etc.," *Arch. Int. Med.*, Vol. 14 (September, 1914), pp. 293–373.

———. "An Experimental Test of the Relation of Sewage Disposal to the Spread of Pellagra," *Arch. Int. Med.*, Vol. 19 (May, 1917), pp. 683–94.

————. "Relation of Pellagra to Location of Domicile in Spartan Mills, S.C. and the Adjacent District," *Arch. Int. Med.*, Vol. 19 (August, 1917), p. 198.

Stannus, H. S. "Pellagra in Nyasaland," *Tr. Soc. Trop. Med. and Hyg.*, Vol. 7 (1913), p. 32.

Sydenstricker, E. "The Prevalence of Pellagra: Its Possible Relation to the Rise in the Cost of Food," *Public Health Reports* (Washington, D.C.), Vol. 30 (October 22, 1915), pp. 3132–48.

Vedder, E. B. "Dietary Deficiency as the Etiological Factor in Pellagra," *Arch. Int. Med.*, Vol. 18 (August, 1916), pp. 137–72.

Wood, E. J. "The Diagnosis of Pellagra," *Arch. Diagnosis* (New York), April, 1917.

6. The Transmissibility of Pellagra. Experimental Attempts at Transmission to the Human Subject[1]

JOSEPH GOLDBERGER

There is a very widely held belief, at least in the United States, that pellagra is a communicable disease. The evidence in support of this is almost wholly indirect and consists, in the main, of certain analogies to infectious diseases presented by some features of its epidemiology. When critically examined one finds that this evidence either completely falls or that it is susceptible of an entirely different interpretation.[2] The only direct evidence in favor of this view that calls for serious consideration is the report by Harris (1913), of New Orleans, of a successful inoculation of a monkey with a filtrate from pellagrous lesions.

The very extensive and comprehensive monkey inoculations by Lavinder and Francis (1914), like those of a number of other workers, including the later (unpublished) work[3] of Harris himself, have failed to confirm this report.

In order to throw further and, if possible, conclusive light on this subject the writer planned to test the question of the infectivity of the disease by experiment on an animal species known to be susceptible, namely, man himself.

This was made possible by the cooperation of a number of my colleagues and associates who, after being informed of the problem, freely volunteered to submit themselves to experiment. It was originally planned to carry out this test during 1915 concurrently with a test of the rôle of diet in the production of pellagra (Goldberger and Wheeler, 1915) to which a group of convicts were at that time being subjected. The pressure of other work, however, made it necessary to defer this phase of the investigation until the spring of the present year.

1 *Public Health Rep.*, Vol. 31, No. 46 (November 17, 1916), 3159–73.
2 A discussion of the literature is reserved for a later communication. In the meantime the reader will find the following of interest: Goldberger, 1915; Vedder, 1916; and Voegtlin, 1914.
3 Communicated at a meeting of Louisiana health officers, New Orleans, July, 1915.

General Considerations

Some 20 individuals volunteered to submit themselves to experimentation. It was not practicable, however, to utilize more than 16 of them. These included 1 woman.

They varied in age from 26 to 42 years. Four were 26 to 29, 9 from 30 to 39, and 3 from 40 to 42 years. Thirteen were physicians. They resided in various localities: Eight at Washington, D. C.; 1 at Columbia, S.C.; 2 at Spartanburg, S.C.; 1 at Milledgeville, Ga.; and 4 at New Orleans, La.

No restraint of any sort was imposed. They were advised to continue their customary habits of life and diet, and were permitted to travel freely in attending to their personal or official business.

No attempt was made to avoid "natural infection." Indeed, it should be noted that five of the volunteers by reason of their official duties came into frequent and intimate contact with pellagra in its natural environment. Three, including the woman, have come into known contact with cases of the disease, while four others have lived for considerable periods in a locality (New Orleans) where casual contact with the disease was at least a possibility.

In the appended list (see p. 106) of the volunteers will be found the age, location of residence, and an indication of the experiment or experiments in which each participated.

The materials used were blood, nasopharyngeal secretions, epidermal scales from pellagrous skin lesions, urine, and feces. The blood was administered by intramuscular or subcutaneous injection, the secretions by application to the mucosa of the nose and nasopharynx, scales and excreta by mouth.

In order to reduce gastric acidity and thus minimize the possibly germicidal effect of the gastric juice, the ingestion of scales and excreta was preceded by a dose of from 10 to 20 grains of sodium bicarbonate. The ingesta were always taken on an otherwise empty stomach.

The materials whose infectivity was tested were obtained from 17 cases of pellagra of various types and of different grades of severity, including three fatal cases. A list is appended (see pp. 106–10) in which the pertinent data relating to each case are given.

The patients were seen and the experiments performed at different places. One, a fatal case, was seen at the Washington Asylum Hospital, Washington, D.C.; 1 at the Charity Hospital, New Orleans, La.; 3 at the State Hospital for Insane at Columbia, S.C.; and 12, including 2 fatal cases, at Spartanburg, S.C. The volunteers participating did not in all instances reside at the place where the experiment was performed, but assembled there at a specified time. This applies particularly to the experiments at Spartanburg, S.C.

Details

As will appear from the details next to be presented, the infectivity of the blood was tested twice, of nasopharyngeal secretions twice, of scales three times, and by reason of the alleged controlling influence of methods of sewage disposal in the propagation of the disease the infectivity of both urine and feces was tested six times. Two or more of these tests were made on seven different occasions. In presenting the details of the experiments it seems best to consider the individual experiment under the group of which it formed a part on one of these seven occasions. The groups are considered in their chronological sequence. A tabular summary is appended (see pp. 98–99).

Experiment Group No. 1

On April 25, 1916, blood and nasopharyngeal secretions were obtained from a patient (case No. 1) with a moderately acute first attack of the disease at the United States Pellagra Hospital, Spartanburg, S.C., and administered to two volunteers, G–J and W–GA.

(*a*) *Blood.*—The blood was drawn from a vein at one of the elbows, defibrinated, and 5 cc. were injected without delay into the left deltoid of W–GA and 6 cc. into that of G–J.

(*b*) *Secretions.*—Secretions were obtained by wiping out the nose and nasopharynx of the patient with a cotton swab and transferred by at once rubbing this over the mucosa of the nose and nasopharynx of the volunteer. A separate swab was used for each.

Effects.—Both men felt some soreness and stiffness for a day or two in the muscle into which the blood was injected; otherwise nothing was observed.

Experiment Group No. 2

On April 28, epidermal scales and urine were obtained from each of two patients and feces from a third at the State Hospital for Insane at Columbia, S.C.

Of the two patients furnishing both scales and urine, one (case No. 3) was a severe first attack and the other (case No. 4) a mild second attack. The patient furnishing the feces (case No. 2) was suffering from a severe attack and was having four soft bowel movements a day.

(*a*) *Scales.*—The scales were obtained by scraping the affected

Tabular summary of experiments

Date	Locality	Material Kind	Material Source (case)	Amount	Manner of administration	Volunteer subject	Remarks	Result
							Time interval.	
1916.								
April 25.	Spartanburg, S.C.	Defibrinated blood	No. 1	5 c.c. / 6 c.c.	Intramuscular injection.	W-GA / G-J	The blood was injected intramuscularly within a few minutes after defibrination.	No pellagra.
		Nasophar. secretions.	....do....	(?)	Applied to mucosa of nose and nasopharynx.	W-GA / G-J	Secretions obtained on cotton swab and at once rubbed over mucosa of subject. Fresh swab used for each subject.	Do.
April 28	Columbia, S.C.	Scales / Urine / Feces	No. 3 and No. 4 / No. 2	0.1 to 0.2 gm. 8c.c. / 4 c.c.	Swallowed.	G-J	Scales taken as "powder." Feces and urine made up into pilular mass with wheat flour and ingested. The quantities are minimal estimates. Interval 1 to 1½ hours.	Do.
		Defibrinated blood	No. 5, No. 6, and No. 7.	7 c.c.	Subcutaneous injection.	G-J / G-MHF / S-E / T-WF / W-DG / W-GA	Case No. 5 furnished 10 c.c. No. 6 furnished 15.5 c.c., and No. 7 furnished 20 c.c. of defibrinated blood. Of the pooled blood 7 c.c. were subcutaneously injected into each subject. The time between drawing and injecting the blood was under two hours.	Do.
May	Spartanburg, S.C.	Nasophar. secretions.	No. 1, No. 5, No. 6, and No. 7.	(?)	Rubbed into mucosa of nose and nasopharynx.	G-J / S-E / T-WF / W-DG / W-GA	Secretions freshly obtained by swabbing out the nose and nasopharynx in each case with a set of 5 cotton swabs and soaking these in saline solution. Six fresh swabs wet with this secretion were rubbed over nasal and nasopharyngeal mucosa of each volunteer. Interval less than 2 hours.	Do.
		Scales	No. 1 and No. 7.	0.06 gm.	Swallowed.	G-J / S-E / T-WF / W-DG / W-GA	Case No. 1 furnished 0.1 gm. and No. 7, 0.22 gm. of freshly scraped scales. These were mixed and divided into five approximately equal parts and swallowed about 7 hours after they were collected.	Do
		Urine / Feces	No. 5, No. 6, and No. 7.	6 c.c. / 3 gms.	....do....	G-J / S-E / T-WF / W-DG / W-GA	Urine and feces rubbed up into a pilular mass with wheat flour. Each volunteer swallowed a portion representing 3 gms. of feces (1 gm. from each case) and 6 c.c. of urine (2 c.c. from each case). Urine and feces 3 to 9 hours old when swallowed.	Do.

Tabular summary of experiments (Continued)

Date	Locality	Material				Volunteer subject.	Remarks.	Result
		Kind.	Source (case).	Amount.	Manner of administration.			
June 7	Washington, D.C.	Urine...........	No. 8...........	2 c.c.	....do........	C-RH.... D-WF.... McC-GW. G-J..... S-AM....	Urine and feces worked up into a pilular mass with cracker crumbs and a little flour. The urine was not over 4 hours old when ingested; each volunteer received 2 c.c. The feces consisted of two specimens, one 15 hours and the other about 5 hours old. Of the former each volunteer took 0.2 gm., of the latter 1 gm.	Do.
		Feces...........	No. 8...........	1.2 gms..				
June 8	....do.........	Urine...........	No. 8...........	2 c.c.	....do........	G-J..... L-JP.... S-EA....	Urine and feces prepared with cracker crumbs and a little flour. Urine was 3 hours old. The feces included 3 specimens; one 39 hours old, the second 12 hours, and the third about 5 hours old. Each volunteer took 2 c.c. of urine and 1 gm. of each fecal specimen.	Do.
		Feces...........	No. 8...........	3 gms....				
June 13	New Orleans, La.	Urine...........	No. 9...........	2 c.c.	....do........	A-CV.... G-J..... L-JB.... M-MB.... W-CL....	Urine and feces prepared with cracker crumbs and flour. Urine was about 5½ hours old. Feces were liquid, following saline purge. Each volunteer took 2 c.c. of urine with 2 c.c. of feces.	Do.
		Feces...........	No. 9...........	2 c.c.				
June 25	Spartanburg, S.C.	Scales..........	No. 14 and No. 17.	0.004 gm.	....do........	G-J.... S-E.... W-GA....	Scales, urine, and feces were worked up into a pilular mass with cracker crumbs. The scales were not over 4 hours old and each volunteer took about 0.004 gm. The urine and feces were not over 6 hours old. Of the urine each volunteer took about 1 c.c. from each case; of the feces 1 gm. from each of six cases and 2 gms. from the seventh (case No. 13).	Do.
		Urine...........	Nos. 10,11,12,14, 15,17,............	6 c.c.				
		Feces...........	Nos. 10,11,12,13, 14,15,16,.........	8 gms....				

areas of the skin and, combined, weighed, it is estimated, about 0.1 to 0.2 gms.

(b) *Urine.*—The urine was a fresh catheter specimen in each case.

(c) *Feces.*—The feces specimen was obtained with the aid of a simple water enema and was liquid.

The scales with about 4 cc. of each specimen of urine and with about the same quantity of the liquid feces were worked up into a pilular mass with wheat flour and in this form swallowed by volunteer G–J, 30 minutes after taking 20 grains of sodium bicarbonate and about 1 to 1½ hours after collecting. After swallowing this mass another dose of 20 grains of sodium bicarbonate was taken. The alkali, as already stated, was intended to reduce gastric acidity and thus perhaps favor infection.

Effects.—For several days after the ingestion of the foregoing materials this volunteer experienced some slight epigastric fullness and eructations of gas after a meal. On the third day a diarrhea with frequent, painless, watery, and rather gaseous evacuations developed. The diarrhea lasted about a week. It was still present on May 7, on which date, as will presently appear, this volunteer participated in another experiment which included the ingestion of scales, urine, and feces.

Experiment Group No. 3

On May 7 blood, nasopharyngeal secretions, scales, urine, and feces were obtained from some patients at the United States Pellagra Hospital, Spartanburg, S.C., and used for the inoculation of each of a group of five volunteers, G–J., S–E., T–WF., W–DG., and W–GA. A sixth volunteer, G–MHF., received blood only.

(a) *Blood.*—The blood was drawn from the general circulation of each of three patients, defibrinated and then pooled. Of this, 7 cc. were injected subcutaneously into each of the six volunteers mentioned. The time elapsing between drawing and injecting the blood was under two hours.

To the pooled blood, one of the patients (case No. 5), with a mild ninth recurrent attack, contributed 10 cc.; one (case No. 6), with a moderately acute second attack, 15.5 cc.; and one (case No. 7), with a severe acute second attack, 20 cc. The patients furnished, therefore, 1.5 cc., 2.5 cc., and 3 cc., respectively, of defibrinated blood for the inoculation of each volunteer.

(b) *Secretions.*—Secretions were obtained from four patients and, after mixing, used for the inoculation of the five men above mentioned. One of the patients (case No. 1) was the same as the one that furnished the secretions for the first experiment (experiment group No. 1, *b*). The three others are cases No. 5, No. 6, and No. 7, already briefly characterized in describing the immediately preceding blood inoculation.

The nose and nasopharynx of each of the four patients were carefully wiped out with a separate set of five cotton swabs. The secretions thus obtained were mixed by rinsing and soaking the swabs in some normal salt solution.

The inoculation was made by rubbing over the mucosa of each side of the nose and nasopharynx each of a set of three swabs soaked in the mixture just described. In this way a fresh set of six swabs was used for each volunteer. The time elapsing between collecting and inoculating was less than two hours. Incidentally it should perhaps be noted that some of the secretions applied to the nasopharynx must have been, eventually, swallowed.

(*c*) *Scales.*—Scales were freshly scraped from affected areas of skin of two patients, cases No. 1 and No. 7, previously characterized. Case No. 1 furnished 0.1 gm. and No. 7, 0.22 gm.

These were mixed and then divided approximately equally among the five volunteers, each of whom swallowed his portion in the form of a "powder" about seven hours after they were collected and shortly after taking the dose of urine and feces next to be described.

(*d*) *Urine; feces.*—A specimen of urine and one of feces was obtained from each of the same three patients (cases No. 5, No. 6, and No. 7) as furnished the blood. In order to make sure of having the feces when wanted a simple water enema was used to get the specimens, none of which was diarrheal.

Ten cubic centimeters of urine and 5 grams of solid feces from each of the three corresponding specimens were worked up into a pilular mass with flour. About 15 minutes after taking 20 grains of sodium bicarbonate each of the five volunteers ingested an approximately equal portion of the mass. Each took therefore the equivalent of about 2 cc. of urine and 1 gram of feces from each of the three patients.

The urine and fecal specimens were between 3 and 9 hours old when ingested.

Effects.—About 10 days after inoculation, one of the volunteers, T–WF, noted a slightly enlarged and somewhat tender lymph gland above the Poupart's ligament of the side of the abdomen that was the site of the blood injection. This gradually subsided. None of the other volunteers experienced any inconvenience, although, as will be recalled, one of them (G–J), on the date of this experiment, had not yet completely recovered from a rather marked attack of diarrhea following a previous ingestion experiment.

Experiment Group No. 4

On June 7, 1916, urine and feces were obtained from a patient (female) at the Washington Asylum Hospital, Washington, D.C. The patient (case No. 8) had a typhoidal first attack, from which she died 10 days later (June 17, 1916).

The urine was a catheter specimen, drawn at 8.45 a.m., June 7.

The fecal matter consisted of two specimens; one, fairly liquid, was passed at about 9 p.m., June 6; the second, of soft puttylike consistency, was passed about 7 a.m., June 7.

Ten cubic centimeters of the urine, 1 gram of the first and 5 grams of the second fecal specimen were worked up into a pilular mass with cracker crumbs and a little flour. Gelatin capsules were filled, approximately equally divided, and at 12.30 p.m. ingested by five volunteers, C–RH, D–WF, McC–GW, G–J, and S–AM. Fifteen minutes before this each volunteer took 10 grains of sodium bicarbonate.

Effects.–Some hours after ingesting the above one of the volunteers, S–AM, developed abdominal discomfort accompanied by abnormal, gaseous evacuations. The movements increased in frequency, developing into a marked diarrhea, which lasted about two weeks. He has been well since.

Another, McC–GW, experienced a little temporary gastric discomfort immediately after taking the material; nothing of note since.

None of the others of this group experienced any appreciable effects.

Experiment Group No. 5

On June 8, 1916, another experiment was made with urine and feces from the patient (case No. 8) furnishing these materials for the preceding experiment, No. 4.

On this occasion the fecal matter consisted of three specimens. One of these, now 39 hours old, was passed at 7 a.m., June 7, and had served in experiment No. 4; it had been kept at room temperature. The second was passed at 11.30 p.m., June 7, and the third at 7.15 a.m., June 8. Both of these latter specimens were liquid.

A urine specimen was drawn by catheter at 8.45 a.m., June 8.

Three grams of the first, 3 cc. of the second, and 3 cc. of the third fecal specimen, with 6 cc. of urine, were prepared as in the preceding experiment, and at 12 o'clock equally divided among the three volunteers G–J, L–JP, and S–EA. Each received, therefore, the equivalent of 1 gram of each of the three fecal specimens and of 2 cc. of the urine. About 20 minutes before taking this material each volunteer had taken 10 grains of sodium bicarbonate.

Effects.—Although two of these volunteers (L–JP and S–EA) had temporary attacks of looseness of the bowels immediately preceding the experiment, neither they nor the third who had participated in each of the preceding ingestion experiments experienced any inconvenience following the ingestion of this experimental material.

Experiment Group No. 6

On June 13, 1916, urine and feces were obtained from a patient at the Charity Hospital, New Orleans, La. This patient (case No. 9) had a mild first attack.

The urine was obtained by catheter at 8 a.m. The stool, a liquid one, was passed at about 7.15 a.m., after a dose of magnesium sulphate.

Measured quantities of this material were prepared as in experiments No. 4 and No. 5 at 1.20 p.m. and ingested by five volunteers, A–CW, G–J, L–JB, M–MB, and W–CL, each one getting the equivalent of 2 c.c. of feces and 2 c.c. of urine. Twenty-five minutes before taking this material each volunteer took 20 grains of sodium bicarbonate.

Effects.—None of this group of volunteers experienced any appreciable effects.

Experiment Group No. 7

On June 25, 1916, material was obtained at Spartanburg, S.C., for a final experiment.

(a) *Scales.*—Epidermal scales were scraped from pellagrous skin lesions of two patients (cases No. 14 and No. 17) at the United States Pellagra Hospital. They were not over four hours old when ingested.

(b) *Urine.*—Urine was obtained from three patients (cases No. 10, No. 11, and No. 12) at the county farm and from three (cases No. 14, No. 15, and No. 17) at the Pellagra Hospital.

(c) *Feces.*—Feces were obtained from four patients (cases No. 10, No. 11, No. 12, and No. 13) at the county farm and from three (cases No. 14, No. 15, and No. 16) at the Pellagra Hospital. Two of the fecal specimens were from patients (cases No. 12 and No. 13) with diarrhea.

The seven patients who furnished the material for this experiment were suffering from attacks of varying grades of severity (see list of pellagra cases), including two fatal cases (No. 12 and No. 13).

Measured quantities of the materials mentioned were worked up with cracker crumbs and a little flour into a pilular mass. Fifteen minutes after taking a dose of 20 grains of sodium bicarbonate this was ingested by each of the three volunteers, G–J, S–E, and W–GA, each taking the equivalent of about 4 milligrams of scales, 6 cc. of urine (1 cc. from each patient), and 8 grams of feces (2 grams from case No. 13 and 1 gram from each of the other six patients). The feces and urine were not over six hours old when ingested.

Effects.—Volunteer G–J, who participated in all of the preceding experiments and who, as was noted, had an attack of indigestion and diarrhea for about one week following the first ingestion experiment, experienced some mild dyspeptic symptoms for a number of days immediately after this.

Within two or three hours after the experiment volunteer S–E began to feel nauseated. The following morning he had three watery evacuations and 12 hours later a diarrhea began that lasted about a week. Nausea persisted for about the same period.

Volunteer W–GA had some slight ill-defined dyspeptic symptoms for about 24 hours following the experiment.

Aside from these immediate, temporary disturbances none of the volunteers has experienced any appreciable effects.

Results and Conclusions

The first experiment was made on April 25 and the last on June 25, so that the volunteers have now (Nov. 16, 1916) been under observation for from four and one-half to six and one-half months approximately. Observation has been maintained by association with a majority of the volunteers, by visits of inspection to the others, supplemented by reports from the volunteers themselves, or in the case of the laymen from medical officers with whom they are associated.

In four or five instances, as above noted, there were more or less marked immediate, but temporary gastrointestinal reactions following and probably due to the ingestion of the large doses of excreta. When one considers the relatively enormous quantities of filth taken the reactions experienced were surprisingly slight.

One of the volunteers, S–EA, had an attack of renal colic of eight to nine days' duration, from August 14 to August 22, 1916. Aside from this he, as well as the other volunteers, has enjoyed his usual health. None has developed any evidence justifying even a suspicion of pellagra.

It is not my present purpose to enter into a discussion of the etiology of pellagra. I may be permitted, however, to recall by way of contrast the result of the feeding experiment carried out last year (Goldberger and Wheeler, 1915). In that experiment, of 11 convicts subsisting on a one-sided diet not less than 6 developed definite evidence of pellagra, while of over 30 controls not one showed any evidence that would justify even a suspicion of the disease.

It would appear, then, that while the opinion that pellagra is a communicable disease gains no support from the work here reported, the conclusion, elsewhere drawn (Goldberger, 1916), that it is a disease essentially of dietary origin, brought about by a faulty, probably "deficient," diet is materially strengthened.

Summary

Sixteen volunteers were subjected to experiment. With one exception all were men and varied in age from 26 to 42 years. No restraints were imposed on their customary habits or activities.

Seventeen cases of pellagra of various types and of different grades of severity furnished some one or more of the experimental materials.

The materials were blood, nasopharyngeal secretions, epidermal scales from pellagrous lesions, urine, and feces. Blood was furnished by 4 of the cases, nasopharyngeal secretions by 4, epidermal scales by 5, and urine or feces by 16, of whom 10 furnished both urine and feces, 3 urine without feces, and 3 feces without urine.

Blood was administered by intramuscular or subcutaneous injection; secretions by application to the mucosa of the nose and nasopharynx; scales and excreta by mouth.

Both urine and feces were ingested by 15 of the volunteers, 5 of whom also took blood, secretions, and scales.

The experiments were performed at four widely separated localities (Washington, D.C.; Columbia, S.C.; Spartanburg, S.C.; and New Orleans, La.), at which different groups of the volunteers were assembled.

Observation has been maintained by association with a majority of the volunteers and by visits of inspection, supplemented by reports from the volunteers themselves, 13 of whom are physicians, and by reports from other medical officers of the service with whom they are associated. During a period of between five and seven months none has developed evidence justifying a diagnosis of pellagra.

These experiments furnish no support for the view that pellagra is a communicable disease; they materially strengthen the conclusion that it is a disease essentially of dietary origin, brought about by a faulty, probably "deficient," diet.

Volunteers

A–CV.—Medical officer, 26 years. Stationed at New Orleans, La. Participated in experiment No. 6.

C–RH.—Medical officer, 37 years. Stationed at Washington, D.C. Participated in experiment No. 4.

D–WF.—Medical officer, 32 years. Stationed at Washington, D.C. Participated in experiment No. 4.

G–J.—Medical officer, 42 years. Stationed at Washington, D.C. Major part of the time spent in field work in Southern states. Participated in all seven experiments.

G–MHF.—Housewife, 35 years. Resides at Washington, D.C. The only woman among the volunteers. Participated in experiment No. 3 at Spartanburg, S.C.

L–JB.—Medical officer, 28 years. Stationed at New Orleans. Participated in experiment No. 6.

L–JP.—Medical officer, 35 years. Stationed at Washington, D.C. Participated in experiment No. 5.

McC–GW.—Medical officer, 40 years. Stationed at Washington, D.C. Participated in experiment No. 4.

M–MB.—Technical assistant, 33 years. Stationed at New Orleans, La. Participated in experiment No. 6.

S–AM.—Medical officer, 39 years. Stationed at Washington, D.C. Participated in experiment No. 4.

S–E.—Statistician, 35 years. Stationed at Spartanburg, S.C. Participated in experiments No. 3 and No. 7.

S–EA.—Medical officer, 39 years. Stationed at Washington, D.C. Had an attack of renal colic August 14–22, 1916. Participated in experiment No. 5.

T–WF.—Medical officer, 28 years. Stationed at Columbia and Spartanburg, S.C. Participated in experiment No. 3.

W–CL.—Medical officer, 28 years. Stationed at New Orleans, La., up to September 12; at San Francisco after that date. Participated in experiment No. 6.

W–DG.—Assistant epidemiologist, 42 years. Stationed at Milledgeville, Ga. Participated in experiment No. 3.

W–GA.—Medical officer, 31 years. Stationed at Spartanburg, S.C. Participated in experiments No. 1, No. 3, and No. 7.

Pellagra Cases

Number 1

W–S.—White female admitted to United States Pellagra Hospital, Spartanburg, S.C., April 14, 1916. Hospital No. 191.

Salient clinical features.—Weakness, moderate skin lesions which first appeared April 7, 1916, moderate diarrhea.

Severity.—Rated by Dr. R. M. Grimm, the medical officer in charge, as a moderately acute first attack.

Experimental material.—Furnished blood and nasopharyngeal secretions on April 25 and epidermal scales and nasopharyngeal secretions on May 7.

Number 2

M–FN.—White male, Ward 4, Columbia State Hospital, Columbia, S.C. Service of Dr. J. T. Munnerlyn. Admitted February, 1916.
Salient clinical features.—History of illness of two years. Insane. Presents marked seborrhea of nose and lips. Dermatitis on both elbows, with encircling "areola" on left. Has about four soft movements a day.
Severity.—Rated by Dr. Munnerlyn as a "severe" case.
Experimental material.—Furnished feces on April 28, 1916.

Number 3

L–JL.—White female, Ward A12, Columbia State Hospital, Columbia, S.C. Service of Dr. D. W. Register. Admitted February, 1916.
Salient clinical features.—Mental manifestations, eruption, red tongue.
Severity.—Rated by Dr. Register as a "severe" first attack.
Experimental material.—Furnished epidermal scales and urine April 28, 1916.

Number 4

M–MC.—White female, Ward A12, Columbia State Hospital, Columbia, S.C. Service of Dr. D. W. Register.
Salient clinical features.—Mental manifestations, extensive eruption. History of an attack in 1914.
Severity.—Rated by Dr. Register as a "mild" second attack.
Experimental material.—Furnished epidermal scales and urine on April 28, 1916.

Number 5

E–EA.—White male, admitted to United States Pellagra Hospital, Spartanburg, S.C., May 5, 1916. Hospital No. 24, 24a, 24b.
Salient clinical features.—History of first attack in 1908; present is ninth attack and is said to have begun about April 15, 1916. Presents mild skin and minor nervous manifestations, marked weakness, constipated.
Severity.—Rated by Dr. Grimm as a mild, acute ninth recurrence.
Experimental material.—Furnished nasopharyngeal secretions, urine, feces, and blood on May 7, 1916.

Number 6

O–I.—White female, admitted to United States Pellagra Hospital, May 6, 1916. Hospital No. 195.
Salient clinical features.—Weakness, moderately severe skin manifestations, moderate "nervousness," vertigo, mild salivation. History of first attack April, 1915.

Severity.—Rated by Dr. Grimm as a moderately acute second attack.

Experimental material.—Furnished nasopharyngeal secretions, urine, feces, and blood on May 7, 1916.

Number 7

S–H.—White male, 8 years old. Admitted to United States Pellagra Hospital, April 26, 1916. Hospital No. 193.

Salient clinical features.—Severe extensive skin manifestations, some of moist type. Mentally dull and depressed. History of a first attack in spring of 1915.

Severity.—Rated by Dr. Grimm as a severe acute second attack.

Experimental material.—Furnished nasopharyngeal secretions, blood, urine, and feces on May 7, 1916.

Number 8

S–M.—White female, 48 years old. Admitted to Washington Asylum Hospital, Washington, D.C., April 27, 1916. Service of Dr. W. M. Barton; resident physician, Dr. Reiss.

Salient clinical features.—Mild skin manifestations, beefy tongue, diarrhea, involuntary evacuations, disoriented, typhoidal.

Severity.—A typhoid-pellagra, fatal; died June 17, 1916.

Experimental material.—Furnished two specimens of feces for experiment on June 7, 1916. One, fairly liquid, was passed at 9 p. m., June 6; the second, more nearly solid, at 7 a. m. June 7. Also a specimen of urine drawn at 8.45 a. m. June 7.

For the experiment of June 8, besides the second of the preceding fecal specimens, which was preserved at air temperature, this patient furnished two additional stools, both fluid, one passed at 11.30 p. m. June 7 and the other at 7.15 p. m. June 8. Also a specimen of urine drawn at 8.45 a. m. June 8, 1916.

Number 9

B–M.—Colored male, 74 years. Admitted to Charity Hospital, New Orleans, La., June 11, 1916, ward No. 31, bed 405. Service of Dr. I. I. Lemmon; resident physician, Dr. C. Dean.

Salient clinical features.—Minor nervous manifestations, mild dermatitis, history of loose bowels.

Severity.—a mild first attack.

Experimental material.—Furnished feces and urine. Stool, liquid, after saline purge, passed about 7.15 a. m.; urine drawn at 8 a. m., June 13, 1916.

Number 10

K–L.—White male, 11 years. Admitted to Spartanburg County Farm June 16, 1916. Service of Dr. O. W. Leonard.

Salient clinical features.—Extensive marked skin manifestations; mild gastrointestinal symptoms.
Severity.—A well-marked first attack of moderate grade.
Experimental material.—Furnished urine and feces June 25, 1916.

Number 11

K–OB.—White male, 43 years. Admitted to Spartanburg County Farm June 16, 1916. Service of Dr. O. W. Leonard.
Salient clinical features.—Extensive severe skin manifestations; mild buccal and gastric symptoms; constipated.
Severity.—A well-marked first attack of medium grade.
Experimental material.—Furnished urine and feces June 25, 1916.

Number 12

K–O.—White female, 9 years. Admitted to Spartanburg County Farm June 16, 1916. Service of Dr. O. W. Leonard.
Salient clinical features.—Extensive severe skin manifestations; marked diarrhea.
Severity.—A fatal first attack. Died August 25, 1916.
Experimental material.—Furnished urine and feces June 25, 1916.

Number 13

S–JE.—White male, 37 years. Admitted to Spartanburg County Farm June 10, 1916. Service of Dr. O. W. Leonard.
Salient clinical features.—Has a history of pellagra extending over six to seven years; mental manifestations winter 1915–16.
Presents well-marked eruption; marked buccal and severe intestinal symptoms (watery diarrhea).
Severity.—A chronic pellagra, fatal. Died August 1, 1916.
Experimental material.—Furnished feces June 25, 1916.

Number 14

J–M.—White female, 33 years. Out patient No. 43, United States Pellagra Hospital, Spartanburg, S.C. Came under observation June 19, 1916.
Salient clinical features.—Weak, tongue slightly red, constipated; moderately extensive, active eruption. History of attack in 1912 and 1915.
Severity.—Rated by Dr. Grimm as a moderately acute third recurrent attack.
Experimental material.—Furnished epidermal scales, urine, and feces June 25, 1916.

Number 15

H–V.—White female, 21 years. Admitted to United States Pellagra Hospital, Spartanburg, S.C., June 24, 1916. Hospital No. 212.
Salient clinical features.—Presents moderately extensive, acute skin mani-

festations; mild mental symptoms (apathetic, confused). History of a first attack in June, 1915.

Severity.—Dr. Grimm rates this as a moderately acute second attack.

Experimental material.—Furnished urine and feces June 25, 1916.

Number 16

S–S.—White female, 30 years. Admitted to United States Pellagra Hospital, Spartanburg, S.C., June 24, 1916.

Salient clinical features.—History of an attack, 1915, and of a recurrence in March, 1916, followed by improvement in April, but with retrogression during May and June. On admission felt weak, nervous, without nausea, but with burning and pain in stomach and with burning of feet. No other gastrointestinal manifestations. No eruption nor residuals of one.

Severity.—Mild second attack in posteruptive stage (or in interval) with mild suggestive symptoms.

Experimental material.—Furnished urine and feces June 25, 1916.

Number 17

Q–LV.—White female, 25 years. Admitted to United States Pellagra Hospital, Spartanburg, S.C., June 24, 1916. Hospital No. 216.

Salient clinical features.—Presents definite skin eruption and mild suggestive symptoms (nervousness, weakness).

Gives history of an attack in 1913 and of one in 1915.

Severity.—Rated by Dr. Grimm as a mild third recurrent attack.

Experimental material.—Furnished epidermal scales and urine June 25, 1916.

References

Goldberger, J. "Discussion of Some Phases of the Work of the Thompson Pellagra Commission," *J. Am. Med. Assn.,* Vol. 65 (December 11, 1915), pp. 2115–16.

———, "Pellagra: Causation and a Method of Prevention," *J. Am. Med. Assn.,* Vol. 66 (February 12, 1916), pp. 471–76.

———, and Wheeler, G. A. "Experimental Pellagra in the Human Subject," *Public Health Rep.* (Washington, D.C.), November 12, 1915.

Harris, W. A. "The Experimental Production of Pellagra in the Monkey," *J. Am. Med. Assn.,* Vol. 63 (September 26, 1914), pp. 1093–94.

Lavinder, C. H., Francis, E., etc. "Attempts to Transmit Pellagra to Monkeys," *J. Am. Med. Assn.,* Vol. 63 (September 26, 1914), pp. 1093–94.

Vedder, E. B. "Dietary Deficiency as the Etiological Factor in Pellagra," *Arch. Int. Med.* (Chicago), August, 1916.

Voegtlin, C. "Discussion of Summary of Second Progress Report of Thompson-McFadden Commission," *J. Am. Med. Assn.,* Vol. 63 (September 26, 1914), p. 1098.

PART THREE

Community Studies

7. The Prevalence of Pellagra. Its Possible Relation to the Rise in the Cost of Food[1]

EDGAR SYDENSTRICKER

Among the recent observations that have been made on the relation of diet to the incidence of pellagra is that in the diet of those developing the disease there is a disproportionately small amount of meat or other animal protein food and a disproportionately large amount of carbohydrates and fats. It has also been observed that the disease is chiefly prevalent in the South and is especially prevalent in mill communities, and that it is closely associated with the condition of poverty. Observation apparently tends to indicate a considerable increase in the prevalence of pellagra during the last seven or eight years.

Thus the possible relation of the incidence of pellagra to certain conditions of an economic character is at once suggested. The purpose of this paper is to present, in a brief and tentative manner, some of the more significant data available from investigations of economic conditions. It should be stated that the economic investigations were made and the collection of the data relating to diet that they furnished was done without any thought of their possible bearing on the question of the prevalence of any specific disease. It was only after these data were compiled that their possible significance in this connection was suggested. It should also be stated that the data summarized in the following pages refer to only some of the conditions that may be relevant, and that further examination of existing data and further investigation may contribute more definitely and completely to the determination of the possible relation of the incidence of pellagra to economic conditions. Assuming, however, that this relation does exist, it is believed that these preliminary statements of economic facts will suggest a partial answer to certain questions of interest at present in the discussion of the prevalence of the disease.

With these qualifications in mind, it is purposed to summarize

1 *Public Health Rep.*, Vol. 30, No. 43 (October 22, 1915), 3132–48.

briefly some conclusions afforded by industrial and budgetary investigations regarding:

1. The relation of the wageworker's family income to diet, with
certain data relating to wages and income of workingmen's families
in the South, and to the adequacy of wages and family income,
measured by the cost of living, of wage earners in the South as compared with wage earners in other sections of the United States.

2. Some factors affecting the availability of the food supply in
southern industrial localities.

3. Differences in the diet of workingmen's families in northern and
southern states.

4. Some factors having a possible effect on the diet of southern
wageworkers' families in recent years, including the source of the
recent labor supply in southern factories and mills and the urban
movement of population, changes in the character of the food supply, changes in the status of southern wage earners' families, and the
recent rise in the retail prices of foods.

Family income and diet.—It is of course apparent that the economic status of the wage earner's family, as indicated by its gross
annual income, bears a very direct relation to the character and the
sufficiency of its diet, but in order to state this relation in as definite
terms as possible it is pertinent to review the results of budgetary
studies affording data (1) as to the proportion of family income available for food expenditures, and (2) as to variations in diet of families
of different incomes.

Studies of the budgets of large numbers of families in the United
States have shown that the smaller the family income the larger is
the proportion of income spent for food and fuel. It also seems to be
established that the smaller the income the smaller is the proportion
spent for clothing, rent, and sundries. Expenditures for food were
found by the Federal Bureau of Labor's study of workingmen's
families in 1901, for example, to constitute only 36 per cent of total
family expenditures when the family income was $1,200 or more a
year, but to reach 46 per cent and over where the income was less
than $600. [Tabulation of per cent of expenditure for various pur-
poses deleted. ED.]

In other words, the smaller the family income, the smaller can be
the expenditures for housing, clothes, decencies, and comforts, in
order to provide food. The fact that progress in civilization is constantly raising the standard of decency and comfort, and creating
new wants and desires, renders the surrender or the lack of means of
obtaining them more and more difficult. Studies of budgets of newer

immigrant families from southern and southeastern Europe, who are accustomed to lower standards of living than American families, have shown that they spend a considerably larger proportion for food and less for other purposes than American families. The tendency is thus for an increasing pressure to be exerted upon the poorer American families to make every possible sacrifice in their diet. Inadequate family income means not only inadequate funds for providing a nutritious diet, but the bringing into play of other forces that tend to cause sacrifices in diet in order to satisfy in some degree other wants and desires.

The actual variations in the character of the food consumed by workingmen's families of different incomes, as they have been ascertained by important budgetary investigations in the United States by the British Board of Trade and in New York City by Prof. R. C. Chapin, illustrate this tendency and afford significant data on the relation of economic status to diet. These studies showed that the higher the family income the greater was the variety and, up to a certain limit of income, the greater the quantity consumed per capita. Without discussing in detail all of the specific variations, it may be said that the most important variation in the diet was a smaller consumption of milk, eggs, and meats in the lower ranges of income. The British Board of Trade's budgets of a large number of American white and British wage earners' families in the United States in 1909 showed that the average per capita consumption of milk was 30 per cent, of eggs 52 per cent, and of meat 33 per cent greater in families where the range of family income was between $19.50 and $25 than in families with less than $10 a week. [Tabulations, compiled from the British report, of average weekly consumption deleted. ED.]

Other differences were chiefly in variety, the tendency being toward a greater increase of baker's bread, cakes, breakfast cereals, coffee, cocoa, chocolate, and the like, as income increased. The conclusion is pointedly suggested, therefore, that the quantity of meat purchasable by poorer families was insufficient to satisfy the craving of the individual. If the natural appetite of the individual can be regarded as an index of his physical needs, then the conclusion is suggested that the meat prices prevailing at that time (1909) prevented this class of families from having a sufficient amount of this article of diet.

Wages and family income in the South.—It is a generally accepted fact that wages in the southern states are generally lower than in the northern or middle western states. In fact, every investigation involving a comparison has shown this to be true. The Federal Bureau of Labor's extensive cost of living study in 1901 secured data as to annual income of 25,440 families of representative workingmen in the principal industrial area of the United States, which showed that the average southern white workingman's family income was between $650 and $690, or approximately 10 per cent lower than in the northern states and 20 per cent lower than in the western states. These data were for all occupations and industries.

In some occupations and industries the difference is considerably greater. The same authority's later investigations found that iron and steel workers in the South were earning considerably lower wages than in other districts.[2] Similar conclusions for this industry were afforded by the industrial investigations of the Federal Immigration Commission.[3] Of greater interest here are the results of the Federal woman and child labor investigations of cotton-mill workers in New England and southern states. While slightly over half of the workers in New England mills were found to be earning under $7 a week, nearly nine-tenths of the southern mill workers were in that group.[4] [Tabulations deleted. ED.]

The average annual income of the southern cotton-mill family was found to be $822, as contrasted with $1,002 for New England cotton-mill families, the southern family income being 20 per cent lower.

The adequacy of wages and income as measured by prices in the South.—The real test of the adequacy of wages or income, however, is in its purchasing power as measured by prices of commodities ordinarily used by wageworkers' families. Using this test, the statement is warranted by all available data that the cost of living of wage earners in the South is not lower in the same proportion as wages or family income. In fact, there is evidence of the contrary. While workingmen's rents are approximately the same or slightly lower in the South than in the North, food prices in industrial localities are, as a general rule, higher in the South. The British Board of Trade's inquiry into the cost of living in American towns in 1909, for example, developed the fact that the food-price level in southern

2 *Report on Conditions of Employment in the Iron and Steel Industry in the United States,* Vol. III (1913), 223–28.
3 *Reports of the Immigration Commission,* Vol. 8 (1911), 70.
4 *Report on Condition of Women and Child Wage Earners in the United States,* Vol. I (1910), 305. Similar differences for workers in the cotton-goods industry in the United States were found by the Tariff Board in its examination of the pay rolls of northern and southern mills. See Cotton Manufactures, Message from the President of the United States transmitting the Report of the Tariff Board on Schedule I of the Tariff Law, Vol. II, House Doc. 643, 62d Cong., 2d sess. (1912), 653–58.

towns, weighted according to actual consumption in wage earners' families, was above the average of the rest of the country, the southern towns being from 2 to 9 per cent higher than New York City.[5]

Prices of the cheaper cuts of beef and of milk were in nearly every instance higher in southern towns than in the North. The conclusion indicated by the available evidence, and in accordance with the principles of family income and expenditure already referred to, are that the wage earner's family in the South is at a greater economic disadvantage than in the northern states, and that there is a greater pressure exerted in favor of sacrifices in diet in order to maintain an otherwise comfortable standard of living.

Food supply in southern industrial communities.—The availability of the supply of various kinds of foods in different sections of the country is another important factor in determining the character of the diet, especially the diet of those whose income is close to the margin of subsistence. To ascertain the full influence of this factor, more extensive and detailed studies of statistics of production, efficiency of food distribution, the prevalence of markets, stores, and other selling agencies, etc., than has been possible to make for these preliminary observations will be necessary. It may be tentatively stated, however, that food production, particularly of beef and several other important animal protein foods, has until recent years lagged behind and is still very far below that of the rest of the country, even when calculated on a per capita basis. The same situation has been observed in the distribution of foods. Lean meat, fresh or salt, for example, is not so generally sold in the southern industrial town and village as in similar localities in the North and Middle West, and where it is sold its prices, as already pointed out, are generally higher. For example, the Federal investigation of woman and child wage earners in 1907 and 1908 found that in over a third of the cotton-mill communities in the South there were stores operated directly or indirectly by the cotton-mill companies which were patronized almost exclusively by the workers. It was found that few company stores sold fresh meat even irregularly or infrequently, in spite of the fact that company stores were generally better stocked with all kinds of articles of ordinary consumption than the private stores in the same localities. Vegetable gardens in the southern mill

5 Cost of living in American towns, report of inquiry by Board of Trade of London (Board of Trade of Great Britain) into working-class rents, housing, and retail prices, with rates of wages in certain occupations in principal industrial towns of United States as presented to British Parliament. 1911. (S. Doc. 22, 62d Cong., 1st sess. Reprint of original edition, London, 1911.)

town and village were found to be over three times as prevalent as in New England mill communities. Except in distinctly rural communities, hogs, cows, and poultry were rarely kept by the cotton-mill families, the practice being discouraged in thickly settled localities.

Budgetary data showing differences in diet according to geographical divisions or sections.—How far each or all of these factors have contributed to the differences in diet that have been found to exist between families of wage earners in the South and in the North, and how far the differences are due to less tangible and measurable influences affecting habits of consumption, cannot be stated at this stage of our study. But the actual differences in diet are unquestioned facts and constitute a condition which is of special interest here. These differences, as determined by budgetary investigations of wage earners' families, may now be briefly stated.

The principal sources of data are the Federal Bureau of Labor's cost of living investigation in 1901, including 2,567 white working-men's families, and British Board of Trade's inquiry into the cost of living in American towns in 1909, including 1,036 white working-men's families. The data obtained by these two investigations are for both quantities and cost of foods and are generally comparable so far as the race and economic status of the families and conditions governing their diet are concerned. They are corroborated by other local budgetary studies.

These budgetary studies indicate marked differences in the diet of wage earners and their families in the northern and southern states. The consumption of lean meats and other protein foods is considerably greater in the North than in the South, and of hydrocarbons and carbohydrates is considerably greater in the South than in the North. For example, beef and milk are much more important articles of diet in the North, while salt hog products and lard are important in the South. The Bureau of Labor's data for 1901 showed that southern wage earner's families consumed over 25 per cent less protein foods, over 45 per cent more hydrocarbons, and over 10 per cent more carbohydrates. While data for the carbohydrate group included only bread, flour and meal, potatoes, sugar, and rice, and thus indicate rather the trend than the total actual consumption of articles of this food group, it is possible that statistics of total consumption would have indicated an even higher percentage in favor of the southern families. [Detailed statistics of quantities consumed in a year by families grouped according to geographical divisions deleted. ED.]

For the "meats and other proteins" group of foods the geographical differences in consumption are significant. In the northern states the average family was found to consume between 1,000 and 1,100 pounds of proteins, while in the southern states the protein consumption averaged between 700 and 800 pounds. The southern family consumed nearly a pound a week less of fresh beef, nearly half as much milk, very much less of "other meats," and hardly any salt beef, as compared with northern families. For the "fats and hydrocarbon" group of foods even more significant differences are shown. While families in northern states were found to consume larger quantities of butter, families in southern states consumed over 60 per cent more lard and nearly three times as much salt hog products. Some of the variations in specific foods are interesting, such as the large consumption of flour and meal in the southern states and of bakers' bread in the North Atlantic states.

The chief differences shown by the Bureau of Labor's 1901 budgets are corroborated by the British Board of Trade's inquiry of 1909.[6] The latter's data is for weekly instead of yearly consumption, and for northern and southern families alone. [Detailed tabulations of quantities consumed deleted. ED.]

The British inquiry was more detailed in its examination of family diet, the quantity purchased, and the cost of practically every article of food being taken into consideration. It furnishes more specific data as to the differences in diet of northern and southern workingmen's families than the Bureau of Labor investigation. The following may be set forth as some of the most significant differences:

1. The quantity of wheat bread and wheat flour consumed by southern families is considerably larger than by northern families. This is only very slightly balanced by the greater quantity of rolls and cakes consumed by the northern family. Taking flour and flour products of all kinds, the average northern family of this group consumed 22.46 pounds weekly as against 26.85 for the southern family. Southern families consume larger quantities of corn and corn meal, rice, and molasses and sirups than the northern families. This is true of families of all incomes.

2. The southern consumption of fats is very much larger than the northern. This is seen chiefly in the fact that the southern family of this group consumes twice as much bacon and ham and more than twice as much lard, suet, and dripping. Butter, oleomargarine, and

6 The data available for geographical comparison in the British inquiry is confined to American-British families; but it is in the main comparable to the Bureau of Labor's data, since the great bulk of nationalities included in both are native white, British and Canadian born.

olive oil are practically the same. Unfortunately, salt pork is not given separately in the budget; it is safe to say that this would show a considerable increase in the amount of fats consumed by southern families.

3. Contrasting sharply with the larger quantities of starches and fats consumed by the southern families is their low consumption of proteins as compared with northern families. With the exception of cheese, sausage, dried peas and beans, and condensed milk—all of which are comparatively unimportant so far as quantity actually consumed is concerned, and of which sausage may almost be said to belong to the fatty foods—the average northern family of this group consumes more proteins of all varieties. This is also true of all families considered in the British-American budgets. In instances where separate data is available for southern native whites, as distinguished from the other families composing the southern American-British group, it is seen that the tendency to consume small quantities of meats on the part of native-born families is further accentuated.

In this connection data obtained from typical budgets of southern cotton-mill workers' families are of interest, and the Federal report on woman and child wage earners, summarizing the dietary data for southern families, says:

> The menus which appear with the family studies show better than can any description the character of the food eaten by the cotton-mill operative. It will be seen that corn bread, biscuit, pork, and coffee form a large part of the diet of all families. No tea is used, but one family substituted Postum for coffee. When pork is mentioned without qualification it means "fat pork," which is fat pork dry salted. This kind of meat contains very little lean. Other kinds of pork are always specified, as ham, pork chops, or bacon. . . . No yeast bread is used. Corn bread or biscuit is used by all families. . . . One family had chicken twice and another had salt herring twice. In all other cities pork in some form was the only meat used. Unless the family owned a cow milk does not appear in the diet, not even for coffee.[7]

Recent economic factors affecting the diet of wage earners' families in the South.—With these marked differences in the diet of wage-earning families in the South as compared with similar families in other industrial areas of the United States, so unmistakably indicated by all of the available data, the question suggests itself, Has the situ-

7 *Report on Condition of Women and Child Wage Earners in the United States*, Vol. XVI. Family Budgets of Typical Cotton-Mill Workers, p. 23. The families studied were in Atlanta, Ga.; Greensboro, N. C.; and at a mill near Burlington, N.C.

ation shown any tendency toward a change in recent years? Or, if there has been a change, Has the situation been mitigated or intensified?

While it has been impossible in a preliminary survey of this phase of the subject to give detailed consideration to all of the possible factors that might affect the situation, at least four important factors should be mentioned. Those are: (1) The changes in diet of families in the South who, in response to the increased demand for white labor, have come from rural districts to live under urban conditions; (2) the trend of wages in the South as indicating possible changes in the economic status of wage earners' families; (3) the trend in the production of food; and (4) the advances in retail food prices.

The change from farm to mill town.—The increase in urban population as compared with the increase in total population, according to the Federal census, was greater in the southern states than in other sections of the United States during the last census decade. There has been a tremendous and an unprecedented movement from rural districts in the South. To a large degree this movement is composed of farmers and their families, or the children of farmers, who are relinquishing country life for life as workers in the rapidly developing factory and mill towns and villages. The average number of wage earners in the South increased 50.8 per cent in the 10 years from 1899 to 1909, the actual average number of wage earners in the South being over 380,000 greater in 1909 than in 1899.

The cotton-goods industry affords perhaps the best illustration of this movement. While the number of active producing spindles in the New England cotton mills increased only 19.7 per cent in the last census decade, it increased 139.9 per cent in the South Atlantic states. The increase in number of wage earners in cotton mills for the principal southern cotton-manufacturing states was as follows: North Carolina, 56 per cent; South Carolina, 50.5 per cent; Georgia, 52.1 per cent. Going back another decade, the number of spindles in southern cotton mills increased from 1,600,000 in 1889 to nearly 10,400,000 in 1909. "This enormous increase," said the Federal report on the condition of woman and child wage earners in 1910, "created a tremendous demand for white labor, which has been supplied almost entirely by the farms of the South. The Negro population has contributed little to this industrial development, as Negroes are employed only as general labor about cotton mills and occasionally for the heavy work in the picker and opening rooms."[8] It

8 *Ibid.*, Vol. I, p. 119.

was found in the same investigation that the percentage of operatives coming from mountain sections was very much smaller than
those from farms surrounding the cotton-mill villages, and that the
so-called "mountaineer" element in the mills was slight.[9]

Hence the transition was from the farm to the industrial village
and town. It was found that in the southern states over 75 per cent
of a large number of representative operatives had spent their childhood on farms, less than 21 per cent in villages, and only 4 per cent
in cities. In New England mills it was found that only 27.3 per cent
of the operatives had spent their childhood on farms, but that over
44 per cent had been reared in cities and about 20 per cent in villages, the last named being principally the children of cotton-mill
operatives who had moved from farms to cotton-mill communities.

The exact dietary effects of this change from farm to industrial
communities cannot be stated, of course, until intensive comparisons can be made of the diet of the farm population in the sections
from which the exodus has taken place with the diet of industrial
wage workers. General observation suggests that the rural population has a better balanced diet than that indicated by the results of
budgetary investigations of southern workingmen's families, particularly in the purely industrial localities.

*The present trend of wages and of income of wage earners' families
in the South.*—While there has been a gradual increase in the rates of
wages in the principal industries in the South during the last 10 or
12 years, the wage level continues to be lower, certainly in similar
industries, in the South than in the North. For example, the wage
statistics of the Federal Bureau of Labor Statistics show that there
has been an increase in the rates of wages of South Carolina cotton-
mill workers of less than 5 per cent during the five-year period 1907–
1912, while wages of lumber-mill workers in the southern states
remained practically stationary. In the years of acute industrial depression, 1908 and 1909, there was an actual decrease in the rates
of wages in cotton mills, and the level of 1907 was not again reached
until 1911. A more marked drop in wage rates occurred in the lumber
mills, and decreases were also shown in wood and furniture manufactures.

The collection and compilation of wage statistics for the South
covering the period from 1900 to the present time have not pro-
ceeded far enough to enable a presentation of them here in proper
form, but it may be stated that these statistics indicate what general

9 *Ibid.*, p. 120.

and familiar observation has shown—that the recent industrial depression caused wage workers and their families in the principal
southern industries to be placed at a very serious economic disadvantage. Not only were the rates of wages lower in some instances,
but the opportunity for earning wages was greatly lessened by the
closing down and curtailment of mills and factories. This meant that
the annual incomes of a very large proportion of the workingmen's
families were considerably reduced, as well as rendered extremely
uncertain and irregular, because of unemployment and irregular
employment. This depression began in the latter part of 1907 and
has continued with varying intensity until the present. The significance of this condition, so far as the diet of wage earners and their
families is concerned, is, of course, apparent in the light of the principles underlying the relation of family income to diet. It will be
seen to possess additional significance when certain facts relating to
the availability of the food supply and the retail prices of food are
considered.

The trend in the availability of the food supply in the South.—
While methods of food distribution in the South have improved with
the development of urban communities in that section, and thus an
apparent advantage has resulted in the better facilities for supplying
all kinds of foods in the average locality, a serious question may be
raised as to whether this advantage is not offset by certain disadvantageous factors affecting the food supply. Without attempting to
make exact statements of their effects on the diet of wage earners'
families in the South, it may be pertinent to suggest some of these
disadvantageous factors.

Although the movement for crop diversification and beef and
milk production in the South has been begun, the trend of actual
food production has not yet been such as to improve materially the
balance in the southern wage earner's diet. The familiar statistics of
the decline in beef production in the United States show that the per
capita production in 1900 was 211 pounds and only about 160 in
1914. The per capita meat consumption fell, in the three years from
1909 to 1912, according to the Federal Bureau of Animal Industry,
from 162 to 152 pounds. The beef supply in southern urban and
industrial centers continues to be chiefly, if not altogether, furnished
by other sections of the country. It has not yet been aided very
materially by increased beef production in the South itself. Without
stating the figures in detail, the census statistics show that population growth in the South during the last decade has been at a more
rapid rate than the increase in the number of cattle, poultry, and

swine, and has only about kept pace with the increase in the number of dairy cattle and the production of eggs.

It is probable that these disadvantageous factors have been augmented by other conditions of a local nature, such as the enactment of "no-fence" laws and the tendency, which was noted in southern mill towns by investigators of the Federal Bureau of Labor in 1907 and 1908, toward prohibiting the keeping of dairy cows as a part of stricter sanitary regulations. It is obvious that both of these conditions would affect the poorer families the most.

The increase in retail prices of foods.—Regardless, however, of the possible results of conditions affecting the availability of a well-balanced food supply, the extent to which the available food supply is actually utilized and a properly balanced diet is actually maintained is determined not so much by the actual presence of such a supply in local markets as by the financial ability of the wage earner and his family to purchase it. This is a matter not only of the size of the family income, but also of retail prices of food. We must therefore regard the increase in food prices as probably the most important of all of the factors affecting the diet of the wageworking population, especially of those whose economic status is close to the margin of subsistence.

If we remember that wages advanced in the period 1900–1913 only about 25 per cent, and probably at a slower rate in the South, particularly of cotton and lumber-mill workers, and that there was a serious industrial depression from 1907 until almost the present time, which was possibly more marked in the South than in other sections, the significance of a rise in the retail prices of foods of over 60 per cent must be at once apparent. It is of peculiar interest to note that the increase in food prices in the South Atlantic states during the six years 1908–1913 was about 50 per cent greater than in the seven years, 1901–1907, and even more pronounced in the South Central states.[10] Not only must a larger proportion of family income have been necessary for food in order to maintain an adequate diet, but unless family income kept pace with food prices there must have been a greater number of families whose incomes were insufficient to provide an adequate diet. This pressure of subsistence upon income has been greatest since about 1908.

There are, however, more specific reasons for believing that the increase in retail food prices has been particularly severe on working-men's families in the South. Since the Federal Bureau of Labor's cost of living investigation in 1901 is used as the basis for weighting price

10 U. S. Bureau of Labor Statistics: Retail Prices 1890–1913, Bull. 140, p. 11.

index figures, that year instead of 1900 will be used here for comparison with 1913 (the latest year for which continuous index figures are
at present available), although the increase in prices will be thus
arbitrarily curtailed by nearly 10 per cent.

1. The retail prices of foods show approximately a 5 per cent
greater increase in the South Atlantic states than in the North
Atlantic states and approximately a 10 per cent greater increase in
the South Central states than in the North Central states. The general percentage of increase for the southern states was greater than
for the northern or western states. [Tabulation of statistics deleted.
ED.]

The southern wageworker's family has been placed at a somewhat
greater economic disadvantage by the advance in retail prices of
foods than the wageworker's family in the North or in the West.

To illustrate the effect of such an increase of food prices upon
family income, the approximate cost of a year's food supply, based
on actual consumption as determined by the Bureau of Labor's cost
of living investigation, for 1900 and 1913, may be compared. In
order to maintain the same diet in 1913 as in 1900, the average workingman's family in the South Atlantic states, for example, would
have had to spend $155 more a year, and in the South Central states
$192 more a year. Since wages have not increased in proportion, it is
impossible to assume that this diet has been maintained. Comparing
1913 with 1907, thus including a period in which wages of cotton-mill
workers in South Carolina (for instance) advanced less than 5 per
cent and in which an industrial depression occurred, the wageworker's family would have had to spend $75 more a year in 1913 than
in 1907, or an increase of nearly 20 per cent. Sacrifices in variety,
quality, and quantity must have been necessary as the result of the
increased cost of food, since it has been found in the course of industrial investigations in 1901 that fully half of the workingmen's families were already living on a very close margin of subsistence.

2. What have been these sacrifices in diet that increased food prices
have necessitated? A partial answer is to be found in the statistics of
increases in prices of specific articles of diet, since the natural tendency is toward the substitution of the cheaper for the more expensive
foods.

The Bureau of Labor Statistics' index figures for 15 principal articles consumed by workingmen's families, on the basis of the 1901
investigation, are given in the table p. 126, for 1901 and 1913
in order to exhibit the relative increase or decrease in the 12 years.

These statistics indicate that there were wide variations in the rate
of price increase of the different articles of food. It is important to

Relative prices of the principal articles of food consumed by workingmen's families in 1901 and 1913.*

(Average price for 1890–1899 = 100.)

Article of food.	1901	1913	Relative increase.
Sirloin steak..........	109.4	171.3	61.9
Round steak............	114.0	199.5	85.5
Rib roast..............	112.7	172.0	59.3
Pork chops.............	119.0	213.8	94.8
Bacon, smoked..........	121.3	225.9	104.5
Ham, smoked............	111.1	181.2	70.1
Lard, pure.............	119.6	166.6	47.0
Hens..................	105.0	171.8	66.8
Flour, wheat...........	94.9	128.4	33.5
Corn meal..............	107.6	160.4	52.8
Eggs, fresh............	107.7	174.8	67.1
Butter, creamery.......	103.0	153.2	46.2
Potatoes, Irish........	114.0	151.2	37.2
Sugar, granulated......	102.1	95.3	6.8[+]
Milk, fresh............	101.4	140.2	38.8

*The foregoing list is illustrative more of the kinds of food constituting the diet of the average working-man's family in 1901 than in 1913, as will easily be seen. Since January, 1912, the bureau has added cold storage eggs and chuck steak to the list. But the foods included in the above list fairly indicate the rise in the prices of the principal varieties of food, although they do not, of course, compose as great a proportion of the workingman's diet now as they did in 1901.
[+]Decrease.

note that the greatest increases have been in the prices of meats, including poultry and eggs, and that the smallest increases have been in the prices of vegetables and cereals. Unfortunately, salt pork, which is so important an article of diet in southern workingmen's families, is not included in the Bureau of Labor Statistics' list, but unofficial statistics indicate that the price of this article of diet has increased only 25 or 30 per cent as compared with percentages for lean fresh meats of from 60 to 100 per cent. But even excluding this item from consideration, and grouping the bureau's list in the three classes—proteins, starches, and fats (including smoked ham and bacon as fats)—we have an average percentage of price increase from 1901 to 1913 as follows:

Proteins	61
Hydrocarbons	38
Carbohydrates	37

The meats and other protein foods have thus increased about 40 per cent more than the other two groups, and very probably at more than that rate as compared with the hydrocarbon group had salt pork been included.

It seems to be clearly shown from available statistics that the trend of food prices has been to intensify the maladjustments in the diet of southern wageworkers' families. Comparisons of actual budgets of wageworkers' families in 1901 with budgets in later years, so far as comparisons are possible, tend to corroborate this conclusion.

Conclusions.—A preliminary review of some of the more important data relating to the diet of workingmen's families afforded in the results of industrial and budgetary investigations appears to point to the following conclusions:

1. The lower the economic status of the white American family, the greater is the pressure for sacrifices in diet, particularly in animal protein foods, since animal protein foods are the most expensive.

2. The economic status of wage earners' families in the southern states, particularly of cotton-mill families, is lower than that of wage-earners' families in other sections of the country.

3. Certain factors have tended to restrict the supply of protein foods in southern industrial localities that do not restrict, at least to the same extent, the supply of carbohydrates and hydrocarbons.

4. Budgetary studies of a large number of native white wage earners' families, generally comparable as to annual family income and size, indicate that the proportion of proteins in the diet of southern families is considerably less and of carbohydrates and of hydrocarbons considerably greater than in the diet of northern families.

5. Certain factors have tended to intensify this condition in recent years, particularly since the industrial depression began in the latter part of 1907. While the supply of a better-balanced diet in southern industrial localities has apparently not been improved materially, the economic status of wage earners' families, especially in the cotton goods and lumber industries, has been lowered, and retail prices of foods have greatly increased, this increase being more pronounced, particularly since 1907, than in other sections of the country. The increase in retail food prices has been at least 40 per cent higher in proteins than in carbohydrates or in hydrocarbons.

The available data thus point to a lessened financial ability of southern wage earners' families to provide a properly balanced diet, as well as a decrease in the availability (measured by retail prices) of an animal protein food supply for the wageworking population, particularly since about 1907 or 1908.

8. A Study of the Relation of Diet to Pellagra Incidence in Seven Textile-Mill Communities of South Carolina in 1916[1]

JOSEPH GOLDBERGER
G. A. WHEELER
EDGAR SYDENSTRICKER

Introduction

From the earliest history of pellagra a more or less important rôle has been assigned to diet in its relation to the disease. This has been forcibly expressed by Lavinder (1915): "Ever since Casal's day students are convinced that pellagra is associated with a poor diet, and volumes of research and arguments have been offered on the subject. The Italians have done little more, Roussel somewhat sarcastically observed many years ago, than to ring changes on Casal's views. Yet they and all others must continue to study the relations between poor food and pellagra. For, among all the complexities and discordant things that surround this disease, this is the one outstanding *fact* [italics in original] that most urgently needs explanation."

It was fundamentally with the view of finding the explanation of this *fact*, current theories being unacceptable, that a series of investigations of pellagra was begun in the spring of 1914 under the direction of one of the present writers (J. G.).

In a paper published June 26, 1914, Goldberger called attention to the significance of certain epidemiological observations which showed that at some institutions at which pellagra was either epidemic or had long been endemic among the inmates, the nurses and attendants, though drawn from the class economically identical with that most affected in the population at large, appeared uniformly to be immune, although living in the same environment and under the same conditions as did the inmates, and many of them also in frequent and intimate contact with cases of the disease. Neither contact nor insect transmission seemed capable of explaining this remarkable exemption of one of the two classes of residents. The suggestion was made that the explanation was to be found in a difference in the diet

1 *Public Health Rep.*, Vol. 35, No. 12 (March 19, 1920), pp. 648–713.

of the two groups, for it was observed that although the nurses and attendants appeared to receive exactly the same food as did the inmates, there was, nevertheless, a difference in the diet of the two groups, in that the nurses and attendants, being in a favorable position to choose from what was provided, selected the best for themselves. They were also free to supplement the institution diet in any manner they pleased. Furthermore, from a study of the dietaries of certain institutions in which pellagra prevailed, the impression was gained that cereals and vegetables formed a much greater proportion in these than they did in the dietaries of well-to-do people, that is, people who, as a class, are practically exempt from pellagra. Accordingly, the tentative suggestion was made that the prevention of the disease be attempted by improving the dietary of those among whom it is most prevalent by reducing the cereal and vegetable component and increasing the fresh animal foods (fresh meats, eggs, and milk) of the ration.

The indications on which this suggestion was based were strikingly confirmed by other findings. Preliminary to an experimental test of the preventability of the disease by diet (Goldberger, Waring, and Willets, 1915; Goldberger, 1916) at an orphanage at Jackson, Miss., a study of the epidemiology of the disease was made at this institution and the singular fact was quickly discovered that the disease was practically exclusively confined to those between 6 and 12 years of age. After a detailed inquiry the only significant difference that suggested itself as an explanation of the exemption of a considerable group of inmates under 6 years and of another over 12 years of age was a difference in the diet. In the diet of the affected group as contrasted with that of the exempt groups, there was noted a disproportionately small amount of lean meat or other animal protein food. Subsequent inquiry at other institutions developed analogous conditions, and, as a whole, in the light of the then recent advances in our knowledge of beriberi, these findings strongly suggested the idea that the disease was dependent for its development on a diet that was for some reason faulty, and that this fault was in some way either prevented or corrected by including in the diet larger proportions of the fresh animal protein foods.

The indications for a possible method of prevention thus confirmed and more clearly defined, were put to a practical test at two orphanages and at an asylum for the insane. At orphanages "M. J." and "B. J.," for several years endemic foci of pellagra, the diet was modified in September, 1914, leaving hygienic and sanitary conditions unchanged. Following the change in diet, no recognizable evidence of a recurrence of the disease was observed at orphanage "M. J." in any of the pellagrins of 1914, 67 of whom remained under observation at least until the anniversary date of their attack. Nor were any new cases observed among the nonpellagrin residents of 1914, 99 of whom remained under observation for not less than a year. At orphanage "B. J.," subsequent to the change in diet, but a single case of a recurrence was observed among the pellagrins of 1914, 105 of whom remained under observation at least until the anniversary date of their attack. At the same time, not a single new case was observed among the nonpellagrin residents, 69 of whom remained under observation for not less than one year.

At the Georgia State Asylum, an endemic focus of the disease, the diet of two wards of pellagrins was modified—one in October and the other in December, 1914—leaving unchanged hygienic and sanitary conditions and the institution routine. Following this change in diet and up to October 1, 1915, the end of the period for which the report was made,[2] no recognizable evidence of a recurrence in any of the pellagrins in these wards was observed, although 72 (36 colored and 36 white females) remained continuously under observation throughout this period, or at least until the completion of the anniversary date of their 1914 attacks. Whereas during the corresponding period not less than 15 (47 per cent) of 32 control female pellagrins presented definite recurrences. This experiment clearly showed that pellagra may be prevented by an appropriate diet without appreciable alteration in the environment, hygienic or sanitary.

While the experiments designed to test the preventability of the disease by suitable additions to the diet were under way, another experiment was carried out to test the possibility of producing pellagra by means of a presumably faulty diet in which the foods which, for the reasons stated, might be assumed to have preventive or corrective power, were at a minimum. This experiment was carried out on convict volunteers at the Mississippi State Penitentiary Farm, near Jackson, Miss., between February 4 and November 1, 1915 (Goldberger and Wheeler, 1915; Goldberger, 1916; Goldberger and Wheeler, 1920). Of 11 men subsisting on a diet consisting of maize, wheat, rice, and pork fat with sweet potatoes, sugar, and some green vegetables, not less than 6 developed clearly marked evidence of pellagra at the end of 5½ to 6 months; while of a large number of controls living under poorer hygienic conditions and working harder,

---

2 These orphanage and asylum studies were continued to the end of 1916 and 1918, respectively, with results that coincided with those of the first year.

but subsisting on a different diet, none showed any evidence of the disease.

Thus, the results attained by the end of 1915 clearly showed the controlling influence of diet in both the prevention and the causation of the disease.[3] Accordingly, with the view of developing as broad a basis as possible for the eventual formulation of practical measures of control, it was planned during the winter of 1915–16 to supplement these (in part epidemiologic, but chiefly experimental) investigations by a study, in different types of industrial and rural communities, of the relation of factors of a dietary, sanitary, and economic character to the incidence of the disease.

For various reasons it was decided to begin with a study of conditions in cotton-mill villages, these villages representing one of the types of communities in which pellagra was believed to be more than ordinarily prevalent. The study was begun in the spring of 1916 and is still in progress. At this time we desire to report the results of the first year's work with respect to the relation of household diet to the incidence of pellagra. Some of these results have already been presented in a previous paper (Goldberger, Wheeler, and Sydenstricker, 1918).

Review of the Studies of Other Workers

Before going on with an account of our work, it seems desirable to review the studies of other workers in this field. An examination of the literature bearing on the relation of diet to pellagra would involve practically all of the very voluminous literature of the disease and would be beyond the scope of the present paper. We propose to confine ourselves, therefore, to a consideration of those recent studies which may be regarded as in some sense comparable to our own, particularly as it is planned to consider the etiology of the disease in a separate paper subsequent to the publication of the results of the series of studies of which the present is a part.

To Grimm (1913) would seem to belong the credit of the first attempt at a modern, comprehensive, unbiased, epidemiological study of pellagra. This study was carried out during the summers of 1911 and 1912 in various localities in Kentucky, South Carolina, and Georgia. The method followed was to visit pellagrous communities and interview health officers and physicians, and with their assistance data were collected by interviewing pellagrins, securing reports of

3 During 1916, Goldberger attempted without success to transmit the disease by a series of inoculations in human volunteers, with blood, naso-pharyngeal secretions, feces, urine, and desquamating epithelium.

cases and deaths and reports of facts and conditions pertaining to the disease.

Grimm reports that upward of 200 physicians were interviewed and information relating to a total of 1,426 cases was obtained. He himself visited 290 pellagrous houses and personally interviewed 323 pellagrins. He found that the collection of accurate and detailed data on the subject of food used by pellagrins previous to the onset of the disease presented insurmountable difficulties. The systematic collection of information concerning the items of food most commonly used, kinds, sources, quantity, and quality had to be abandoned, as it was found that this information could be obtained in too few instances. "In many cases it was impossible to get even a meager account of what had been eaten, as the memory and powers of observation of these people seemed extremely defective when the character of their diet was inquired into. . . ." The character of the data secured did not, in Dr. Grimm's opinion, warrant any conclusions. So far as his observations went, however, no constant difference was found to have existed between the diets of the pellagrous and the non-pellagrous members of the families. In the closing remarks of the report of this pioneer investigation, Grimm states that from his observations "the relationship between food and pellagra seems to be a real one," but gives no indication of the evidence on which this opinion is based.

In June, 1912, a commission (Thompson-McFadden), consisting of J. F. Siler, P. E. Garrison, and W. J. MacNeal, began an elaborately planned study in South Carolina, which has resulted in adding materially to our knowledge of the disease. We shall, in the present connection, concern ourselves only with the part of their investigations dealing with diet.

The study of the first year (Siler and Garrison, July, 1913), extending from June 1 to October 15, 1912, carried out in Spartanburg County, S. C., was of a preliminary character. Their data were based on information obtained from statements of patients, physicians, storekeepers, millers, and others. "In order to determine the relative frequency with which the more important foodstuffs were used, patients and their families were closely questioned as to how often certain articles of food would appear on the family table, and with regard to the patient's particular fondness for any particular dish." This information was of a general nature and dealt with the habitual dietary of pellagrins and their families. The tabulated data submitted by them for the year studied represent, it would seem, the habitual dietary of the pellagrins occurring in three groups of the population of the county studied, namely, mill village, urban, and rural. Among the foods considered, it is interesting to note the finding that fresh beef was not a staple article of diet of any of these groups during the summer months. On the other hand, they report that fresh fowl was used quite extensively during the summer months in all three groups. The actual percentages of those using fowl, either daily or habitually, are reported to have been as follows: Urban cases, 66 per cent; rural cases, 65 per cent; and mill village cases, 41 per cent. With respect to milk, it is reported that 72 per cent of the mill village cases, 67 per cent of the rural cases, and 54 per cent of the urban cases used this food either daily or habitually. The interesting observation is also recorded that, in the locality studied, in contrast to northern Italy, wheat flour is the principal breadstuff.

Summarizing the results of this study, the commission states that "observations upon the habitual use of the more common foodstuffs failed to discover any points of difference between pellagrins and nonpellagrins in the county." It does not appear, however, that the data presented relate to any but pellagrins, and so it is not clear on what this statement is based. They state further (Siler, Garrison, MacNeal, Jan. 3, 1914) that careful consideration was given to the possible relation of an insufficient diet to the occurrence of pellagra, and that they are inclined to ascribe considerable importance to it, not as the sole or essential cause of pellagra, but as a predisposing factor. They state that the foods rich in animal protein, namely, meat, milk, and eggs, although apparently used in abundance by a few individual pellagrins in their series were, nevertheless, conspicuous by their deficiency in many of the cases.

In evaluating the significance of this study one will have to take into consideration (1) the very general character of the data which apparently related only to the diet of pellagrins, and (2) the absence of any evidence of appreciation of the importance of the seasonal factor in relating diet to the incidence of the disease.

This study was continued by the commission during 1913, when they undertook "a careful investigation of the dietary habits, not only of pellagrins and their families, but also of all the remaining population of the same class living under the same conditions, in certain selected industrial communities." Data were secured for each family by personal interview with a member of the family. The investigators recorded the diet served in the family as a whole, and each member of the household was considered as belonging to the dietary group of his family. In obtaining the data, a record was made of the frequency of use in the family of various foods, recognizing

7 classes of frequency: "First, daily use, which is self-explanatory;
second, habitual use, meaning as often as twice a week on the average; third, part time daily, which means daily use during certain
seasons of the year; fourth, part time, habitually, or habitual use
during certain seasons; fifth, rarely, which means used less frequently
than twice a week; sixth, part time rarely, and, seventh, never."

In analyzing these data the population as represented first by the
family as the unit and then by the individual as the unit was divided
into several groups distinguished from each other by the frequency
with which the particular food was used in the family, and then the
relative number of cases of pellagra in the different groups was compared. As the data related to family and not to the individual use
of various foods, the analyses, using the individual as a unit, do not
seem to us to have been permissible as involving danger of a confusion of ideas, of which, indeed, there is repeated evidence throughout the report of this interesting study. Thus, in discussing the
relationship of the frequency of use of fresh meat to pellagra they
state that "in the total population of the six villages the pellagra
morbidity is actually highest in the group of 82 persons who used
fresh meat daily," when all that could properly have been meant was
that the morbidity was highest in the group *of households* (composed
of 82 persons) who used fresh meat daily.

They analyzed their data in relation to corn meal, fresh meat,
canned goods, milk, and eggs, and state that they found that the
theory that pellagra is caused by the excessive use of corn meal, or
that it is caused by a deficiency of fresh meat in the diet, was not
supported. On the contrary, it appeared to them quite certain that
in the population studied, *those avoiding fresh meat contracted this
disease the least.* ([Italics are ours.] It is interesting to note in this
connection that they state the lowest morbidity from pellagra was
observed by them in the two of the six villages in which the local
market sold fresh meat throughout the year.) Similarly, the frequent,
even daily use of fresh eggs afforded no relative protection from pellagra. With respect to canned goods they state that their study failed
to discover any evidence that the use of canned goods causes pellagra.
From the analyses presented on the use of milk it seemed to them
"evident that in the whole population those persons using milk daily
contracted pellagra the least." "In every one of the six villages
[studied], the group using milk daily showed a lower incidence than
the average for that village, and the group never using milk showed
a higher incidence than the average. The correlation is quite inconsistent in the groups using milk habitually and rarely. The tendency

toward correlation between the occurrence of new cases of pellagra and the deficiency of milk in the diet is nevertheless distinctly evident, on the whole, and suggests that the use of milk (including buttermilk) as a food has some value in the prevention of pellagra." Summarizing this study, the commission states (Siler, Garrison, MacNeal, Sept. 26, 1914) that a "house-to-house canvass of the homes of over 5,000 people living in six endemic foci of pellagra failed to disclose any definite relation of the disease to any element of the dietary."

In evaluating the significance of this, as of their preliminary investigation, account must be taken of the fact (1) that the data are again of a very general character; (2) that there is no evidence of appreciation on the part of these workers of the importance of the seasonal factor in relating diet to the incidence of the disease; (3) that the data relate to family, not to individual use of foods; (4) that the term "pellagrin" is not defined, leaving one in doubt whether, in some of their analyses, this includes only active cases or whether, as seems not improbable, it also includes some quiescent cases; and (5) that an error, the magnitude of which it is impossible to estimate from the data published, probably entered as the result of the relative incompleteness, for the purpose of such study, of the pellagra incidence data that is certain to arise unless cases are systematically and continuously sought for by personal canvass (see also criticism by Vedder, 1916, p. 152). Finally, some account should perhaps also be taken of their methods of statistical interpretation, best illustrated in connection with the analysis relating to the use of milk. Here, in considering the distribution of families according to the frequency of use of this food, they point out (Siler, Garrison, MacNeal, Sept., 1914, p. 357) that the groups using milk "habitually, rarely, and never" were well represented, and that the percentage table suggests "that pellagra was, on the whole, somewhat less common in families using milk daily."

The table they cite actually shows that the rate of incidence for those families using milk rarely (13.6 per cent) was practically identical with those using it daily (13.5 per cent), and was therefore much lower than those using it habitually (22.5 per cent), the rate for the latter group being but little below that for the group using it never. This would seem to indicate that if the table under discussion suggests anything, it suggests that pellagra was, on the whole, somewhat less common in families using milk daily and rarely than in those using it habitually, etc., a paradox which would seem to point quite clearly to the need of extreme reserve in attaching significance to such indications if, indeed, any significance whatever can be attached to them.

A consideration of the relation of pellagra to diet was included in a study by Jobling and Petersen (1916 and 1917) of the epidemiology of the disease in Nashville, Tenn., during 1915 and 1916. During the first year's work, which was commenced August 1, 1915, "inquiries were made of the patients and of their friends as to whether there had been any definite change in the general character of food consumed during the two years previous to the onset of the disease, and whether there had been times during this period when they had not had sufficient food." Of 320 white people, 14.4 per cent, and of 101 colored, 11.8 per cent are reported to have stated that there had been times during the two years preceding their first attack when they had not had sufficient food. These statements, it is pointed out, had reference to a deficiency of all foods, not of any particular constituent. In only five instances, they report, were they able to obtain information that there had been a definite change in diet for the worse during the two years previous to the onset of the disease. In the remaining instance the patients and their friends are reported to have asserted that the food consumed had been the same or better in both quality and quantity than they had been accustomed to previously.

With reference to protein, Jobling and Petersen state that of the 421 patients considered, 66.8 per cent gave histories which indicated that they had been getting considerably more than 40 grams a day. They refer to the possibility that the deficiency in protein may be in quality, not in quantity. This, they state, was possible in certain cases; but in the majority of the patients they considered the diet sufficiently varied to make it improbable.

In discussing the results of their study they state that "the inhabitants of the South consume excessive amounts of carbohydrates, and fats," but no data on which this statement is founded are presented. In considering the theory of a vitamin deficiency advanced by Funk, and his suggestion that the disease might be prevented by the addition of vitamin-containing substances, such as potatoes, milk, butter, fruit, etc., they state that people in their section eat a great deal of potatoes, fruits, and other green foods, both cooked and raw, during the spring and summer. "It seems strange," they remark, "if this theory is correct, that pellagra should be rare in winter when green foods are scarce, and so frequent in the spring and summer when green foods and fruits are plentiful and cheap." It is evident that these workers have overlooked the significance of the strikingly similar seasonal behavior of endemic scurvy in relation to the avail-ability of green foods and fruits—known preventives of the disease.

In weighing the significance of this study it will be noted (1) that the dietary data are of a most general character, and (2) that, seem-ingly, it is the judgment of the pellagrin, or that of his family, with respect to the pellagrin's diet, that constitutes the basic data, rather than quantitative statements or actual records of food supplies or of food consumption for a specific period or season of the year.

The second year's study was an amplification of the first. Appar-ently the method of inquiry of the patient or of his family with respect to the pellagrin's diet was continued. In the second year's study it is stated that the pellagrins fell into two groups: One with active symptoms, acute skin changes, etc., "and one with chronic symptoms, in which the characteristic atrophy of the skin of the hands or feet, with occasional diarrhea, or in which evidence of degenerative changes in the central nervous system are apparent, cases in which the disease process is more or less quiescent." In a certain number of cases, constituting in effect a third group, this information, it is stated, was not clearly obtained. Of the white cases, 42 per cent of the males and 33 per cent of the females are reported to have had active lesions, and 47 per cent of the males and 60 per cent of the females were classed as "more or less quiescent" cases. Their examiners, "from questions and observations, reported that a deficiency in quantity probably existed in 15 per cent of the whites and in 28 per cent of the colored cases." Of 576 white pellagrins "90 per cent positively denied any deterioration in either the quan-tity or quality of the diet in the years immediately preceding the first attack (which seemingly may have been several years before the date of the survey), and only 18 per cent of the colored cases had changed their diet in a manner that would indicate a lowering of its value."

Furthermore, "in order to obtain an accurate idea of the balancing of the diet" statements were obtained "as to the variety of the foods consumed, their quantity, and an average daily menu." "In this way" they are able, they state, "to approximate in a fairly satisfactory way the food value and the quality." How the quantity of the food consumed was actually determined is not described, but would seem to have been by the simple statement of the patient or of a member of the family. What period this statement of food consumption covered or the average daily menu represented, is likewise not en-tirely clear; presumably it was either (1) for "the years immediately preceding the first attack" (which, in some instances, must have been several years anterior to the date of the survey), or (2) for the current period at the time of the survey. In either event the assumption of accuracy in such data would imply, in view of Grimm's experience, unusual powers of observation and surprisingly good memories in these people; furthermore, if these were statements of current consumption, approximately 50 per cent of the menus were those of "more or less quiescent" cases—cases, that is, that from the point of view of diet may be considered as possibly subsisting on a diet favoring convalescence or recovery from the disease (see also p. 142).

A classification of pellagrins on the basis of certain diets designated as high, medium, and low protein, and one on the basis of "partaking regularly" of certain protein foods, namely, eggs, meat, milk, and legumes, are given. No definition of the phrase, "partaking regularly" is presented. From the chart in which the latter analyses are presented it would seem that between 40 and 50 per cent of the white female pellagrins and between about 25 and 45 per cent of the white male pellagrins claimed to have partaken regularly of milk. Of meat, apparently some 40 to 50 per cent of white female pellagrins and some 40 to 60 per cent of the white male pellagrins claimed to have partaken regularly; while of the colored pellagrins some 35 to 65 per cent of the females and 50 to 70 per cent of the males claimed to have partaken regularly of this food.

In estimating the significance of the reported results of this study, note will be taken of the facts (1) that the data are of a very general character, apparently uncontrolled statements of patients or friends covering an undefined period of the "years" immediately preceding the first attack, which itself may have occurred several years before the date of the survey, and (2) that the statements of the quantity of the foods consumed appear to have been made from memory by the patient or member of the family represented, and it would seem, represented either an undefined period preceding the first attack (in some instances, a year or more anterior to the date of the survey) or an undefined current period at the time of the survey; in the latter event approximately 50 per cent of the menus would represent the diet of more or less quiescent (conceivably convalescent or recovered) cases.

In closing our review of these interesting studies it may be worth noting that in all of them the primary purpose seems to have been the discovery of the cause of the disease; in contrast, our own investigations have, from the outset in the spring of 1914, had as their immediate objective the determination of some method of prevention and control. Such light as we have been able to throw on the question of etiology has been, in the main, incidental. This mode of attack appeared to us preferable because of a number of considerations, chief among which were (1) the lack of conclusiveness of all previous studies and (2) the promise of practically very valuable results by an indirect mode of attack, suggested by the many striking epidemiologic analogies to endemic scurvy and beriberi for which, it will be recalled, methods of prevention and control were developed long before their etiology was determined.

Plan and Methods of Present Study

In planning the study, with one phase of which the present communication deals, it was our purpose to make as accurate observations as possible relating to the diet, the economic conditions, and the sanitary environment of a population in which pellagra was endemic, and to correlate the results with the incidence of the disease in this population. In such study, account must be taken of many factors which might seriously influence the character of the results. The importance of such factors as racial customs and habits in affecting diet, and season and locality in affecting food availability, is readily appreciated.

More elusive, yet of equal fundamental importance, is the character of the etiological conception of the disease, the relations of which it is proposed to study. Thus, vital differences of method are involved in the study of certain important correlations according as to whether the disease is conceived of as of microbial (infectious) or of dietary origin, and as to whether it is conceived of as a disease, the periodic exacerbations or recurrences of which are or are not due to periodically repeated externally acting causes.

Accordingly, as will appear, in planning our study and in selecting methods of analyzing our data, we sought, as far as possible, to eliminate or minimize the effect of disturbing or confusing factors. In spite of this, however, the indications afforded by our data must be interpreted with caution.

Locality.—Seven cotton-mill villages situated in the northwestern part of South Carolina were selected for study. Four (*At., In., Sn.,* and *Wy.*) are in Spartanburg County, two (*Sa.* and *Ny.*) in Oconee County, and one (*Rc.*) in Chester County. In selecting these localities we were influenced, in some measure, by the fact that they had previously been studied more or less intensively by the Thompson-McFadden Commission, with whose results we thought our own would therefore be more directly comparable than if our work were done elsewhere. A further consideration was that all these places were readily reached from the city of Spartanburg where the United States Public Health Service had already established a hospital and laboratory for the clinical and biochemical study of pellagra.

Population.—The selected villages, quite typical of such communities, were of about average size; none had over 800 or less than 500 inhabitants. Each constituted a distinct, more or less isolated community, surrounding or immediately adjacent to cotton-cloth manufacturing plants, and each was composed practically exclusively of the mill employees and their families. With the exception of a few Negro families which were not considered, all were white, and, with hardly a single exception, of Anglo-Saxon stock, born in this country of American-born parents.

The families of the mill officials, store managers, and Negro employees were not considered. The exclusion of these families had the drawback of correspondingly reducing the total number of families available for study. The number thus excluded, however, was relatively small, and thus unimportant. It had the compensating advantage of leaving for study a group exceptionally homogeneous with respect to racial stock, dietary custom, and also, we thought, to economic status. Subsequent experience, however, has shown that this last premise was not entirely justified.[4]

Pellagra incidence.—For the study of the relation of household diet to pellagra, it is of fundamental importance to determine as completely as possible the household incidence of the disease. In order to supply this vital need we adopted the expedient of a house-to-house canvass. The search for cases was begun about the middle of April, 1916, and carried on by one of us (G. A. W.) every two weeks to the end of that year. So far as we are aware, this is the first time that this expedient has been applied systematically and continuously on so large a scale and over so long a period to the study of this disease.

At each canvass every family was visited and an effort was made to see and question all individuals in or about the house. At first considerable reluctance was displayed by some of the people in

---

4 As compared with certain other classes of the general population, all of the mill-workers' families in the seven villages studied were on a distinctly low economic level; in this sense, therefore, they may be considered homogeneous with respect to economic status. Among them, however, and thus within their own range of income, quite marked differences in economic status were found to exist. These differences, considered in relation to differences in food supplies and in pellagra incidence, will be presented in a later paper.

speaking of any condition which they believed or suspected to be pellagrous; but, as we became better known to the village people, this reserve in large measure disappeared, so that from time to time cases were brought to our attention which might otherwise have escaped us.

In order to see as many as possible of those at work in the mill (i. e., not at home at the time of the canvass), the time of the canvass was so varied as to utilize more or less of the lunch hour and Saturday half-holidays in different villages and in different sections of the same village in rotation. At each visit inquiries were made as to the health of absent members of the household and as to the existence of any suspicious illness or condition in the village, particularly in members of neighboring households. Reports regarded as suggestive were investigated; at times trips to the mill were made for this purpose.

Information with respect to the occurrence of cases of pellagra was also sought from local physicians. Although we believe we enjoyed the full cooperation of the local medical profession, the number of cases coming to our attention in this way formed a very small proportion of the total recorded by us. This is interesting as indicating that but a small percentage of cases occurring in any season come to the attention of a physician.

Criteria of pellagra.—Only patients with a clearly defined, bilaterally symmetrical dermatitis were recorded as having pellagra. In the course of the canvass, cases with manifestations more or less suggestive of the disease were encountered from time to time but, in the absence of a clearly marked bilaterally symmetrical eruption, were recorded at most as "suspects" and are excluded from present consideration. We think it important to invite attention to what, for the purpose of this study, constituted pellagra. The criterion adopted is in harmony with conventional clinical requirements; but we believe that it operated to exclude some cases without or with only poorly defined eruption that might properly have been included. Practically, this was of importance only with respect to those instances that escaped notation as "suspects." Households of which such individuals were members, unless they also included "suspects" or cases with eruption, would, as a consequence, appear in our records as nonpellagrous and thus in some degree constitute a disturbing element in the study of the diet of this class of households.

The classification adopted is not without importance in another connection. We (J. G. and G. A. W.) have been increasingly impressed by the suspicion that, as conventionally defined, pellagra probably includes at least two commonly related (what for want of a better term may be designated as) syndromes; namely, (1) the syndrome that is comprehended by the phrase "pellagra sine pellagra," and (2) the dermatitis, or pellagra without or with only very slight other manifestations. According to this idea both syndromes are dependent primarily on a faulty diet; but the factor, complex of factors, or balance (whatever it may prove to be) constituting the fault responsible for one is essentially distinct though probably very closely related to that responsible for the other.[5] The chief basis for this suspicion is the fact, many times observed by clinicians, that, on the one hand, the syndrome without eruption frequently occurs and recurs and, each season, may persist for months without recognizable eruption, and, on the other, that the eruption frequently occurs without or with only very slight other manifestations. The major portion of all of our cases belongs in this latter class.

In relating pellagra incidence to dietary conditions all active cases were considered without regard as to whether they were first or recurrent attacks. So-called inactive or quiescent cases—that is, individuals who had had the disease in a previous year, but during 1916 presented no eruption or evidence sufficient to be classed as "suspects"—were placed in the group of nonpellagrins. For if it is conceived that diet plays a rôle in pellagra in some sense analogous to that played by it in scurvy or in beriberi, then it must be recognized that the assumption of "once a pellagrin always a pellagrin," implied by considering "inactive" cases as pellagra, may be as erroneous as would be a similar conception in relation to beriberi or scurvy. In other words, the freedom from recurrence in pellagra must be recognized as possibly due to the same cause as that responsible for the like phenomenon in beriberi or in scurvy, namely, a change in diet. It follows, therefore, that to attempt to relate the diet of the household of such an individual to pellagra, as would, in effect, be done if quiescent were classed with active cases, carries with it possibilities of error and confusion such as would arise if we were to attempt to associate with beriberi or scurvy the diet of one who once had had one or other of these diseases but who now presented but residuals, stigmata, or sequelæ of such attack.

Onset of attack.—The date of the appearance of the eruption was assumed to mark the onset of the attack. This date could be fixed

---

5 Of interest in this connection is the suggestion advanced by Goldberger and Wheeler (1920) that the site of the initial skin lesion in pellagra is bound up with a specific quality of the diet and that the latter differs in some essential detail with differences in localization of the initial dermatitis.

fairly accurately in most adults, but was frequently rather difficult of determination in children, for it often happened that in them the existence of an eruption was not recognized until attention was called to it in the course of the canvass. In such instances the date could frequently be placed as within the period of the immediately preceding two weeks by the fact of the absence of the eruption at the date of the preceding examination; or, in the event of the individual not having been seen at the immediately preceding visit, the date could, as a rule, be placed as falling within the preceding four weeks. A definite date, however, so far as possible, was always assigned, even in such instances. In selecting it the appearance and stage of the eruption, with such other circumstances as the history of the case might bring out, were used as a guide. In general it may be said that in the vast majority of our cases the date of "onset" is probably correct within less than a week, and in practically all cases it may be said that the eruption appeared "not later than" this date. It is possible that some of the cases recorded as occurring late in the year were really relapses, the eruption in the early part of the year having escaped our observation.

It is recognized that in assuming that the appearance of the eruption marks the onset of the attack of pellagra a certain error is involved. In many of our cases a definite history of symptoms antedating the eruption was obtained; in much the greater proportion, however (children for the most part), such history either could not be elicited or it was so vague as to be of no value in fixing the date of onset. In the latter event the assumption that the first appearance of the eruption marks the onset of the disease was, therefore, practically unavoidable. For the sake of uniformity and in order to eliminate any possible bias, this rule was adopted and applied in all cases. It follows, therefore, that our "date of onset" should be interpreted as indicating that the attack began "not later than" that date.

Assignment of cases to households.—As a considerable proportion of the population of any mill village is of a transient character, and as much of the pellagra occurs in this class, some rule was necessary for assigning cases to households and villages.

From the point of view that diet is the primary controlling factor in the causation of the disease, it may be assumed that a minimum of several months is required in a previously normal person before the disease manifests itself in recognizable form. During such a period an individual (boarder) may have lived in a number of households in succession in the same or different villages, the diet in all of

which may have been equally contributory to the eventual development of the disease. On the other hand it is conceivable that, at
the time of the development of the dermatitis, the individual may be
living in a household the diet of which is not or is no longer
pellagra-producing, i.e., a diet which is not responsible for the
attack, and which indeed, given a sufficient time, may favor recovery
from the attack.

Our studies had taught us that in the average case very definite
clinical improvement may be observed after about 10 days or 2
weeks on an appropriate diet. It seemed to us reasonable to assume,
therefore, that, in most cases at least, the progress of an incipient
case to full development (of the eruption) would be halted and the
dermatitis prevented from appearing after, say, 30 days of a suitable
diet and, as a corollary, that the fact of a case developing might be
interpreted as indicating that the diet during at least the earlier
part of the immediately preceding period of 30 days had been of a
relatively poor quality and might be studied in relation to the disease
as a pellagra-producing diet.[6] Accordingly a case was assigned to a
household only if the individual had been a member of that household for not less than 30 days immediately preceding the beginning
of the attack. In practically all instances, however, the pellagrins had
been members of their respective households all their lives and may
be assumed to have been living under the conditions of the same
household, so far as diet was concerned, during the entire spring of
1916 or longer.

Season.—In order that dietary data may properly be related to
pellagra incidence, it is clearly necessary that they be representative
of the season immediately anterior to the greatest incidence of the
disease; that is, the season when, more than at any other time, the
diet, if it has any relation to the incidence of the disease, may be
expected to be distinctively pellagra-producing, just as it may reasonably be expected that the diet at the season immediately anterior
to and coincident with the rapid decline in incidence and the clinical
improvement of active cases, is distinctively pellagra preventing.
Curiously enough, in no previous study of which we have knowledge
has this vitally important seasonal factor been given due recognition,
and we venture to suggest this, along with the very general character

6 We have here a source of possible confusion and error in that it is conceivable (indeed probable) that a diet just sufficient for maintenance may
still be somewhat lacking in that which is necessary to prevent the progress
of an incipient case (especially when well along in its development) to a
confirmed attack.

of the data and the inclusion of "inactive" or "quiescent" cases, as among the most important contributing elements in the failure of previous American workers to discover any definite significant relationship between diet and the incidence of the disease.[7]

Such statistics of pellagra morbidity as were available indicated that the height of the seasonal curve of pellagra incidence in the southern states began in the late spring and reached its peak in June. In accordance with the principle enunciated in the preceding paragraph, it seemed permissible to assume that the distinctively pellagra-producing dietary season began sometime in the late winter or early spring and continued up to or possibly somewhat into June. The period actually selected for which dietary observations were made by us extended from April 16 to June 15. Cooperating to fix the limits of this period was the circumstance that we found it impracticable to organize and begin the collection of dietary data sooner than April 16, nor could the available personnel complete the collection of the desired data before June 15. The accompanying graph (see p. 146) shows the relative position of this period with respect to the monthly incidence of pellagra as subsequently actually found in the seven villages studied in 1916.

It will be seen that the selected period coincides with the steepest portion of the up-curve of pellagra incidence. It may be noted also that the incidence of the disease dropped very sharply in July, suggesting that the diet of an increasing number of families may be regarded as having been pellagra preventing for some time during the month of June. The possibility must, therefore, be kept in mind that the portion of the selected period extending into June may no longer have been fully representative of the pellagra-producing dietary season.

Dietary data.—Our data with respect to diet relate to households and do not indicate any difference that might have existed, and in all probability did exist, in the diets of the individual members. The ideal procedure, it might seem, would be to secure a record of individual consumption. This has been the procedure frequently adopted in previous studies. The practical difficulty, however, of securing an accurate statement of individual consumption from a sufficiently large number of individuals for a period sufficiently long to be fairly

---

7 In the study of the individual case this seasonal factor in relation to that individual attack is all too commonly overlooked. In relating the diet of the individual to a particular attack, attention should primarily be given to the diet of the period of two or three months immediately preceding the onset of the attack.

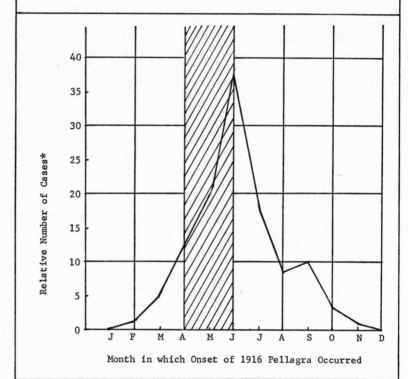

Seasonal Incidence of Pellagra in Seven Cotton Mill Villages
of South Carolina during 1916 in Relation to the Specific
Period for which Records of Household Food Supplies were
Secured

Month in which Onset of 1916 Pellagra Occurred

 Period During which Data Relating to the Household
Food Supplies were Secured

*Based on the monthly average of attacks during the year, the
number occurring each month having been adjusted to a 31-day
month.

representative of the pellagra-producing dietary period seemed to us so great as to preclude its adoption. Of necessity, therefore, we adopted the household as the unit, assuming that with a knowledge of the diet of a considerable number of them the outstanding characteristics of the diet of groups of households would be suggested, in a general way at least, when classified according to the occurrence or nonoccurrence of pellagra, economic status, or other basis.

As it was manifestly impracticable to secure a record of the complete food supply of each household for the entire period selected as the pellagra-producing season, it was necessary to content ourselves with a record for such portions of the selected period as might properly be assumed to be fairly representative of the whole, and for which an accurate record would be practicable. For these reasons and because nearly all of the households purchased the great bulk of their food supplies at semimonthly or more frequent intervals, a 15-day sample or cross-section period for which a record of the diet of each household was to be secured was decided upon as meeting the exigencies of the situation.

Information with respect to diet was secured by arranging with the principal stores at which the families dealt, for a record to be kept for us of every purchase of food by mill workers and members of mill workers' households during a specified 15-day period. Immediately at the close of such period trained enumerators, under the immediate direction and supervision of one of us (E. S.), were sent to the village to ascertain the composition of each household with respect to the age and sex of the individuals included during the period, to secure information relative to the economic status of the family, and to determine the quantity and value of the articles of food obtained from sources other than the stores where purchase records were secured. Such articles included those produced at home or given to the household, those purchased from neighbors, from farmers and hucksters, and from all other sources. With the exception of fresh milk and, to some extent, butter, eggs, and fresh meats, very few of the articles of food came from sources other than the stores. The great majority of the households dealt almost altogether at the stores at which purchase records were kept.

As it was not feasible with the limited personnel available to cover all seven villages in the same 15-day period, the record of the food supply was secured in successive periods, as follows: For village *Sa.*, April 16–30; villages *At.* and *Sn.*, May 1–15; villages *Ny.* and *In.*, May 16–30; and villages *Rc.* and *Wy.*, June 1–15.

With rare exceptions such information as it was necessary to obtain from the households was given willingly and frankly by the informants. Care was taken to secure the information from the housewife or other responsible member. The simple household economy prevailing in the households aided the enumerator in securing replies to the definite queries made, which gave very distinct impressions of accuracy in all except a comparatively few instances. The questionnaires or schedules, as soon as they were filled out and completed from the purchase records, were scrutinized carefully, and missing data, apparent inconsistencies, and indefinite entries were in all cases rectified as far as possible by further visits to the households within a few days. All completed schedules on which the data for any reason appeared to be of doubtful accuracy were discarded. Thus, where the informant was uncertain as to the amount of an article or articles of food, or where it appeared that the informant was unable to make accurate statements, the condition was noted by the enumerator and the schedule for the household discarded. Likewise, a schedule for which the store record was for some reason incomplete would be discarded. In a few instances where the data were incompete or indefinite in relation to one or two articles of food, the schedule was utilized for the other items. In general, however, the practice was to select for final consideration only those completed schedules which appeared to be reasonably accurate from every point of view.

As has been stated, our dietary data are assumed to be samples of the food supply of the pellagra-producing season, so that the limitations upon the representativeness of samples in general apply in a measure to these data. The principal limitation lies, of course, in the fact that the record of the use of a given article of food during the 15-day period may not be fairly representative of its use during the entire season of which the 15 days' record is assumed to be a sample. The importance of this limitation is greatly minimized, however, for several reasons. One is that the food supply of the population studied was made up largely of a few principal articles of food which were purchased regularly and by practically every household. These staple foods constituted what may be termed the "basic" portion of the diet of all or nearly all households. Other foods entered into their diet as variables, appearing in the diet of some households and not at all or in much less degree in others. It is with respect to these foods that the "sampling" method might have proved inadequate; but certain conditions existed which, we believe, largely eliminated the possibility of serious error.

The most important of these variable foods were milk, meat, fruit, and vegetables. Milk appeared in the food supply of a household either regularly or hardly at all for the reason that being almost altogether home-produced or purchased from a cow-owning neighbor the supply within certain limits was fairly constant for the milk-consuming households. Meat, particularly fresh meat, was used at fairly regular, though in different households at varying, intervals during the season when available. With respect to fruit and fresh vegetables it is to be noted that practically the total supply of these was purchased from stores, the period being too early for home-produced foods from the summer gardens and the spring gardens yielding but small quantities of onions, lettuce, and greens, and these for only a minority of the households.

The statement of the average quantity of the foods constituting the household supply seems to us therefore to be fairly representative of the importance (quantitatively) of the individual food at that season.

Some irregularities in the data for households when considered without regard to locality necessarily were caused by the gradual change in the availability of certain foods during the two months from April 16–June 15. For example, in the households surveyed for the period June 1–June 15, fresh vegetables were a more important article of diet than in the households surveyed for the period April 16–30. The contrary was true of eggs, the supply of these becoming smaller and their prices increasing in the latter part of May and in June.

It is to be emphasized that our dietary data are not records of consumption but, rather, records of household food supply for a 15-day sample period. Since, however, but few of the households purchased in quantities large enough to constitute a supply for more than a 15-day period, the data, for practical purposes, may be considered as records of consumption plus refuse and waste. The exceptional households were usually the small ones, and the articles purchased in quantities larger than the ordinary were staples, principally flour and cornmeal and occasionally lard and sirup. This should be held in mind, for, although we attempted to minimize irregularities from this source by using averages of as large groups as possible as a basis for comparison, it is probable that in some instances they have not altogether been eliminated.

In the computation of these data, the supply of any article or group of articles of food obtained by a household or group of households has been expressed in quantity per adult male unit, the Atwater (Atwater, 1915, p. 33) scale of food requirements for the sexes at different ages being used for the purpose. The factors selected were on the basis of adults "at moderately active muscular work." The following scale was used:

Age.	Equivalent "adult male units."		Age.	Equivalent "adult male units."	
	Male.	Female.		Male.	Female.
Adult (over 16)..	1.00	0.80	10-11.......	0.60	0.60
15-16.............	.90	.80	6-9.........	.50	.50
13-14.............	.80	.70	2-5.........	.40	.40
12................	.70	.60	Under 2.....	.30	.30

The results of recent studies suggest that some modifications of this scale should be made, particularly with respect to males between the ages of 12 and 16. Such modifications, however, would not have affected materially the results presented in this report except that because of the age distribution of the population in the various groups of households considered, the tendency of the modifications would have been to make the contrasts between the groups somewhat more sharp. Such contrasts as our analyses bring out are, therefore, all the more significant.

In analyzing our data our aim has been to ascertain (1) such outstanding differences as might exist between the diets of households in which no pellagra was observed and the diets of those in which one or more cases occurred, and (2) to test the significance of the differences thus found by determining the variation, if any, in pellagra incidence among households having varying supplies of certain single foods and groups of foods.

Comparison of Diets

(a) *Nonpellagrous versus pellagrous households.*—With the view of ascertaining in what respect, if any, the diet of households in which no pellagra was observed differed from that of households in which one or more cases of the disease occurred, we began with a general comparison of the average diet of the nonpellagrous with that of the pellagrous households of the villages studied. This is presented in Table 11.

A glance at this table at once discloses decidedly suggestive differences in the food supply of the two groups of households, the average supply of most articles of food being decidedly lower in the diet of

TABLE 11—*Approximate average daily supply of various foods during a fifteen-day period, between April 16 and June 15, 1916, compared for nonpellagrous households and households in which pellagra occurred during the year 1916 in seven cotton-mill villages of South Carolina.**

Article of food.	Average supply per adult male unit in grams per day.		Ratio of supply of pellagrous to non-pellagrous households.
	Households not affected with pellagra.+	Households affected with pellagra.#	
Meats:			
Fresh...........................	26.7	15.2	0.57
Cured (lean)....................	23.4	16.3	.70
Canned.........................	14.2	14.2	1.00
Eggs...............................	43.5	40.2	.92
Milk:			
Fresh...........................	517.6	223.5	.43
Preserved.......................	2.9	1.5	.52
Butter.............................	31.7	22.3	.70
Cheese.............................	2.5	.5	.20
Pork (salt)........................	51.0	64.0	1.26
Lard and lard substitutes...........	48.0	41.7	.87
Peas and beans:			
Dried.",........................	32.0	34.4	1.07
Canned".........................	5.0	1.7	.34
Wheat flour........................	420.4	363.6	.86
Wheat bread, cakes, and crackers...	14.2	12.4	.87
Corn meal..........................	152.8	158.8	1.04
Grits..............................	5.3	11.2	2.11
Corn (canned)......................	6.1	10.4	1.70
Rice...............................	5.2	4.1	.77
String beans:			
Green...........................	12.3	4.1	.33
Canned..........................	5.1	2.0	.39
Other vegetables:			
Green...........................	51.0	42.3	.83
Canned..........................	36.2	31.7	.88
Fruits:			
Fresh...........................	29.7	18.0	.61
Dried...........................	9.6	6.2	.65
Canned..........................	18.9	16.6	.88
Potatoes:			
Irish...........................	71.9	99.3	1.38
Sweet (fresh)...................	5.9	2.8	.47
Sweet (canned)..................	5.5	2.3	.42
Sugar..............................	47.1	35.3	.75
Sirup..............................	18.5	18.4	.99
Jellies and jams...................	7.7	9.9	1.29
All other foods (cost in cents)....	3.6	3.1	.86

*An explanation of the articles and groups of articles of food in this and succeeding tables is presented in the Appendix.
+692 households composed of 2,769.3 adult male units. Data were available for the following number of adult male units for the articles of food specified: Fresh meats, 2,760.2; canned meats, 2,771.8; fresh milk, 2,694.2; butter, 2,775.3; Irish and fresh sweet potatoes, 2,764.7; salt pork, 2,742.6; lard, 2,765.1; green vegetables, 2,764.9; dried fruits, 2,756.0; canned fruits, 2,760.1.
#51 households composed of 288.9 adult male units. Data were available for the following number of adult male units for the articles of food specified: Canned meats, 286.4; fresh milk, 256.7; butter, 274.2.
"Exclusive of canned string beans.

the pellagrous households than in that of the nonpellagrous. The significance of these differences is obscured and the value of this general comparison is materially affected by certain circumstances, not previously considered, relating to the character of the data presented in Table 11. Thus, some households for which we secured food records moved away soon thereafter and so passed from observation. Such might appear to have been free from pellagra, when, in reality, one or more cases may have developed shortly after passing from observation. This, obviously, might also be true of individual members of those households that remained under observation. The moving of individual members of households was very slight in the case of boarders who were not members of the families. The fact, however, that among boarders who remained, as well as among the members of families which had boarders (not members of families) and which had an income from this source, practically no pellagra occurred, would appear to reduce this possible element of error in pellagra incidence to a negligible quantity.

Again, by restricting the diagnosis of pellagra to cases presenting a definite eruption, cases with poorly defined eruption, and cases clinically pellagra but without eruption were, as previously stated, not included as such, but, when noted, were designated simply as "suspects" so that some of the households appearing in our records as nonpellagrous should perhaps more truly have been classed as pellagrous. Another element of error which, like the preceding, would lead to the inclusion of some, probably very few, households as nonpellagrous, that were in reality pellagrous, arises from the fact that some few cases may have been, and probably were, unavoidably missed.

Finally, and perhaps most important of all, there is to be noted the circumstance that in a few of the households classed as pellagrous the pellagra occurred later in the year, that is, at a considerable time after the "sample" period. In these it is manifestly possible that the diet records were not representative of the conditions in the period immediately preceding the onset of the attack. Accordingly, in order to minimize these possible sources of error we have included in the comparisons about to be presented only those nonpellagrous households which continued under observation from April 15 to October 1, 1916, and in which no one with suspicious symptoms was observed, and only those pellagrous households in which one or more cases of pellagra with clearly defined, bilaterally symmetrical dermatitis occurred before August 1, 1916.

(b) *Nonpellagrous households of highest income versus pellagrous households, each with at least two cases.*—In order to bring out possibly significant differences in the diets of nonpellagrous and those of pellagrous households as definitely as possible, not only must the various possible sources of error affecting the data be eliminated, or at least minimized, but so far as may be, the diets to be compared should be those of households of as markedly contrasting pellagra incidence as the available data afford. With this in mind, the comparison that next suggested itself was that between the food supply of nonpellagrous households of the highest income class and that of pellagrous households in each of which at least two cases of the disease were observed.

By restricting the group of nonpellagrous households in this comparison to those of the highest income not only have we a group in which no pellagra was actually observed, but it is also one in which, by reason of the economic factor, the chance of the occurrence of the disease in the first place may be considered to have been relatively at a minimum. It is a group, therefore, that actually is more nearly free from pellagra, or the chance of its occurrence, than any other included in our study, and, accordingly, the diet of the group may be regarded as being more surely pellagra preventive, or having a wider margin of safety, than that of any other of our household groups.

Similarly, by restricting the group of pellagrous households to those having at least two cases each, the possible error arising from considering as associated with pellagra the diet of borderland households or that of a household in which a case developed as the result of individual dietary eccentricity is believed to be minimized, as the chance of two cases arising in a household under such circumstances may be regarded as negligible. The average food supply of this group of pellagrous households may therefore be regarded as more closely approximating a pellagra-producing diet than that of any other of our groups.

In comparing the food supplies of these two groups, then, we are comparing a sample of what may be regarded as a relatively highly preventive diet with a sample closely approximating a surely pellagra-producing one. The comparison is presented in Table 12. By reference to this table it will be seen that here, as in the general comparison between the diet of all our nonpellagrous and that of all our pellagrous households, shown in Table 11, the food supply of the nonpellagrous appears decidedly more liberal than that of the pellagrous households.

In this connection it must be noted that while the nonpellagrous households in the present comparison are all of the highest income

TABLE 12—*Approximate average daily supply of various foods during a fifteen-day period, between April 16 and June 15, 1916, compared for nonpellagrous households with highest incomes and households in which two or more cases of pellagra occurred during the period March–July, 1916, in seven cotton-mill villages of South Carolina.*

Article of food.	Average supply per adult male unit, in grams per day.		Ratio of supply of pellagrous to nonpellagrous households.
	Higher-income households not affected with pellagra.*	Households affected with pellagra.+	
Meats:			
Fresh..........................	48.9	16.3	0.33
Cured (lean)...................	54.0	8.1	.15
Canned.........................	25.1	15.7	.63
Eggs..............................	69.5	31.1	.45
Milk:			
Fresh..........................	379.3	126.9	.33
Preserved......................	4.5	1.8	.40
Butter............................	27.2	11.2	.41
Cheese............................	3.6	.2	.06
Pork (salt)......................	38.6	65.2	1.69
Lard and lard substitutes..........	52.8	34.7	.66
Peas and beans:			
Dried..........................	31.1	34.1	1.10
Canned#........................	12.1	1.6	.13
Wheat flour.......................	445.4	351.5	.79
Wheat bread, cakes, and crackers...	18.1	9.4	.52
Corn meal.........................	127.1	144.3	1.14
Grits.............................	9.4	5.2	.55
Corn (canned).....................	11.5	6.3	.55
Rice..............................	4.5	5.5	1.22
String beans:			
Green..........................	31.7	3.4	.11
Canned.........................	9.1	0.0	.00
Other vegetables:			
Green..........................	90.6	57.4	.63
Canned.........................	56.2	19.9	.35
Fruits:			
Fresh..........................	42.3	10.1	.24
Dried..........................	9.7	9.5	.98
Canned.........................	37.4	15.7	.42
Potatoes:			
Irish..........................	48.9	53.1	1.00
Sweet (Fresh)..................	7.9	3.9	.49
Sweet (Canned).................	7.9	3.1	.39
Sugar.............................	55.6	32.0	.58
Sirup.............................	7.9	22.6	2.86
Jellies and jams..................	10.9	6.0	.55
All other foods (cost in cents)....	1.7	.9	.53

*60 households composed of 209.4 adult male units.
+22 households composed of 117.5 adult male units.
#Exclusive of canned string beans.

class (from $14 to about $20 per adult male unit per 15-day period), the pellagrous households all fall in the lower ranges of income—in fact, fully three-fourths of them belong in the lowest income class studied by us (less than $6 per adult male unit per 15-day period). While, therefore, it may be, and, as we shall see, actually is the case, that the greater liberality in the food supply of the nonpellagrous households is (in some measure at least) significantly related to their freedom from pellagra, before this may be properly assumed the influence of the marked difference in economic status of the households of the two groups must be eliminated, for it may well be that the greater liberality in supply of the nonpellagrous groups is simply a reflection of their decidedly better economic status.

(c) *Nonpellagrous households of lowest income versus pellagrous households, each with at least two cases.*—In order to eliminate the influence of the economic factor from consideration, the nonpellagrous households must be of the same, or at least of no higher economic class than those of the pellagrous group, with the diet of which that of the former is to be compared. This requirement is believed to be fulfilled by comparing with the diet of those of our pellagrous households in each of which at least two cases occurred, the diet of the nonpellagrous households of the lowest income class. For, as has already been pointed out, all of the households of the former group belong in our lower income classes—fully three-fourths, indeed, falling in the lowest—the same class, that is, as that in which this nonpellagrous group belongs. The two groups may therefore be regarded as rather close together economically, or, if anything, it is the pellagrous group that has a slight advantage. Consequently, any greater liberality in the food supply that the nonpellagrous may be found to have cannot be attributed to a better income status.

This comparison is presented in Table 13, examination of which shows that here again, as in the preceding comparisons, the nonpellagrous appear to have a distinctly more liberal food supply than do the pellagrous households.

In connection with a detailed examination of the differences suggested by this comparison it will, we believe, be helpful to consider also the average food supply of the pellagrous households of our lowest income class. This group differs from the group of pellagrous households with at least two cases each in this, that some of the former households have but one case, that is, possibly borderland households, and all of the group are in the lowest income class. It may be assumed, therefore, that the average food supply of this group does not represent quite as close an approximation to a

TABLE 13—*Approximate average daily supply of various foods during a fifteen-day period, between April 16 and June 15, 1916, compared for nonpellagrous households with lowest incomes and households in which two or more cases of pellagra occurred during the period March–July, 1916, in seven cotton-mill villages in South Carolina.*

| Article of food. | Average supply per adult male unit, in grams per day. | | Ratio of supply of pellagrous to non-pellagrous households. |
	Nonpella-grous with lowest in-comes.*	Pellagrous multiple cases, ma-jority with lowest in-comes.+	
Meats:			
Fresh....................	19.9	16.3	0.82
Cured (lean).............	11.8	8.1	.69
Canned..................	10.6	15.7	1.48
Eggs......................	38.9	31.1	.80
Milk:			
Fresh....................	554.0	126.9	.22
Preserved................	2.3	1.8	.78
Butter....................	30.2	11.2	.37
Cheese...................	2.0	.2	.10
Pork (salt)...............	50.7	65.2	1.27
Lard and substitutes........	37.1	34.7	.94
Peas and beans:			
Dried...................	31.4	34.1	1.09
Canned#.................	1.8	1.6	.89
Wheat:			
Flour...................	398.6	351.5	.88
Bread, cakes, crackers...	10.3	9.4	.91
Corn meal..................	164.9	144.3	.88
Grits.....................	6.6	5.2	.76
Corn (canned)..............	3.5	6.3	1.73
Rice......................	5.4	5.5	1.02
String beans:			
Green....................	6.6	3.4	.52
Canned..................	4.1	0.0	.00
Other vegetables:			
Green....................	33.9	57.4	1.70
Canned..................	32.9	19.9	.61
Fruits:			
Fresh....................	21.1	10.1	.48
Dried...................	9.7	9.5	.98
Canned..................	14.5	15.7	1.08
Potatoes:			
Irish....................	63.7	53.1	.80
Sweet (fresh)............	3.9	3.9	1.00
Sweet (canned)..........	3.1	3.1	1.00
Sugar......................	38.6	32.0	.83
Sirup......................	8.6	22.6	2.63
Jellies and jams............	4.2	6.0	1.43
All other foods............	1.5	.9	.73

*184 households composed of 730.7 adult male units.
+22 households composed of 117.5 adult male units.
#Exclusive of canned string beans.

pellagra-producing diet as that of the group in each household of which at least two cases of pellagra occurred. In other words, we expected to find that the diet of this group would be somewhat less removed from that of the nonpellagrous households than was that of the pellagrous households each with at least two cases. The difference actually found, however, was, as will be seen, rather slight. Accordingly, for purposes of further study we have brought together in Table 14 the diet of these 3 groups and, in order to facilitate comparison between them, also that of the nonpellagrous households of highest income. The diets of the pellagrous households here presented are, so far as known by the authors, the first in the literature giving a detailed quantitative statement of the approximate average supply for a sample period of the season immediately anterior to or coincident with the sharp rise in the seasonal incidence of the disease.

For the sake of simplicity of reference, the diets will be designated as No. 1, No. 2, No. 3, and No. 4, and the corresponding household groups will be similarly distinguished. Diets No. 1 and No. 2 are those of the nonpellagrous, No. 3 and No. 4 of the pellagrous households. Of the diets of the nonpellagrous groups, No. 1 is that of households of the highest of our income classes, while No. 2 is that of households belonging to the lowest class. Of the diets of the pellagrous groups, No. 3 is that of households having one or more cases each, while diet No. 4 is that of households with a minimum of two cases each. As has already been stated, economically the group with diet No. 3 is of the same low class as that with diet No. 2, and of the households constituting group No. 4 fully three-fourths are not only of the same class as are groups No. 2 and No. 3, but actually constitute part of Group No. 3.

An examination of Tables 14 and 15 discloses the same gross differences in supply that have previously been referred to. [Graphic representation deleted. ED.] The large number of single articles, many of them seemingly unimportant quantitatively, constituting the several diets, makes a determination in this manner of anything but very gross outstanding differences difficult or impossible. The difficulty is increased, moreover, by the use, seemingly, of increased quantities of one article in one diet in the place of a related one in another, as, for instance, the substitution of salt pork for lard and of sirup for sugar.

In order to minimize the obscuring and confusing effect of these factors, foods that, in the existing state of knowledge, seemed closely related, have been combined into groups and the fuel value of

TABLE 14—*Approximate average daily supply of various articles of food for groups of nonpellagrous and of pellagrous households in seven cotton-mill villages of South Carolina during a fifteen-day period between April 16 and June 15, 1916.*

Article of food.	Average daily supply, in grams, per adult male unit.			
	Nonpella-grous households whose half month's income per adult male unit was $14 and over.*	Households whose half month's income per adult male unit was less than $6.		Households in which at least 2 cases of pellagra occurred."
		Not af-fected with pellagra.+	Affected with pel-lagra.#	
	(1)	(2)	(3)	(4)
Meats:				
Fresh.......................	48.9	19.9	9.4	16.3
Cured (lean).................	54.0	11.8	11.1	8.1
Canned......................	25.1	10.6	17.5	15.7
Eggs.............................	69.5	38.9	30.6	31.1
Milk (fresh)....................	379.3	554.0	187.2	126.9
Milk (preserved)...............	4.5	2.3	2.8	1.8
Butter..........................	27.2	30.2	16.0	11.2
Cheese..........................	3.6	2.0	.2	.2
Pork (salt).....................	38.6	50.7	69.5	65.2
Lard and lard substitutes........	52.8	37.1	32.0	34.7
Peas and beans:				
Dried..........................	31.1	31.4	31.4	34.1
Canned**.......................	12.1	1.8	3.3	1.6
Flour, wheat.....................	445.4	398.6	323.1	351.5
Wheat, bread, cakes, and crackers	18.1	10.3	13.1	9.4
Corn meal........................	127.1	164.9	149.8	144.3
Grits............................	9.4	6.6	3.3	5.2
Corn (canned)....................	11.5	3.5	4.8	6.3
Rice.............................	4.5	5.4	4.2	5.5
Beans (string):				
Green...........................	31.7	6.6	3.5	3.4
Canned..........................	9.1	4.1	1.3	0.0
Other vegetables:				
Green...........................	90.6	33.9	32.3	57.4
Canned..........................	56.2	32.9	27.8	19.9
Fruits:				
Fresh...........................	42.3	21.1	9.7	10.1
Dried...........................	9.7	9.7	9.7	9.5
Canned..........................	37.4	14.5	16.6	15.7
Potatoes:				
Irish...........................	48.9	63.7	71.0	53.1
Sweet (fresh)...................	7.9	3.9	1.7	3.9
Sweet (canned).................	7.9	3.1	1.4	3.1
Sugar............................	55.6	38.6	37.1	32.0
Sirup............................	7.9	8.6	15.1	22.6
Jellies and jams.................	10.9	4.2	7.5	6.0
All other foods (cost in cents)..	1.7	1.5	1.2	.9

*60 households composed of 209.4 adult male units.
+184 households composed of 730.7 adult male units. Data were available for the following number of adult male units for the articles of food specified: Fresh milk, 713.1; green vegetables, 726.3; dried fruits, 726.6.
#29 households composed of 134.6 adult male units. Data were available for only 117.1 adult male units with respect to fresh milk and butter.
"22 households composed of 117.5 adult male units.
**Exclusive of canned string beans.

TABLE 15—*Relative average daily supply of various articles of food for groups of nonpellagrous and of pellagrous households in seven cotton-mill villages of South Carolina during a fifteen-day period between April 16 and June 15, 1916.*

Articles of food.	Relative average daily supply per adult male unit. (Base: Arithmetic average for nonpellagrous households with highest incomes--100.)			
	Nonpellagrous households whose half-month's income per adult male unit was $14 and over.	Households whose half-month's income per adult male unit was less than $6.		Households in which at least two cases of pellagra occurred.
		Not affected with pellagra.	Affected with pellagra.	
	(1)	(2)	(3)	(4)
Canned string beans.............	100	45	14	0
Cheese.........................	100	56	6	6
Beans, string, green...........	100	21	11	11
Peas and beans, other canned....	100	15	27	13
Meats, cured lean..............	100	22	21	15
Fruits, fresh..................	100	50	23	24
Milk, fresh....................	100	146	49	33
Meats, fresh...................	100	49	19	33
Vegetables, other, canned*.....	100	59	49	35
Potatoes, sweet, canned........	100	39	18	39
Milk, preserved................	100	51	62	40
Butter.........................	100	111	59	41
Fruits, canned.................	100	39	44	42
Eggs...........................	100	56	44	45
Potatoes, sweet, fresh.........	100	49	22	49
Wheat bread, cakes and crackers.	100	57	72	52
Jellies and jams...............	100	39	69	55
Corn, canned...................	100	30	42	55
Grits..........................	100	70	35	55
Sugar..........................	100	71	67	58
Vegetables, other, green.......	100	37	36	63
Meats, canned..................	100	42	70	63
Lard, and lard substitutes.....	100	70	61	66
Wheat flour....................	100	89	73	79
Fruits, dried..................	100	100	100	98
Potatoes, Irish................	100	130	145	109
Peas and beans, dried..........	100	101	101	110
Corn meal......................	100	130	118	114
Rice...........................	100	112	93	122
Pork, salt.....................	100	132	180	169
Sirup..........................	100	109	191	286
All other foods (cost in cents).	100	88	71	53

*Exclusive of canned corn--principally tomatoes.

each group has been used as an index[8] of their relative importance in the respective diets. The resulting groups and the fuel value of the supply of each group of households are shown in Table 16. [Graphic representation deleted. ED.] It is to be noted that the computations of the caloric value of the groups of foods are to be regarded as partaking somewhat of the nature of estimates, since, in certain instances, they are unavoidably based on the fuel values of certain articles assumed to be representative of the group, and since, in a few instances, they are averages after taking into consideration the relative importance (from the point of view of quantity) of the foods composing the group. In one instance assumed equivalents (jellies and jams) were used as the base, inasmuch as the percentage composition of the articles actually appearing in the supplies of the households considered were not available. No chemical analysis of the food supply was attempted. All our computations are based on Bulletin 28, United States Department of Agriculture (Atwater and Bryant, "The Chemical Composition of American Food Materials"). An allowance in accordance with the figures in this publication was made for "refuse," but no deduction except where specified was made for edible waste occurring in the household. In spite of these important qualifications it is believed that our figures are fairly close approximations to actual average values, and will serve satisfactorily for purposes of comparing the relative importance of the corresponding groups of foods in the respective diets.

Proceeding now to an examination of these diets, and considering first of all the total fuel supply represented by each, we find that the diets of the pellagrous groups (No. 3 and No. 4) with approximately 3,290 and 3,310 gross calories, respectively, are essentially identical in this regard, but clearly below that of either of the diets (No. 1 and No. 2) of the nonpellagrous groups, thus confirming the gross indications, previously noted, that the nonpellagrous enjoyed a more liberal food supply than did the pellagrous.

The difference in potential energy value between the diets of the nonpellagrous and the pellagrous groups is probably not quite as great as the figures in the table would indicate. For there is some

8 It is to be understood, of course, that this is far from being completely satisfactory. But that it is sufficiently accurate for the present purpose is shown by the fact that when the protein value of the groups is similarly used as the index, the indications are the same. The ideal would be an index that would take into account and give due weight to all essential dietary factors.

reason to believe that the fuel supply of the nonpellagrous is somewhat exaggerated as the result of an error arising from the fact, already referred to, that in the case of the smaller households which almost without exception were in the nonpellagrous group, the customary purchases of such articles as flour and meal tended in

TABLE 16—*Approximate caloric value of various groups of foods* constituting the average daily supply of specified groups of pellagrous and of nonpellagrous households in seven cotton-mill villages of South Carolina during a fifteen-day period between April 16 and June 15, 1916.*

	Average calories per adult male unit daily.			
	Nonpellagrous households whose half-month's income per adult male unit was $14 and over.	Households whose half-month's income per adult male unit was less than $6.		Households in which at least two cases of pellagra occurred.
Groups of foods.		Not affected with pellagra.	Affected with pellagra.	
	(1)	(2)	(3)	(4)
Meats (exclusive of salt pork) eggs, milk, butter, cheese.....	762	639	338	270
Salt pork, lard, and lard substitutes...................	741	673	748	745
Dried and canned peas and beans (exclusive of canned string beans)......................	126	113	115	123
Wheaten flour, bread, cakes and crackers, corn meal, grits, canned corn, rice.............	2,162	2,082	1,752	1,840
Green and canned vegetables (exclusive of canned corn), green and canned string beans, fruits of all kinds..........	131	71	60	69
Irish and sweet potatoes.......	55	53	53	46
Sugar, sirup, jellies, and jams.	290	205	222	217
Calories from all foods....	4,267	3,836	3,288	3,310
Total calories, after allowing 10 per cent for waste....................	3,840	3,452	2,959	2,979

*Foods as purchased less nonedible portion. The computation of edible portion and the caloric value thereof is according to analyses published in Bulletin 28 (revised edition), U.S. Department of Agriculture (Atwater and Bryant: "The Chemical Composition of American Food Materials.") Because of the form in which it was necessary to obtain the data, the computations are only approximately correct, not absolutely exact.

these households to be somewhat in excess of actual consumption during our 15-day sample period. So that the average supply of these articles, as it appears, is probably somewhat too high.

In passing, it may be of interest to note that as between the non-pellagrous groups the diet of the group of poorer households (No. 2) appears to provide somewhat less energy than that of the group (No. 1) of the highest income class, a difference which appears to be a reflection, in the main, if not altogether, of the difference in economic status of the two groups. The relation of diet to economic status will be considered in a separate communication.

By reference to Table 16 it may be seen that the marked similarity of the diets of the groups of pellagrous households (No. 3 and No. 4) with respect to total fuel value holds good in a general way also with respect to the calories furnished by each of the 7 groups into which the articles of food enumerated in Table 14 have been combined, with the possible exception of the group including the meats, milk, and eggs, etc., with which diet of group No. 3 seems somewhat more liberally supplied. On comparing with diet No. 1 it is found that the lower fuel values of diets No. 3 and No. 4 are due mainly to a smaller supply in three classes of foods,[9] namely, (1) meats, milk, etc.; (2) green vegetables, including fruits; and (3) sugar, sirup, etc. If consideration were given only to the contrast between diets No. 3 and No. 4 on the one hand and No. 1 on the other, the interpretation would seem to be suggested that the freedom from pellagra enjoyed by the nonpellagrous households with diet No. 1 was associated with a more liberal supply of some one or some combination of the foods in the groups in which the pellagrous households with diets No. 3 and No. 4 were notably short.

As has previously been suggested, however, the relative shortage in supply of the pellagrous groups No. 3 and No. 4 may be partly at least a reflection of a lower income status. This view is supported by the fact that we find that the diet (No. 2) of the nonpellagrous households of lowest income at once closely resembles diets No. 3 and No. 4 of the pellagrous groups and differs from the diet (No. 1) of the nonpellagrous households of highest income in substantially the same degree as do diets No. 3 and No. 4 with respect to the supply from all groups of foods but one: this one is the group comprising the animal protein foods, namely, the lean meats, milk, butter, cheese, and eggs, the supply from which in diet No. 2 is notably greater than in diets No. 3 and No. 4 and but little less than

9 A fourth class, the cereals, is not as important as might seem to be the case.

that in No. 1. Clearly, then, the freedom from pellagra of the non-pellagrous households can be considered as significantly associated with a more liberal supply from this one group of foods.[10]

Relation of Pellagra Incidence to Variations in Supply of "Animal Protein" Foods

It now becomes important to test the association so clearly indicated in the foregoing in order that its significance may more satisfactorily be evaluated. Accordingly, we have analyzed our data with respect to the relation of pellagra incidence to variation in the supply of the single foods of this group. In this analysis, as in the preceding comparisons, the household, not the individual, has been considered as the unit with respect to food supply as well as with respect to pellagra incidence.

It is to be noted that for the purpose of this analysis (with respect to single foods) a pellagrous household is one in which one or more cases of pellagra occurred *at any time* during 1916.[11] As has previously been pointed out, this definition carries with it a possible source of error, in that the disease may not have occurred so long after the record of diet was secured that this may have been properly representative. Such relationship as does appear must therefore be regarded as all the more significant.

Milk.—In the study of the relation of varying supplies of milk to pellagra incidence, buttermilk and whole milk were added together without distinction, and 1 pound of preserved milk (almost exclusively evaporated milk) was considered equivalent to 1 quart of fresh milk. It should be noted, also, (1) that home-churned buttermilk was the predominating form in which milk was used by the households (the ratio being about 3 of buttermilk to 1 of whole milk), and preserved milk was used in only small quantities and by a very small proportion of the households; (2) that the use of home-made or country-made butter was fairly concomitant with the use of buttermilk. For practical purposes, therefore, "milk" may be con-

---

10 Both nonpellagrous groups appear to have a slightly more liberal supply from the cereal group (wheat, corn, rice). This, we believe, is very largely if not entirely due to the practice of certain (small) households of purchasing flour and corn meal in relatively large quantities, these households being almost without exception in the nonpellagrous group.

11 In our preliminary report we restricted our pellagrous households in this analysis as in the preceding comparisons to those in which pellagra occurred between March 1 and August 1, so that the figures there given are not quite the same as those here to be presented. The indications, however, are in no way affected.

sidered as fresh whole milk, since it was used either whole or in the form of buttermilk and butter. The proportion represented by preserved milk was so small that it may be considered as a practically negligible element. It may be noted further that our "sample" was more accurately representative with respect to regularity in use of milk during the season in question than with respect to regularity in use of other of the variable articles of food, for the reason that households using milk were either owners of cows or purchased milk regularly from cow-owning neighbors or nearby farmers.[12]

In order to eliminate as far as possible households which were exceptional in this respect, those whose cows had become fresh within less than a month previous to the enumerator's visit and were at that time giving abnormally large quantities of milk were not considered. The few instances where it was definitely established that milk had been consumed by pellagrins for therapeutic reasons and had not been an article of household diet, have, however, not been excluded, but are indicated in the table to be presented. The results of our study in relation to milk are shown in Table 17. [Graphic representation deleted. ED.] By reference to this it will be seen that the incidence of pellagra declined markedly as the milk supply of the households increased, and that among households having a supply of less than one quart per adult male unit for the 15-day period (approximately 65 grams per day), the incidence was three times as great as in households which had larger supplies of milk.[13] The significance of this indication becomes clearer when it is recalled that the presence of a large milk supply in a household was not a mere reflection of a better economic status and therefore of an ability to buy other possibly preventive articles of diet since, as may be seen by reference to Table 14, nonpellagrous households

12 It is probable that the informants' statements of quantity of milk supply tended toward slight exaggeration, especially in the case of cow-owning households. Inexact measurements of milk produced (e.g., a "gallon" of milk as stated was probably a gallon bucket not quite full at milking time), the habit of stating quantities in round numbers, coupled with a not unnatural disposition, to exaggerate the yield of a home-owned cow, undoubtedly resulted in overstatements, rather than understatements, of the household milk supply.

13 It may be worth noting, however, that pellagra was observed in households with a milk supply, as reported, averaging approximately one quart per adult male unit per day. As pointed out in the preceding footnote, there is a probability that this amount is somewhat overstated. We have no information, moreover, as to the distribution of the milk among individual members of the households other than the general but frequently made observation that wide variations in the amount consumed by individuals do occur.

(No. 2) with lowest incomes had an even larger average supply of milk than did those with highest incomes (No. 1).

Further evidence that pellagra was relatively rare among households having a liberal supply of fresh milk is afforded in a classification of households according to the ownership of milk-giving cows. [Tabulation of these statistics deleted. ED.] The incidence of pellagra among households having milk from such a source was less than 3 per cent as against nearly 10 per cent in households without a supply from such a source. The contrast in incidence of two or more cases in a single household is even more striking. The significance of this indication is enhanced when we note that in the group of no-cow-owning families some enjoyed a liberal supply of milk by purchase.

In connection with the foregoing, Bouchard's observation (Bouchard, 1862, p. 186), over half a century old, is of great interest. He closes a discussion of the relation of occupation to pellagra with a statement of what he justly characterized as a "remarkable fact," namely, "Shepherds are almost all pellagrous (in the endemic area of southwestern France); cowherds are hardly ever such. They have the same occupation, the same manner of life, but the cowherd nourishes himself in large part with milk." Quite characteristically, however, a milk diet had been accused by some previous observers as the cause of the disease (Roussel, 1845, p. 161).

TABLE 17—*Pellagra incidence during 1916 among households of cotton-mill workers in seven villages of South Carolina, classified according to the household milk supply per adult male unit for a fifteen-day period between April 16 and June 15, 1916.*

Household milk supply in quarts per adult male unit, for a 15-day period.	Total number of households.	Number of households affected with pellagra.	Per cent of households affected with pellagra.
All amounts............	727	56	7.7
Less than 1.0.........	154	28	18.0
1.0-6.9...............	262	16*	6.2
7.0-12.9..............	163	8	4.9
13.0-18.9.............	90	4	4.4
19.0 and over.........	58	0	.0

*Includes one household using milk at the time of canvass by advice of family physician attending pellagrin, but not using milk previously so far as it could be ascertained.

Fresh meats.—In the present analysis the item "fresh meats" includes the same varieties as were included in this item in the tables already presented. The incidence of pellagra in relation to varying supplies of fresh meat is shown in Table 18. [Graphic representation deleted. ED.] It will be observed that as the fresh meat supply increased, the incidence of pellagra declined in almost as marked a manner as in the case of milk; the incidence among households having a fresh-meat supply of less than 1 pound per adult male unit per 15-day period (approximately 30 grams per day) was more than three times as great as in households with a larger supply.

Inasmuch, however, as the average supply of fresh meat per household was considerably higher, and a large supply appeared more frequently among households with the highest than among those with the lowest incomes (Table 14), the possibility is suggested that a relatively large supply of fresh meat may have been merely a reflection of better economic status, and thus of the ability to purchase other possibly preventive articles of diet. The data were further analyzed, therefore, in order to determine whether the variation in the fresh-meat supply within household groups of different economic conditions showed a relation to pellagra incidence similar to that just observed.

For this purpose the households were divided into three income classes, and each in turn subdivided into groups of households with varying meat supply and then the incidence of pellagra was com-

TABLE 18—*Pellagra incidence during 1916 among households of cotton-mill workers in seven villages of South Carolina, classified according to the household fresh-meat supply per adult male unit for a fifteen-day period between April 16 and June 15, 1916.*

Household supply of fresh meats in pounds per adult male unit, for a 15-day period.	Total number of households.	Number of households affected with pellagra.	Per cent of households affected with pellagra.
All amounts...........	741	61	8.2
Less than 1.0.........	495	54	10.9
1.0-1.9...............	131	4	3.1
2.0-2.9...............	61	2	3.3
3.0-3.9...............	36	1	2.8
4.0 and over..........	18	0	.0

puted for each of these groups. The results appear in Table 19. While the subdivision of the households in each income class necessitates the consideration of rather small numbers, nevertheless it seems fairly clearly indicated that, while there is a decline in incidence with increased income, the supply of fresh meat remaining the same, there is quite a sharp and fairly regular decline in pellagra incidence as the supply of fresh meat increases in the lower two of the three income classes, no definite effect being appreciable in that of the highest income. If the use of fresh meat were merely a concomitant of high income, the tendency to a diminution of the incidence rate with an increase in the fresh-meat supply in households of the same income class should practically disappear. The fact, however, that a clearly marked tendency to a decline in incidence with increase in supply is present among households whose half-month's incomes were between $6 and $10 as well as among those with less than $6 appears to confirm and strengthen the previous indication that pellagra incidence was materially lower when the

TABLE 19—*Pellagra incidence during 1916 among households of cotton-mill workers of different incomes in seven villages of South Carolina, classified according to the household fresh-meat supply, per adult male unit for fifteen-day period between April 16 and June 15, 1916.*

Household supply of fresh meats in pounds per adult male unit, for a 15-day period.	Family income during a 15-day period per adult male unit.		
	Under $6.	$6 to $9.99	$10 and over.
Total number of households:			
Less than 0.5......................	124	159	81
0.5-0.9...........................	27	51	35
1.0-1.9...........................	35	68	45
2.0 and over......................	26	41	48
Number of households affected with pellagra:			
Less than 0.5......................	19	20	2
0.5-0.9...........................	3	6	1
1.0-1.9...........................	3	2	1
2.0 and over......................	1	2	0
Per cent of households affected with pellagra:			
Less than 0.5......................	15.3	12.6	2.5
0.5-0.9...........................	11.1	11.8	2.9
1.0-1.9...........................	8.6	2.9	2.2
2.0 and over......................	3.8	4.9	0.0

average daily household supply of fresh meat was more than approximately 30 grams per adult male unit per day.

Milk or fresh meats.—Our analyses having indicated in a definite manner that pellagra occurred less frequently or not at all in households having a daily minimum average supply of approximately a pint of milk or of 30 grams of fresh meat per adult male unit, it becomes important to ascertain whether these associations are independent each of the other. Accordingly we have attempted to determine this by observing the variation in the pellagra rate for households having but a small supply of the one when grouped according to variations in supply of the other. This analysis is shown in Tables 20 and 21. [Graphic representation deleted. ED.] The households having a supply of fresh meat exceeding 1 pound per adult male unit per 15-day period (approximately 30 grams daily) are discarded in the former table, and those having a supply of milk of over 7 quarts per adult male unit per 15-day period (approximately 1 pint daily) are discarded in the latter.[14] The results of this analysis clearly indicate that an increasing supply of each of these foods, independently of the other, was definitely associated with a decreasing pellagra incidence.

TABLE 20—*Pellagra incidence during 1916 among households of cotton-mill workers in seven villages of South Carolina, whose supply of fresh meats was less than one pound per adult male unit per fifteen-day period, classified according to the household supply of milk, per adult male unit, for a fifteen-day period between April 16 and June 15, 1916.*

Household supply of milk in quarts per adult male unit, for a 15-day period.	Total number of households.	Number of households affected with pellagra.	Per cent of households affected with pellagra.
All amounts..............	464	46	10.0
Less than 1.0............	103	23	22.3
1.0-3.9..................	63	5	7.9
4.0-6.9..................	90	7	7.8
7.0-12.9.................	102	7	6.9
13.0-18.9................	67	4	6.0
19.0 and over...........	39	0	0.0

14 The mass of our data was too small to permit of restricting this analysis to households with a still smaller milk supply.

Other "animal protein" foods.—Analyses with respect to the other individual foods of the "animal protein" group were attempted but proved unsatisfactory by reason of the insufficient mass of the available data. It is to be noted, however, that the indications afforded by the analysis presented with respect to fresh milk should be regarded as, in a general way, also representative of butter, for, as has already been mentioned, fresh milk appeared in the diet of the mill people in the form, for the most part, of home-churned buttermilk and butter.

Foods of the Groups Associated with Increased Pellagra Incidence

As has been seen (Table 16) the diet of our group of nonpellagrous households of the lowest income (No. 2) closely resembles the diets of our pellagrous groups with respect to the supply from all but one of the classes of foods, namely, the "animal protein" foods, a liberal supply of which is associated with a relative or absolute freedom from the disease. Conversely, a reduced or minimal supply of the foods of this group *in relation to the type of diet under consideration* may be considered as associated with an increased pellagra incidence.[15] Or, viewed in another way, one may regard

TABLE 21—*Pellagra incidence during 1916 among households of cotton-mill workers in seven villages of South Carolina, whose supply of fresh milk was less than seven quarts per adult male unit per fifteen-day period, classified according to the household supply of fresh meats per adult male unit, for a fifteen-day period between April 16 and June 15, 1916.*

Household supply of fresh meats in pounds per adult male unit, for a 15-day period.	Total number of households.	Number of households affected with pellagra.	Per cent of households affected with pellagra.
All amounts..............	435	45	10.3
Less than 1.0...........	282	40	14.2
1.0-2.9.................	114	4	3.5
3.0 and over...........	39	1	2.6

15 This is not to be interpreted as meaning that a restricted supply of the "animal protein" foods is necessarily the cause of pellagra or that only foods of this group are pellagra preventive.

the portion of these diets (i.e., the diets here considered) exclusive of the "animal protein" group as approximating a pellagra-producing diet.[16] Analyses were therefore made of the relation to pellagra incidence of variations in supply of a number of the more conspicuous (quantitatively) foods included in what may be regarded as the pellagra-producing combination.

Corn meal.—In Table 22 are shown the results of an analysis of our data in relation to corn meal. As might have been anticipated from the indications afforded by the statistics of average quantities shown in Tables 14 and 15 and by the frequency figures in Tables 28 and 29, no consistent correlation is apparent. This is of great interest when the etiological rôle that has for so long been attributed by Italian students of the disease to spoiled maize is recalled. It is quite exceptional for mill-village stores to have on sale at one time more than one grade of meal; and so all households in any one village using this cereal are supplied with the same quality of this product. If, therefore, spoiled corn is, as Lombroso and his pupils have taught, the cause of pellagra, then it would seem reasonable to expect some indication of an increasing incidence with an increase in supply. This our tables do not show to be the case; on the

TABLE 22—*Pellagra incidence during 1916 among households of cotton-mill workers in seven villages of South Carolina, classified according to the household corn* meal supply† per adult male unit for a fifteen-day period between April 16 and June 15, 1916.*

Household supply of corn meal in pounds per adult male unit, for a 15-day period.	Total number of households.	Number of households affected with pellagra.	Per cent of households affected with pellagra.
All amounts.............	742	61	8.2
0-3.9....................	304	20	6.6
4.0-7.9.................	260	24	9.2
8.0-11.9................	117	13	11.1
12.0 and over...........	61	4	6.6

*Maize.
†Includes grits.

16 This was one of the indications followed in formulating the experimental diet used in the Rankin Farm (Mississippi) prison experiment (Goldberger and Wheeler, 1915 and 1920; also Goldberger, 1916).

TABLE 23—*Pellagra incidence during 1916 among households of cotton-mill workers in seven villages of South Carolina, classified according to the household wheat flour supply per adult male unit for a fifteen-day period between April 16 and June 15, 1916.*

Household supply of wheat flour in pounds per adult male unit, for a 15-day period.	Total number of households.	Number of households affected with pellagra.	Per cent of households affected with pellagra.
All amounts............	748	61	8.2
0-3.9.................	61	7	11.5
4.0-7.9................	46	4	8.7
8.0-11.9...............	182	15	8.2
12.0-15.9..............	199	16	8.0
16.0 and over..........	260	19	7.3

contrary it appears (Tables 14, 28, and 29) that this cereal was used quite as liberally in the nonpellagrous as in the pellagrous households. Our results cannot, therefore, be interpreted as affording any support to the etiological theory which up to within the past few years had all but universally been the accepted one. This lack

TABLE 24—*Pellagra incidence during 1916 among households of cotton-mill workers in seven villages of South Carolina, whose supply of fresh meats was less than one pound, and of fresh milk less than four quarts, per adult male unit per fifteen-day period, classified according to the household supply of wheat flour per adult male unit for a fifteen-day period between April 16 and June 15, 1916.*

Household supply of wheat flour in pounds per adult male unit, for a 15-day period.	Total number of households.	Number of households affected with pellagra.	Per cent of households affected with pellagra.
All amounts............	175	29	16.6
0-3.9.................	15	5	33.3
4.0-7.9................	8	0	0
8.0-11.9...............	44	8	18.2
12.0-15.9..............	49	6	12.2
16.0 and over..........	59	10	17.0

TABLE 25—*Pellagra incidence during 1916 among households of cotton-mill workers in seven villages of South Carolina, classified according to the household supply of dried peas and beans per adult male unit for a fifteen-day period between April 16 and June 15, 1916.*

Household supply of dried peas and beans in pounds per adult male unit, for a 15-day period.	Total number of households.	Number of households affected with pellagra.	Per cent of households affected with pellagra.
All amounts.............	747	61	8.2
Less than 0.5...........	255	18	7.1
0.5-0.9.................	150	12	8.0
1.0-1.9.................	199	18	9.0
2.0 and over...........	143	13	9.1

of indication would seem to be in harmony with the results of the controlled feeding experiment of Goldberger and Wheeler (1915 and 1920), in which at least 6 of 11 convicts subsisting on a diet containing corn of good quality developed pellagra.

TABLE 26—*Pellagra incidence during 1916 among households of cotton-mill workers of the lowest income class* in seven villages of South Carolina, classified according to the household supply of dried peas and beans per adult male unit for a fifteen-day period between April 16 and June 15, 1916.*

Household supply of dried peas and beans in pounds per adult male unit, for a 15-day period.	Total number of households.	Number of households affected with pellagra.	Per cent of households affected with pellagra.
All amounts.............	216	27	12.5
Less than 0.5...........	77	9	11.7
0.5-0.9.................	43	7	16.3
1.0-1.9.................	49	4	8.2
2.0 and over...........	47	7	14.9

*All the households considered had a total cash income of less than $6 per adult male unit in the family during the half month for which dietary records were secured.

Wheat flour.—The results with respect to wheat flour are shown in Tables 23 and 24. In the first of these tables there appears a suggestion of an inverse correlation in pellagra incidence, but when this was tested by eliminating the households having supplies of milk and fresh meat in significant quantities the results, as shown in the second of these tables (Table 24), are irregular and the suggested correlation disappears. This, however, may be due to the rather small mass of data that is thus left for study. Definite determination of this point must be left to further study.

Dried legumes.—With respect to dried legumes,[17] the results of our analyses are presented in Tables 25, 26, and 27. Although a slight suggestion of a direct correlation appears in Table 25 and again in Table 27 it is altogether absent from Table 26; so that, on the whole, we have here no significant variations in incidence with variation in supply. This is in harmony with the indications afforded by the statistics of average quantities presented in Tables 14 and 15 and by the frequency of supply in various amounts shown in Tables 28 and 29, namely, that the use of dried legumes appeared to be quite similar in the case of nonpellagrous and of pellagrous

TABLE 27—*Pellagra incidence during 1916 among households of cotton-mill workers whose supply of fresh meats was less than one pound and of fresh milk was less than four quarts per adult male unit per fifteen-day period, classified according to the household supply of dried peas and beans per adult male unit for a fifteen-day period between April 16 and June 15, 1916.*

Household supply of dried peas and beans in pounds per adult male unit, for a 15-day period.	Total number of households.	Number of households affected with pellagra.	Per cent of households affected with pellagra.
All amounts...........	169	28	16.6
Less than 0.5.........	44	6	13.6
0.5-0.9..............	29	4	13.8
1.0-1.9..............	46	9	19.6
2.0 and over.........	50	9	18.0

17 The dried legumes principally used were "white" beans, "pink" beans, and field, or cowpeas. Beans were used in considerably larger quantities than peas.

TABLE 28—*Percentages of households having supplies of various articles of food in different quantities per adult male unit per day, in seven cotton-mill villages of South Carolina, during a fifteen-day period between April 16 and June 15, 1916, compared for non-pellagrous households and for households in which one or more cases occurred in March–July, 1916, all households being in the lowest income class.*

| | | Per cent of households whose average daily supply per adult male unit was-- | | | |
Article of food and group of household.	Average daily supply per adult male unit.	None.	None or less than one-third average of all households.	One-third but less than average of all households.	Average or more than average of all households.
Fresh meats:	Grams.				
All households..........	26.6	......	......	......	......
Nonpellagrous..........	19.9	47.8	52.2	16.7	30.6
Pellagrous..............	9.4	64.3	67.9	17.9	14.3
Cured lean meats:					
All households..........	22.8	......	......	......	......
Nonpellagrous..........	11.8	58.6	62.5	12.8	24.4
Pellagrous..............	11.1	53.6	53.6	39.3	7.1
Canned meats:					
All households..........	14.0	......	......	......	......
Nonpellagrous..........	10.6	49.2	54.6	17.5	27.9
Pellagrous..............	17.5	33.3	33.3	33.3	33.3
Eggs:					
All households..........	43.1	......	......	......	......
Nonpellagrous..........	38.7	31.8	41.7	26.4	31.9
Pellagrous..............	30.6	17.9	39.3	35.7	25.0
Fresh milk:					
All households..........	493.4	......	......	......	......
Nonpellagrous..........	554.0	19.1	27.0	32.0	41.0
Pellagrous..............	187.2	42.3	65.4	23.1	11.5
Preserved milk:					
All households..........	2.8	......	......	......	......
Nonpellagrous..........	2.3	85.2	85.2	1.1	13.7
Pellagrous..............	2.8	64.3	64.3	3.6	32.1
Butter:					
All households..........	30.8	......	......	......	......
Nonpellagrous..........	30.2	20.7	33.5	28.5	38.0
Pellagrous..............	16.0	20.0	52.0	36.0	12.0
Cheese:					
All households..........	2.3	......	......	......	......
Nonpellagrous..........	2.0	74.7	74.7	3.3	22.0
Pellagrous..............	0.2	92.8	92.8	3.6	3.6
Salt pork:					
All households..........	52.3	......	......	......	......
Nonpellagrous..........	50.7	4.5	7.8	49.7	42.5
Pellagrous..............	69.5	3.6	7.1	42.9	50.0
Lard and lard substitutes:					
All households..........	47.3	......	......	......	......
Nonpellagrous..........	37.1	10.9	19.7	44.8	35.5
Pellagrous..............	32.0	10.7	17.9	50.0	32.1
Dried peas and beans:					
All households..........	32.3	......	......	......	......
Nonpellagrous..........	31.4	28.4	33.3	27.3	39.4
Pellagrous..............	31.4	17.9	28.6	32.2	39.3

Table 28 *(continued)*

Article of food and group of household.	Average daily supply per adult male unit.	Per cent of households whose average daily supply per adult male unit was--			
		None.	None or less than one-third average of all households.	One-third but less than average of all households.	Average or more than average of all households.
Canned peas and beans:	Grams.				
All households........	4.2	......	......	......	......
Nonpellagrous.........	1.8	89.6	89.6	0.0	10.4
Pellagrous............	3.3	85.7	85.7	0.0	14.3
Wheat flour:					
All households........	415.9	......	......	......	......
Nonpellagrous.........	398.6	7.7	9.3	49.7	41.0
Pellagrous............	323.1	7.1	14.3	53.6	32.1
Wheat bread, cakes, and crackers:					
All households........	14.1	......	......	......	......
Nonpellagrous.........	10.3	42.2	54.6	18.6	26.8
Pellagrous............	13.1	46.4	50.0	17.9	32.1
Corn meal:					
All households........	153.7	......	......	......	......
Nonpellagrous.........	164.9	18.7	21.4	28.6	50.0
Pellagrous............	149.8	10.7	17.9	35.7	46.4
Grits:					
All households........	5.9	......	......	......	......
Nonpellagrous.........	6.6	89.6	89.6	0.5	9.8
Pellagrous............	3.3	89.3	89.3	0.0	10.7
Rice:					
All households........	5.1	......	......	......	......
Nonpellagrous.........	5.4	71.6	72.1	0.0	27.9
Pellagrous............	4.2	75.0	75.0	0.0	25.0
Green string beans:					
All households........	11.6	......	......	......	......
Nonpellagrous.........	6.6	85.2	91.8	6.0	2.2
Pellagrous............	3.5	89.3	96.4	3.6	0.0
Canned string beans:					
All households........	4.5	......	......	......	......
Nonpellagrous.........	4.1	86.8	86.8	0.0	13.2
Pellagrous............	1.3	96.4	96.4	0.0	3.6
Green vegetables (bought):					
All households........	50.1	......	......	......	......
Nonpellagrous.........	33.9	29.4	35.6	31.1	33.3
Pellagrous............	32.3	21.4	42.9	32.1	25.0
Other canned vegetables:					
All households........	35.6	......	......	......	......
Nonpellagrous.........	32.9	35.5	41.0	20.8	38.2
Pellagrous............	27.8	39.3	46.4	17.9	35.7

(Table 28 continued on page 176)

households. The present study therefore fails to confirm deductions from epidemiologic observations made by one of us (J. G.) about five years ago with respect to the apparently important preventive value of the common varieties of dried beans and peas.

Table 28 (*continued*)

Article of food and group of household.	Average daily supply per adult male unit.	Per cent of households whose average daily supply per adult male unit was--			
		None.	None or less than one-third average of all households.	One-third but less than average of all households.	Average or more than average of all households.
Fresh fruits:	Grams.				
All households.........	28.4	......	......	......	......
Nonpellagrous..........	21.1	49.2	52.5	22.1	25.4
Pellagrous.............	9.7	50.0	67.9	17.8	14.3
Dried fruits:					
All households.........	9.2	......	......	......	......
Nonpellagrous..........	9.7	44.0	44.0	2.2	53.8
Pellagrous.............	9.7	46.4	46.4	0.0	53.6
Canned fruits:					
All households.........	18.7	......	......	......	......
Nonpellagrous..........	14.5	67.2	67.7	8.7	23.5
Pellagrous.............	16.6	64.3	64.3	7.1	28.6
Irish potatoes:					
All households.........	74.4	......	......	......	......
Nonpellagrous..........	63.7	42.6	46.4	14.8	38.8
Pellagrous.............	71.0	39.3	50.0	7.1	42.9
Fresh sweet potatoes:					
All households.........	6.3	......	......	......	......
Nonpellagrous..........	3.9	96.7	96.7	0.0	3.3
Pellagrous.............	1.7	96.5	96.5	0.0	3.5
Canned sweet potatoes:					
All households.........	3.9	......	......	......	......
Nonpellagrous..........	3.1	91.2	91.2	0.0	8.8
Pellagrous.............	1.4	85.7	85.7	0.0	14.3
Sugar:					
All households.........	46.2	......	......	......	......
Nonpellagrous..........	39.6	15.3	24.0	50.3	27.7
Pellagrous.............	37.1	14.3	21.4	39.3	39.3
Sirup:					
All households.........	16.3	......	......	......	......
Nonpellagrous..........	8.6	63.4	63.4	2.7	33.9
Pellagrous.............	15.1	64.3	64.3	3.6	32.1
Jellies and jams:					
All households.........	7.9	......	......	......	......
Nonpellagrous..........	4.2	66.9	66.9	8.8	24.3
Pellagrous.............	7.5	53.6	57.2	21.4	21.4

It is important to note, however, that in the light of various recent studies (Daniels and Nichols, 1917; Daniels and Laughlin, 1918; McCollum, 1917; and Osborne and Mendel, 1917) this does not necessarily apply to other species and probably still less to the immature or green stage, namely, the green string bean. Indeed, our observations, indicating as they do that the abundant seasonal supply of the green string bean is associated with the marked seasonal

TABLE 29—*Percentages of households having supplies of various articles of food in different quantities per adult male unit per day in seven cotton-mill villages of South Carolina during a fifteen-day period between April 16 and June 15, 1916, compared for non-pellagrous households with highest incomes and for households in which two or more cases occurred in March–July, 1916.*

		Per cent of households whose average daily supply per adult male unit was--			
Article of food and group of households.	Average daily supply per adult male unit.	None.	None or less than one-third average of all households.	One-third but less than average of all households.	Average or more than average of all households.
Fresh meats:	Grams.				
All households............................	26.6	......	....	......	......
Nonpellagrous (highest incomes)..........	48.9	25.4	25.4	11.1	63.5
Pellagrous (with two or more cases)......	16.3	59.1	63.6	13.6	22.7
Cured lean meats:					
All households............................	22.8	......	....	......	......
Nonpellagrous (highest incomes)..........	54.0	23.8	31.8	6.3	61.9
Pellagrous (with two or more cases)......	8.1	54.6	59.1	27.3	18.2
Canned meats:					
All households............................	14.0	......	....	......	......
Nonpellagrous (highest incomes)..........	25.1	49.2	52.7	6.3	41.3
Pellagrous (with two or more cases)......	15.7	45.5	45.5	22.7	31.8
Eggs:					
All households............................	43.1	......	....	......	......
Nonpellagrous (highest incomes)..........	69.5	3.2	6.3	25.4	68.3
Pellagrous (with two or more cases)......	31.1	18.2	31.8	31.8	36.4
Fresh milk:					
All households............................	493.4	......	....	......	......
Nonpellagrous (highest incomes)..........	379.3	17.5	23.8	50.8	25.4
Pellagrous (with two or more cases)......	126.9	50.0	79.0	15.0	15.0
Preserved milk:					
All households............................	2.8	......	....	......	......
Nonpellagrous (highest incomes)..........	4.5	74.6	74.6	0.0	25.4
Pellagrous (with two or more cases)......	1.8	77.3	77.3	0.0	22.7
Butter:					
All households............................	30.8	......	....	......	......
Nonpellagrous (highest incomes)..........	27.2	14.3	25.4	25.4	49.2
Pellagrous (with two or more cases)......	11.2	25.0	50.0	40.0	10.0
Cheese:					
All households............................	2.3	......	....	......	......
Nonpellagrous (highest incomes)..........	3.6	76.2	76.2	0.0	23.8
Pellagrous (with two or more cases)......	.2	95.5	95.5	0.0	4.5
Salt pork:					
All households............................	52.3	......	....	......	......
Nonpellagrous (highest incomes)..........	38.6	-17.5	23.8	31.8	44.5
Pellagrous (with two or more cases).....	65.2	4.5	4.5	36.4	59.1
Lard and lard substitutes:					
All households............................	47.3	......	....	......	......
Nonpellagrous (with highest incomes)....	52.8	14.3	17.5	25.4	57.2
Pellagrous (with two or more cases).....	34.7	9.1	18.2	68.2	13.6
Dried peas and beans:					
All households............................	32.3	......	....	......	......
Nonpellagrous (highest incomes)........	31.1	31.8	33.3	23.8	42.9
Pellagrous (with two or more cases).....	34.1	9.1	22.7	31.8	45.5

(*Table 29 continued on page 178*)

decline in incidence of the disease, suggest the possibility of a distinctly preventive rôle for this vegetable. It is hoped that the large mass of data collected during 1917 now being analyzed may afford more definite indications on this point.

Table 29 *(continued)*

Article of food and group of households.	Average daily supply per adult male unit.	Per cent of households whose average daily supply per adult male unit was--			
		None.	None or less than one-third average of all households.	One-third but less than average of all households.	Average or more than average of all households.
Canned peas and beans:	Grams.				
All households............................	4.2	......	......	......	......
Nonpellagrous (highest incomes)..........	12.1	71.4	71.4	1.6	27.0
Pellagrous (with two or more cases)......	1.6	90.9	90.9	0.0	9.1
Wheat flour:					
All households............................	415.9	......	......	......	......
Nonpellagrous (highest incomes)..........	445.4	9.5	9.5	44.5	46.0
Pellagrous (with two or more cases)......	351.5	4.5	13.6	45.5	40.9
Wheat bread, cakes, and crackers:					
All households............................	14.1	......	......	......	......
Nonpellagrous (highest incomes)..........	18.1	39.7	42.9	14.3	42.9
Pellagrous (with two or more cases)......	9.4	36.4	50.0	18.2	31.8
Corn meal:					
All households............................	153.7	......	......	......	......
Nonpellagrous (highest incomes)..........	127.1	31.8	31.8	30.2	38.1
Pellagrous (with two or more cases)......	144.3	9.1	18.2	45.5	36.4
Grits:					
All households............................	5.9	......	......	......	......
Nonpellagrous (highest incomes)..........	9.4	81.0	81.0	1.6	17.5
Pellagrous (with two or more cases)......	5.2	95.5	95.5	0.0	4.5
Rice:					
All households............................	5.1	......	......	......	......
Nonpellagrous (highest incomes)..........	4.5	60.3	60.3	1.6	38.1
Pellagrous (with two or more cases)......	5.5	72.7	72.7	0.0	27.3
Green string beans:					
All households............................	11.6	......	......	......	......
Nonpellagrous (highest incomes)..........	31.7	47.6	73.0	23.8	3.2
Pellagrous (with two or more cases)......	3.4	86.4	95.5	4.5	0.0
Canned string beans:					
All households............................	4.5	......	......	......	......
Nonpellagrous (highest incomes)..........	9.1	85.7	85.7	0.0	14.3
Pellagrous (with two or more cases)......	0.0	100.0	100.0	0.0	0.0
Green vegetables (bought):					
All households............................	50.1	......	......	......	......
Nonpellagrous (highest incomes)..........	90.6	27.0	33.0	28.6	38.1
Pellagrous (with two or more cases)......	57.4	9.1	45.5	18.2	36.4
Other canned vegetables:					
All households............................	35.6	......	......	......	......
Nonpellagrous (highest incomes)..........	67.7	19.1	22.2	12.7	65.1
Pellagrous (with two or more cases)......	26.2	31.8	31.8	27.3	40.9

(Table 29 continued on page 179)

Other foods.—Similar single-food analyses were also attempted with respect to potatoes, fruit, and fresh vegetables without significant indications. No weight can be attached to this, however, by reason of the fact that but a small mass of data was available for the study relating to these foods.

Dietary Factors

We have thus far studied the food supply constituting the diets of nonpellagrous and those of pellagrous households with the view,

Table 29 (*continued*)

Article of food and group of households.	Average daily supply per adult male unit.	Per cent of households whose average daily supply per adult male unit was--			
		None.	None or less than one-third average of all households.	One-third but less than average of all households.	Average or more than average of all households.
Fresh fruits:	Grams.				
All households........................	28.4	......	......	......	......
Nonpellagrous (highest incomes)........	43.2	36.5	42.9	19.1	38.1
Pellagrous (with two or more cases)....	10.1	50.0	63.6	22.7	13.6
Dried fruits:					
All households........................	9.2	......	......	......	......
Nonpellagrous (highest incomes)........	9.7	65.1	65.1	6.3	28.6
Pellagrous (with two or more cases)....	9.5	54.6	54.6	4.5	40.9
Canned fruits:					
All households........................	18.7	......	......	......	......
Nonpellagrous (highest incomes)........	37.4	36.5	39.7	7.9	52.4
Pellagrous (with two or more cases)....	15.7	68.2	68.2	9.1	22.7
Irish potatoes:					
All households........................	74.4	......	......	......	......
Nonpellagrous (highest incomes)........	48.9	49.2	50.8	12.7	36.5
Pellagrous (with two or more cases)....	53.1	45.5	50.0	18.2	31.8
Fresh sweet potatoes:					
All households........................	6.3	......	......	......	......
Nonpellagrous (highest incomes)........	7.9	93.6	93.6	0.0	6.4
Pellagrous (with two or more cases)....	3.9	95.2	95.2	0.0	4.8
Canned sweet potatoes:					
All households........................	3.9	......	......	......	......
Nonpellagrous (highest incomes)........	7.9	85.7	85.7	0.0	14.3
Pellagrous (with two or more cases)....	3.1	80.9	80.9	0.0	9.1
Sugar:					
All households........................	46.2	......	......	......	......
Nonpellagrous (highest incomes)........	55.6	14.3	20.6	22.2	57.2
Pellagrous (with two or more cases)....	32.0	22.7	22.7	40.9	36.4
Sirup:					
All households........................	16.3	......	......	......	......
Nonpellagrous (highest incomes)........	17.9	73.0	73.0	3.2	23.8
Pellagrous (with two or more cases)....	22.6	50.0	50.0	4.5	45.5
Jellies and jams:					
All households........................	7.9	......	......	......	......
Nonpellagrous (highest incomes)........	10.9	44.5	47.6	3.2	49.2
Pellagrous (with two or more cases)....	6.0	45.5	45.5	27.3	27.3

primarily, of discovering outstanding differences of a general character, and we have seen that the only difference between them to which significance could properly be attached related to a more liberal supply of the "animal protein" foods which the nonpellagrous enjoyed. It becomes important now to examine the more intimate make-up of these diets with a view to ascertaining in more detail the essential differences between them.

Calories.—Attention has already been called to the caloric value (Table 16) of the diets under discussion. The average energy value of the edible portion of the food supply of the pellagrous households may be taken as approximately 3,300 calories, which is somewhat less than that of the nonpellagrous households of comparable economic status.

These figures represent an estimate of the energy supplied, not that consumed. To determine the latter, some deduction for waste should be made. What this actually was we found it impracticable to attempt to determine, but judging from such general observations as we were able to make we believe that this was on the whole rather small and related mainly to the bread foods (corn meal and wheat flour). The careful dietary studies of the United States Department of Agriculture have shown that in private families the waste may range from practically zero to as high as 8 or 10 per cent (W. O. Atwater, Farmers' Bulletin, No. 142, p. 46). A deduction from our figures of 10 per cent for waste may therefore be considered as a fairly liberal allowance. Deducting this, we find that the average energy value of the diet of the pellagrous households was about 2,970 calories, which will at once be recognized as conforming remarkably well to accepted standards (Lusk, 1917, p. 347; Chittenden, 1907, p. 280), and so the fuel supply of the diet would seem in itself not to be an *essential* factor in relation to the incidence of the disease, although the fact that the average fuel supply of the nonpellagrous households of like income status tended to be somewhat larger would suggest that this factor may not be altogether without significance.

Protein.—The approximate protein content of the total average food supply per adult male unit per day has been computed for each of the four groups compared in the foregoing. The same limitations as to accuracy noted with respect to potential fuel value apply here. The results are therefore estimates of the average total number of grams of protein per adult male unit per day in the edible portion of the food supply of the sample period. [Tabulation of these statistics deleted. ED.] Except for a small allowance that should be made for waste, this very nearly represents the average quantity of protein consumed. Although these quantities cannot be regarded as exact, we believe that, like the caloric values, they are sufficiently close approximations for the present purpose. Diet No. 1 supplies approximately 128; No. 2, 105; No. 3, 84; and No. 4, 85 grams of protein. From this it is evident that the protein supply of the two groups of pellagrous households (No. 3 and No. 4) is identical, and at the same time it is somewhat smaller than that of the groups of nonpellagrous households.

With the exception of the nonpellagrous households of the highest income (No. 1), the protein supply in all these diets is considerably lower than the older American standards (Atwater) call for. Nevertheless, even after allowing for waste, the supply of the pellagrous households exceeds somewhat the allowance of 60 grams considered by Chittenden (1907, p. 272) as being more than sufficient to meet the true needs of the body, and very much exceeds the quantity (25 grams) found by Hindehede (1913, p. 134) to be sufficient. In this connection it may be noted that the proportion of the total caloric supply derived from protein is practically the same in all four diets under consideration. These facts would suggest, therefore, that the quantity of protein supplied is in itself not an *essential* factor in relation to the incidence of pellagra, although as with the caloric supply the greater average supply of protein in nonpellagrous households would suggest that this may not be without significance.

In view of the importance attaching to the biologic quality of the protein, particularly emphasized by the recent studies of McCollum and by those of Osborne and Mendel, we have examined the sources of the protein supply of each of the diets here considered and find that in diet No. 1, approximately 39 per cent, in No. 2, approximately 33 per cent, in No. 3, approximately 28 per cent, and in No. 4, approximately 25 per cent is derived from animal foods. On the other hand, diet No. 1 derives approximately 57 per cent of its protein from cereals (wheat, maize, rice), and the common dried (including the canned) beans and peas, diet No. 2 derived approximately 64 per cent, diet No. 3 approximately 68 per cent, and diet No. 4 approximately 71 per cent of its protein from these sources. [Tabulation of these statistics deleted. ED.] In other words, the protein supply of the nonpellagrous households tends to include, on the one hand, a larger proportion derived from animal foods, and on the other, a somewhat smaller proportion from cereals and dried legumes than does that of pellagrous households.

In the light of such recent work as that of Osborne and Mendel (Mendel, 1915), and of McCollum (1917) and his associates, these facts would suggest that the protein mixture (amino-acid supply) in the diets of the nonpellagrous households is likely to be of a somewhat better character (physiologically adequate) than in the diet of the pellagrous groups. This likelihood is increased by the tendency to a larger intake of protein in the former than in the latter.

Carbohydrate and fat.—Inasmuch as the protein supply in the diets of the two groups of pellagrous households is quantitatively essentially identical, the total calories being the same, the supply of carbohydrate and fat considered together is, of course, likewise identical. By deducting from the total calorie supply of each of the diets the respective calories from protein, we find that the combined supply of carbohydrate and fat, expressed in calories, is for diet No. 1 approximately 3,740, for No. 2 approximately 3,400, for diet No. 3 approximately 2,940, and for No. 4 approximately 2,960. The average supply of carbohydrate and fat combined is, therefore, somewhat less in the diet of the pellagrous than in that of the non-pellagrous households. As may already have been inferred, however, the proportion of the total calories furnished by these constituents is much the same for all four diets under consideration.

Our data are not in a form to permit of satisfactory computation of the exact proportion of the total calories furnished by carbohydrate apart from fat. We may, however, by a study of Table 16 arrive at a fairly satisfactory approximation to it. With the exception of but a negligible quantity the carbohydrate is derived from the foods of other than animal origin, which latter are the principal sources of fat in the diets. Therefore, by deducting the calories derived from (1) the animal protein and (2) the salt pork and lard group from the total calories of the respective diets, we find that diet No. 1 derives approximately 2,765; No. 2, approximately 2,525; No. 3, approximately 2,200; and No. 4, approximately 2,300 calories, or 65, 66, 61, and 61 per cent, respectively, of the total number of calories of the corresponding diets are derived from carbohydrate sources, preponderatingly carbohydrate themselves. The diets of the nonpellagrous households would, therefore, appear actually somewhat more liberally supplied with carbohydrate than those of the pellagrous households. If allowance is made, however, for the probable error, previously referred to, arising from the character of the data in relation to flour and maize meal which tends to make the supply of these foods appear somewhat larger than they probably actually were in the diets of the nonpellagrous households, the difference in carbohydrate supply is somewhat reduced and, perhaps, largely disappears. In any event these data would not seem to bear out the suggestion repeatedly encountered in the literature (Albera, Gherardini, Strambio) and recently particularly emphasized by Deeks (1912 and 1916), that the production of pellagra is dependent on the excessive consumption of carbohydrate.

Sources of fat supply.—It is of interest and importance to consider the sources of the fat supply in these diets. As might have been anticipated from what has gone before, both the nonpellagrous groups enjoy a larger supply from such sources as milk and butter than do the pellagrous. The most important other sources are salt pork and lard, but no significant difference between the diets of pellagrous and nonpellagrous households in the supply from these is discernible.

Vitamins.—In the present state of knowledge we have no means of directly measuring the content of a diet in the factors now commonly designated as vitamins. It is possible, however, to compare the relative richness of diets in vitamins on the basis of the relative supply of the foods known to carry these but recently definitely recognized essential food factors.

Since it appears from a study of Table 16 and from the facts already considered, that the supply in the diets of nonpellagrous and in those of pellagrous households of the South Carolina mill villages studied is substantially the same with respect to all groups of foods except the "animal proteins," of which the nonpellagrous enjoy a notably more liberal supply, it would seem to follow that the diets of the nonpellagrous households are correspondingly richer in the vitamins carried by the foods of this group.

Of the three vitamins at present definitely recognized, this group of foods is believed to be particularly rich in that designated by McCollum as the "fat-soluble A," so that such disparity in vitamin supply as exists between the diets of the nonpellagrous and those of the pellagrous households is particularly marked with respect to the fat-soluble factor.

Inorganic constituents.—With respect to the ash constituents, one may compare the diets on much the same basis as that for vitamins. So far as concerns the sources of supply (quantitatively or otherwise) of essential minerals the outstanding differences between the nonpellagrous and the pellagrous households again relate to the group of animal protein foods of which, in this connection, milk is the most important. Milk being generally recognized as a most valuable source of mineral elements in a diet, this would seem quite clearly to indicate that during the season represented by our data, the mineral make-up of the diets of the nonpellagrous households will tend to be superior to or, at least, is less likely to be deficient as a whole or in any of its elements than that of the pellagrous households.

Discussion

From the data that have been presented it would seem clear that basically the diet of the nonpellagrous and that of the pellagrous households (of comparable economic status) in the communities and at the season studied are much the same, the only outstanding difference being a more liberal supply of the foods of the animal protein group in the diet of the nonpellagrous households. The difference between these diets would seem, therefore, to be one of degree, not of kind. A recognition of this is of great practical importance, for, in the first place, it clearly follows that a mere qualitative statement of the diet, such as most previous workers in this field have contented themselves with may be very misleading, and, further, that a comparison of diets on the basis of data of such character may fail to reveal existing differences of considerable degree and importance, and this all the more when no account is taken of any definite season either in relation to the incidence of the disease or to that in relation to its onset in the individual. These considerations will help to explain many of the seemingly contradictory observations recorded in the literature of the subject, and further will help to make clear how worse than futile are likely to be arguments based on general, more or less hurried, and, therefore, superficial inquiries or surveys.

The significance of the indicated association of a more liberal supply of the animal proteins with a relative or absolute freedom from pellagra is very greatly enhanced by the demonstration of a marked inverse correlation between (1) the supply of milk, (2) the supply of fresh meat, and the incidence of the disease. These results, it may be noted, coincide with those previously reported from the series of studies of which the present is a part, and thus constitute additional evidence of the controlling influence of diet in the prevention and the causation of the disease. It is of interest to note in this connection that, beginning in 1735 with the first pellagrologist, Casal (cited by Lavinder, 1915), one finds in the literature repeated mention of an absence or shortage of fresh meat or animal food in the diet of those most subject to pellagra.

In this regard Strambio's comment on Albera's suggestions for the prevention of pellagra is highly significant: "But," says Strambio (1796, p. 133) "to use milk, butter, and fresh cheese in the place of oil may indeed be practicable in other places, but in the northern part of my country these are wholly lacking."

Accepting the indications of the preventive value of milk and of fresh meat, the question arises as to what element or elements in these foods to credit with their preventive action. The addition of either milk or meat to a diet means, of course, an increase in the content of the diet of the following known dietary factors: (1) Protein of a high biological quality; (2) antiscorbutic, antineuritic, and "fat soluble" vitamins; and (3) ash constituents. The question now becomes, Which of these is to be credited with the preventive action associated with a meat or milk supplement?

With respect to protein, the evidence which has already been considered seems to us to indicate that from the point of view of quantity
alone a deficiency in this factor cannot be considered as essential to
the development of pellagra; considering protein as a combination
of amino-acids, however, the possibility of a deficiency in some one
or more of these, already suggested by Voegtlin in 1914, cannot be
excluded, a possibility that must be seriously considered in view of
the principal sources of the protein and of the tendency to a relatively low level of intake observable in the diets of the pellagrous
households.

It would seem then that while the addition or increase in quantity
of milk or meat in a diet can not be interpreted as operating to prevent pellagra simply through a quantitative increase in protein as
such, it is possible that such an addition or increase is effective by
making good a possibly inadequate intake of some amino-acid or
acids; in other words, a high protein diet may be effective, not because there is any actual need for a large quantity of protein as such,
but because a larger intake is more likely to assure an adequate
supply of all essential amino-acids.

In the course of our study no clinical evidence of a lack of the antiscorbutic or the antineuritic vitamins was observed. This would suggest that at least no gross deficiency in these occurred, an interpretation that is strengthened with respect to the antineuritic vitamin,
when we note that all diets were fairly liberally supplied with the
foods believed to be rich in this factor. The preventive action of a
meat or milk supplement, therefore, would hardly seem to be due,
in any important degree at least, to an increase in quantity of these
factors.[18] It is more difficult to judge of the rôle of the "fat soluble A"
essential, by reason of the meagerness of our knowledge of the symptoms produced by a deficiency in this factor. We observed no inflammation of the eye, such as has been observed to occur in rats on diets
low in this vitamin, nor was there observed in children affected with
the disease a retardation of growth or development analogous to that
observed in rats when subsisting on a diet deficient in this dietary
essential. If the findings in rats may be applied to the human this

18 The failure to prevent the occurrence of the disease in some individuals
consuming a liberal daily supplement of soy beans and a failure to prevent
the disease in two instances after a daily consumption over a considerable
period of seven ounces of California black-eyed peas (Goldberger and
Tanner; unpublished data) would seem quite conclusively to exclude the
antineuritic vitamin, in which these legumes are believed to be rich, from
consideration as an essential factor.

would suggest that a deficiency in the "fat soluble" vitamin is not an essential factor in the production of the disease.

While this, as will be seen, is almost certainly the case it would be premature to draw this conclusion from the considerations mentioned. If, as seems probable, a deficiency in the "fat soluble A" may be expected to show itself in the human (child) as it does in the rat by a retardation of growth, the apparent absence of any notable evidence of stunting in pellagrous children can nevertheless not be interpreted as conclusively showing that a deficiency in this factor is not essential in relation to the production of pellagra. For it must be recalled that the rate of growth in the human is relatively small. Retardation to be recognizable by ordinary observation—that is, without careful weight and height measurements—would therefore have to be marked, and this could not be expected to occur except after a continuous period of deprivation of considerable length.

As under natural conditions the diet of human beings is considerably affected by seasonal changes in availability and price, and as there is in pellagra a well-marked seasonal rhythm, it is manifestly possible that the retardation occurring during one period of the year (the period of deprivation, let us say) may, in large part, if not fully, be made up during the succeeding more favorable season. Thus the effects in the child of a deficiency in this or any other growth-promoting factor might readily escape recognition or become appreciable only after the lapse of a considerable number of years, when the cumulative effects of repeated periods of deprivation, with more or less incomplete recoveries, might become sufficiently marked. The possibility that an increase in the "fat soluble A" contained in a meat or milk supplement may be an essential preventive factor would seem, however, to be eliminated by the recent observation by Goldberger and Tanner (unpublished data) of the failure to prevent the occurrence of the disease in two individuals who, daily, during a period of four to five months before developing the eruption, consumed the fat soluble vitamin contained in three ounces of creamery butter.

Another possibly preventive factor that must be considered relates to the ash constituents. Whether an improvement in any of these is essential to the prevention of the disease and is effected by an adequate meat or milk addition the facts before us do not permit of determination; the possibility that it may be cannot therefore be excluded.

From the foregoing considerations it would seem that the preventive power of a milk or fresh meat supplement may be due to the effect of a correction of a deficiency in supply (*a*) of some amino-acid or acids; (*b*) of the mineral elements; or (*c*) of some combination of these. There remains also the possibility of some as yet unrecognized factor (vitamin?) that is thus supplied and which alone, or in combination with some one or more of the factors just indicated, operates to prevent the disease.

The analogy between the occasional occurrence of pellagra in nursing infants and the same phenomenon in scurvy is very suggestive in this regard. Opposed to this possibility is McCollum's insistence (1) that but two factors of this nature are essential in mammalian nutrition, and (2) his failure to produce in rats a condition resembling pellagra in man or the pellagra-like symptoms reported by Chittenden and Underhill in the dog. (McCollum, Simmonds, and Parsons, 1919.) The force of these objections disappears, however, when the recent work (Chick, Hume, and Skelton, 1918; Cohen and Mendel, 1918; Hess and Unger, 1918; Harden and Zilva, Oct., 1918 and Dec., 1918; and Drummond, 1919) demonstrating the occurrence of a third, a "water soluble C" or antiscorbutic factor is recalled. Evidently we have the possibility that the rat is as unsuitable an experimental animal for pellagra as it is proven to be for scurvy.

Until the essential dietary factor or factors concerned in the prevention of the disease are determined, it would seem warranted to urge for prophylactic purposes an increased consumption of the foods rich in (1) protein (particularly protein of high biological quality), and (2) mineral matter. Besides milk and fresh meat, which our study would seem to indicate provide the essential preventive factor or factors,[19] cheese, fresh green vegetables and fruit may be mentioned as helping to fulfill these requirements.

Summary and Conclusions

1. To supplement the studies, chiefly experimental, of 1914 and 1915, a study was begun in the spring of 1916, in seven cotton mill villages of South Carolina of the relation of factors of a dietary, economic, and sanitary character to the incidence of pellagra. In the present communication the results of the first year's work with respect to the relation of household diet to pellagra incidence is reported.

19 It is not to be assumed that a pellagra-preventive diet—that is, a diet that is not pellagra producing—is necessarily biologically satisfactory in all respects; we believe that quite the contrary may be the case. In other words, a diet may be seriously defective in a number of respects and yet be adequate so far as pellagra-prevention is concerned.

2. The selected communities were typical cotton-mill "villages" and were of about average size; none had over 800 or less than 500 inhabitants. Only the families of white mill operatives were included in the study.

3. Pellagra incidence was determined by a systematic bi-weekly house-to-house search for cases carried on continuously from April 15, 1916, to the end of that year.

4. Only patients with a clearly defined bilaterally symmetrical eruption were recorded as having pellagra. It is suggested that, clinically, pellagra includes at least two commonly associated but etiologically essentially distinct, though closely related, syndromes.

5. Only active cases, without regard to whether they were first or recurrent attacks, were considered; the date of the appearance of the eruption was assumed to mark the onset of the attack.

6. Data relating to household diet were secured by obtaining records of sale from the principal stores, for a 15-day sample period during the season immediately anterior to or coincident with the sharp seasonal rise in incidence of the disease.

7. Comparisons of diets of nonpellagrous with those of pellagrous households revealed that the nonpellagrous enjoyed a more liberal supply of the foods of the "animal protein" group (lean meat, milk, including butter, cheese, and eggs).

8. Increasing supplies of milk or of fresh meat were found associated, one independently of the other, with a decreasing pellagra incidence.

9. No consistent correlation was found between varying supplies of either (1) maize meal, (2) wheat flour, or (3) the common dried legumes, and pellagra incidence. The results of the present study offered no support for the Zeist theory of the etiology of pellagra.

10. The potential energy in the average food supply of pellagrous households, though somewhat less than in that of nonpellagrous households, nevertheless conformed closely to accepted standards so that the fuel supply of the diet would seem in itself not to be an *essential* factor in relation to the incidence of the disease.

11. The quantity of protein in the average food supply of the pellagrous households was somewhat smaller than in that of the supply of nonpellagrous households of comparable economic status; but even after allowing for waste this exceeded somewhat the allowance considered by Chittenden as ample for physiological needs, so that a deficiency in total protein would seem not to be an *essential* factor in relation to the incidence of the disease.

12. The protein supply of the pellagrous households tended to

include, on the one hand, a somewhat smaller proportion derived from animal foods and, on the other, a somewhat larger proportion from cereals and the common mature beans and peas, which would suggest that the protein mixture (amino-acid supply) in the diets of the nonpellagrous households is more likely to be physiologically adequate than that in the diets of the pellagrous groups.

13. The proportion of calories derived from carbohydrate and fat combined is essentially identical in the supply both of pellagrous and of nonpellagrous households. The supply of carbohydrate was, if anything, somewhat smaller in the diets of the pellagrous than in those of the nonpellagrous households, so that the production of pellagra would seem not to be dependent on the excessive consumption of this nutrient.

14. The diets of the pellagrous households have a smaller average supply of the recognized vitamins than do those of the nonpellagrous, the disparity in supply being particularly marked with respect to the "fat soluble A" factor.

15. The mineral make-up of the diets of the nonpellagrous households will tend to be superior to, or, at least, is less likely to be deficient either as a whole or in any of its elements than that of the pellagrous households.

16. The indications afforded by this study suggest that the pellagra-preventive power of a milk or a meat supplement is due to the effect of a correction in the type of diet studied, of a deficiency in supply either (1) of some amino-acid or acids, (2) of the ash or of some of its constituents, (3) of some as yet unknown essential (vitamin?), or (4) of all or of a combination or combinations of some of these. Conversely, they suggest that the pellagra-producing dietary fault is the result of some one or of a combination or combinations of two or more of the following factors: (1) A physiologically defective protein (amino-acid) supply; (2) a defective or inadequate mineral supply; (3) a deficiency in an as yet unknown dietary essential (vitamin?). The somewhat lower plane of supply, both of potential energy and of protein, in the diets of the pellagrous households, though apparently not an essential factor, may, nevertheless, be contributory by favoring the occurrence of a deficiency in intake of some one or more of the essential dietary factors, particularly with diets having only a narrow margin of safety.

17. The indications afforded by this study clearly point to an increase in the availability of milk, particularly by increasing cow ownership, and of fresh meat, by all-year-round meat markets as

important practical measures of prevention and control in communities of the character studied.

Addendum: After our manuscript had gone to press there came to hand a copy of the "Report of a Committee of Enquiry Regarding the Prevalence of Pellagra among Turkish Prisoners of War" in Egypt (published February, 1919). Among the conclusions reached, the following are of most interest in the present connection:

I. "There is no evidence of the presence of any bacterial infection standing in etiological relation to pellagra.

II. "There is no evidence of infection by any protozoal, spirochetal, or ultramicroscopic organism standing in etiological relation to pellagra.

III. "Pellagra is due to a deficiency in protein, as gauged by its biological value."

Appendix

*Explanation of Articles
and Groups of Articles of Food
Presented in Tables 11, et seq.*

In order to lessen the detail of the tables presenting comparisons of the average supply of various groups of households, certain broad groupings of articles of food have been made which are defined in the following.

Fresh meats include all meats not cured, salted, or canned. The great bulk of "fresh meats" was beef. Occasionally sausage (made of beef and pork), poultry, fish, and fresh pork occurred in the household food supplies. All of the beef and pork purchased by the households during the 15-day periods were slaughtered locally and sold without much regard to cut, except with the following general distinctions: Beef was sold as "steak," "roast," and "stew meat," and pork was sold altogether in the form of sausage (mixed with beef), very little pork being slaughtered at the time of the year during which the data were collected. The prices at which steak, roast, and stew meat were sold were fairly generally in the following ratio: Steak 100, roast 75, and stew meat 50. "Stew meat" included rib meat, brisket, and all of the beef not sold as roast or steak. For these reasons this meat rather than steak or roast was more commonly purchased by the poorer households. All poultry was home or locally produced and killed at home. Fish was a local product in two villages which were near streams and, relatively, were unimportant components of the fresh meat groups.

Cured lean meats include all cured and salted meats, except salt pork, and consisted principally of bologna sausage, occasionally pork, shoulders and ham, and, rarely, breakfast bacon. All these articles were packers' products.

Canned meats include a considerable variety of kinds and brands manufactured by well-known packing and canning establishments. Salmon was by far the most important article in this group. For each household purchasing during the 15-day period "Vienna" sausage, "pork" sausage, roast beef, chipped beef, and oysters, two purchased sardines, three purchased tripe and corned beef, four purchased potted meats, and thirty used salmon.

Eggs were all country eggs, no cold storage eggs being sold.

Fresh milk includes sweet whole milk and buttermilk, the greater proportion being buttermilk. In every instance the buttermilk was from churnings made in the mill workers' households or in the households of near-by farmers, the practice being to leave a considerable residue of the butter in the milk because of unimproved methods of butter-making. The sweet milk in all cases was purchased whole or was from home-owned cows. In some households it was skimmed lightly to obtain cream for coffee. Practically all of the cows in this section were of mixed breed, with the Jersey perhaps predominating. In computing the weight of milk the specific gravity was assumed to be about 1.03.

Preserved milk includes evaporated milk and, in a very few cases, condensed milk, of the commonly known brands.

Butter in all instances was homemade or country made, all being produced locally; no butter substitutes were purchased.

Cheese in all instances was "American" pale cheese; none was home or locally produced.

Dried peas and beans include several varieties of each. Beans were principally "pink" beans (*Phaseolus vulgaris*), less frequently "white" beans, and infrequently lima beans. Peas were of the general variety known in this section as "field" peas, for the most part commonly known as "blackeyed peas." Apparently the varieties of either beans or peas were used rather indiscriminately. Beans were purchased by approximately twice as many households as were peas.

Canned peas and beans include the commonly known brands of English peas and "pork and beans." Of the two, beans were more frequently bought, the peas being rarely used. (Canned string beans are given as a separate article of food in the accompanying tables.)

Wheat flour in all instances was standard patent flour. None of it was locally milled. It was sold as "plain" flour or as "self-rising" flour, the latter being a "prepared flour" (of which several brands were available) which required no baking powders in biscuit making. Where "plain" flour was purchased, a preparation known as "Horseford's bread preparations" was usually purchased.

Wheat bread, cakes and crackers include only bakery products. The bread was made from standard patent flour. Crackers were the common "soda crackers." In this group are included a miscellaneous variety of small sweet cakes or cookies sold loose or in 5-cent cartons and manufactured by well-known biscuit companies. Cakes and crackers were purchased only occasionally for household use.

Corn meal. All maize meal used during the period for which records were secured and, so far as could be ascertained, during the winter of 1915–1916 and the entire spring of 1916, was of local production and milling or of the generally adjacent section. None of it was highly milled, much of it only slightly bolted, and most of it was the so-called "water-ground meal" (i.e., ground in water-power mills). In this connection it may be noted that merchants selling to mill workers stated that there was a marked preference on the part of mill workers for the locally milled meal, partly because it was believed to have a better taste and to spoil less quickly, and partly because of a rather general belief that "shipped-in" meals were a cause of pellagra.

Grits (coarsely-ground maize) was not locally produced, and was of the variety generally available at groceries.

Canned corn was corn cut off the cob and canned by well-known manufacturers. A considerable proportion of the canned corn was not "sweet" or "garden" corn, but the ordinary variety of "field" corn.

Rice was the white polished variety commonly purchasable at groceries.

Salt pork. With the exception of a very few households which had salt pork left from home slaughtering of the preceding fall and winter, all of the salt pork was shipped from national packing centers. This salt pork was of two kinds, the "fat back" and "sow belly," cut from the back and the belly of the hog, and the "streaked meat" or "rib meat," cut from under the ribs. The fat back and sow belly contained no lean, but in the rib meat there was a small "streak" of lean. The latter was slightly higher in price and was used to a much less extent than the former. Salt pork is cooked and eaten with greens and green string beans and dried peas and beans, and also fried. When fried, the grease is mixed with flour (occasionally a little milk is added) to make a gravy which is eaten with home-made biscuits and bread, and the remainder of the meat or crackling is eaten as bacon. Much of the grease from frying is used in cooking, and to that extent displaces lard or lard substitutes.

Lard and lard substitutes include the so-called "leaf lards" and the "compound lard" manufactured and sold generally. It was found impracticable to differentiate in many instances between lard and lard substitutes in the purchase records and family statements. From such information as was secured it appeared that lard substitutes were used much more generally than lard, the approximate ratio being 3 or 4 to one.

Green string beans were beginning to be available in the stores during the periods for which data were obtained, only a very few households getting them from home gardens or from other sources. These beans were eaten unshelled. In this group are included a very few households having green English peas.

Canned string beans were the brands commonly purchasable at groceries.

Green vegetables include cabbage, onions, and turnip and mustard greens, purchased at stores. Of the articles named, cabbage was the preponderating one, onions being infrequently used and then only in small quantities, while greens were rarely purchased. These articles were shipped in from other sections of the South.

In some households home gardens were beginning to yield a little lettuce, greens, onions, and cabbage. The amounts were not large, although a fair proportion of the households were "getting a mess" occasionally. The data were not secured in such a form as to permit of the inclusion of home-grown green vegetables in the tabulations, and will be referred to in another connection.

The bought vegetables (or "store" vegetables) may be said to constitute the supply which was available throughout the winter and spring of the year; while the home-produced green vegetables may be said to constitute the supply which began to be available for a proportion of the households in small quantities in the late spring and to an increasing extent after about June 15.

Canned vegetables include all canned vegetables except legumes and potatoes. Practically all of the canned vegetables used were tomatoes, kraut, and beets, the frequency of their purchase being in the ratio of about 1 of beets to 3 of kraut and 15, or more, of tomatoes. These vegetables were of the brands generally purchasable at groceries.

Fresh fruits include bananas, apples, oranges, and lemons. Of these, bananas and apples were the predominating varieties, oranges and lemons being used infrequently. Bananas were consumed principally by mill-working members of the households between meals or at midday lunches, while apples entered more largely into the general household diet.

Dried fruits include only apples and peaches, both being of the "evaporated" variety. The two fruits were used to an approximately equal extent.

Canned fruits include principally peaches and a few blackberries and apples. With rare exceptions these articles were purchased at stores and were of the commonly known brands.

Irish potatoes were purchased in all instances from stores, and, in all except a small proportion of households, were of the preceding season's crop. Spring potatoes began to be sold about May 15, but their price was nearly double that of the fall crop.

Fresh or raw sweet potatoes were purchased in all instances from stores. They were only occasionally available during the periods for which data were secured, and had been scarce during the winter months.

Canned sweet potatoes were from canneries in adjacent sections, principally North Carolina.

Sugar included only the common white granulated variety.

Sirup included only "corn sirup," the most popular brand being the "Karo corn sirup."

Jellies and jams include, with few exceptions, the cheaper varieties commonly purchasable at groceries. The exceptions were homemade jellies and "preserves" which were used by a very small proportion of the households. The jellies purchased at stores were apple jelly with various flavors.

All other foods include principally coffee, tea, baking powder, soda, "bread preparation," and condiments. Their combined average cost was approximately 1 per cent of the total average cost of the purchased household food supply.

References

Atwater, W. O. "Principles of Nutrition and Nutritive Value of Foods," *Farmer's Bull.* (U. S. Dept. of Agriculture, No. 142), Washington, D.C.

Bouchard, C. *Recherches Nouvelles sur la Pellagre* (Paris, 1862).

Chick, H., Hume, E. M., and Skelton, R. F. "The Antiscorbutic Value of Cow's Milk," *Biochem. J.*, Vol. 12 (June, 1918), pp. 131–53.

Chittenden, R. H. *The Nutrition of Man* (New York, 1907).

Cohen, B., and Mendel, L. B. "Experimental Scurvy of the Guinea Pig, etc.," *J. Biol. Chem.*, Vol. 35 (September, 1918), pp. 425–53.

Daniels, A. L., and Loughlin, R. "Feeding Experiments with Peanuts," *J. Biol. Chem.*, Vol. 33 (1918), pp. 295–301.

Daniels, A. L., and Nichols, M. B. "The Nutritive Value of the Soy Bean," *J. Biol. Chem.*, Vol. 32 (1917), pp. 91–102.
Deeks, W. E. "Pellagra in the Canal Zone," *Medical Record* (New York), Vol. 81 (1912), pp. 566–69.
————. "Pellagra, its Etiology and Treatment," *Southern Medical Journal* (Birmingham, Ala.), Vol. 9 (February, 1916), pp. 123–24.
Drummond, J. C. "Note on the Role of the Antiscorbutic Factor in Nutrition," *Biochem. J.*, Vol. 13 (May, 1919), pp. 77–80.
Goldberger, J. "The Etiology of Pellagra," *Public Health Rep.* (Washington, D.C.), Vol. 29 (1914), p. 1683.
————. "Pellagra—Causation and a Method of Prevention," *J. Am. Med. Assn.*, Vol. 66 (Feb. 12, 1916), pp. 471–76.
————, Waring, C. H., and Willets, D. G. "The Prevention of Pellagra," *Public Health Rep.* (Washington, D.C.), Vol. 30 (1915), p. 3117.
————, and Wheeler, G. A. "Experimental Pellagra in the Human Subject, etc.," *Public Health Rep.* (Washington, D.C.), Vol. 30 (1915), p. 3336.
————. "The Experimental Production of Pellagra in the Human Subject by Means of Diet," *Hyg. Lab. Bull.* (Washington, D.C.), No. 120 (February, 1920).
————, and Sydenstricker, E. "A Study of the Diet of Nonpellagrous and of Pellagrous Households, etc.," *J. Am. Med. Assn.*, Vol. 71 (Sept. 21, 1918), pp. 944–49.
Grimm, R. M. "Pellagra—A Report on its Epidemiology," *Public Health Rep.* (Washington, D.C.), Mar. 7 and 14, 1913, pp. 425 and 491.
Harden, A. "Accessory Factors in the Nutrition of the Rat," *Biochem. J.*, Vol. 12 (December, 1918), pp. 408–15.
————, and Zilva, S. S. "Note on the Etiology of Scurvy in Guinea Pigs," *Biochem. J.*, Vol. 12 (October, 1918), pp. 270–74.
Hess, A. F., and Unger, L. J. "The Scurvy of Guinea Pigs," *J. Biol. Chem.*, Vol. 35 (September, 1918), pp. 479–86 and 487–96.
Hindehede, M. *Protein and Nutrition* (London, 1913).
Jobling, J. W., and Petersen, W. "A Preliminary Report upon the Epidemiology of Pellagra in Nashville, Tenn.," *J. Infect. Dis.*, Vol. 18 (January, 1916), pp. 501–67.
————. "The Epidemiology of Pellagra in Nashville, Tenn. (II)," *J. Infect. Dis.*, Vol. 21 (August, 1917), pp. 109–31.
Lavinder, C. H. "The History of Pellagra, etc.," *New York Med. J.* (December 11, 1915), pp. 1169–72.
Lusk, Graham. *The Elements of the Science of Nutrition* (Philadelphia, 1917).
McCollum, E. V. "The Supplementary Dietary Relationships Among Our Natural Foodstuffs," *J. Am. Med. Assn.*, Vol. 68 (1917), pp. 1379–86.
————, Simmonds, N., and Parsons, H. T. "A Biological Analysis of Pellagra-Producing Diets (VI)," *J. Biol. Chem.*, Vol. 38 (May, 1919), pp. 113–46.

Mendel, L. B. "Nutrition and Growth," *J. Am. Med. Assn.*, Vol. 64 (1915), pp. 1539–47.

Osborne, T. B., and Mendel, L. B. "The Soy Bean as Food," *J. Biol. Chem.*, Vol. 32 (1917), pp. 369–76.

Roussel, T. *De La Pellagre, de son Origine,* etc. (Paris, 1845).

Siler, J. "A Statistical Study of the Relation of Pellagra to Use of Certain Foods, etc.," *Arch. Int. Med.*, Vol. 14 (September, 1914), pp. 292–373.

———, and Garrison, P. E. "An Intensive Study of the Epidemiology of Pellagra," *Am. J. Med. Sci.* (Philadelphia), Vol. 146 (July and August, 1913).

———, and MacNeal, W. J. "Pellagra—A Summary of the First Prog. Rep., etc.," *J. Am. Med. Assn.*, Vol. 62 (January 3, 1914), pp. 8–12.

———. "Further Studies, etc.—A Summary of the Second Prog. Rep.," *J. Am. Med. Assn.*, Vol. 63 (September 26, 1914), pp. 1090–93.

Strambio, G. *Abhandlungen über das Pellagra* (Leipzig, 1796).

Vedder, E. B. "Dietary Deficiency as the Etiological Factor in Pellagra," *Arch. Int. Med.*, Vol. 18 (August, 1916), pp. 137–72.

Voegtlin, C. "The Treatment of Pellagra," *J. Am. Med. Assn.*, Vol. 63 (September 26, 1914), pp. 1094–96.

9. Pellagra Incidence in Relation to Sex, Age, Season, Occupation, and "Disabling Sickness" in Seven Cotton-Mill Villages of South Carolina During 1916[1]

JOSEPH GOLDBERGER
G. A. WHEELER
EDGAR SYDENSTRICKER

Introduction

In the spring of 1916 we began a study of pellagra in certain cotton-mill villages of South Carolina. The results of that portion of the first year's study dealing with the relation of diet to pellagra incidence have already been reported (Goldberger, Wheeler, and Sydenstricker, 1920). In the present paper we desire to report the results of the part of the study dealing with the incidence of the disease in relation to certain social factors. Although a number of students have made somewhat similar studies, which we hope to review in a later paper, this, so far as we are aware, is the first time that the actual age and sex incidence of the disease have been determined for a population enumerated in direct connection with the study.

Locality and Population

The study was made in seven representative cotton-mill villages situated in the northwestern part of South Carolina. The population of each was composed almost entirely of mill employees and their families. The few Negro families present and living in a quarter somewhat apart were not considered, so that our study deals with an exclusively white population which, with hardly a single exception, was of Anglo-Saxon stock, born in this country of American-born parents. We also excluded from our study the mill executives, store managers, clerks, and their households. There was, therefore, no significant difference in race or occupation (other than that of employment or nonemployment in the cotton mills) in the population (village people) studied.

1 *Public Health Rep.,* Vol. 35, No. 28 (July 9, 1920), 1650–64.

Methods of Study

Pellagra incidence was determined, as described in a previous paper by a biweekly house-to-house visit and search for cases. This was begun about the middle of April and carried on by one of us (G. A. W.) regularly every two weeks throughout the remainder of the year. This is believed to be the first time this expedient has been applied systematically and continuously over so long a period to the study of this disease.

At each canvass every family was visited and an effort made to see and question all individuals in or about the house. At first considerable reluctance was displayed by some of the people in speaking of any condition which they believed or suspected to be pellagrous; but as we became better known this reserve in large measure disappeared, so that from time to time cases were brought to our attention which might otherwise have escaped us.

In order to see as many as possible of those at work in the mill, the time of the canvass was so varied as to utilize more or less of the lunch hour and Saturday half-holidays in different villages and in different sections of the same village in rotation. At each visit inquiries were made as to the health of the absent members of the household and as to the existence of any suspicious illness or condition in the village, particularly in members of neighboring households. Reports regarded as suggestive were investigated, at times trips to the mill being made for this purpose.

Information with respect to the occurrence of cases of pellagra was also sought from local physicians. Although we believe we enjoyed their full cooperation, the number of cases coming to our attention in this way formed a very small proportion of the total recorded by us. This is interesting as indicating that but a small percentage of cases occurring in any season come to the attention of a physician.

Only those patients with a clearly defined bilaterally symmetrical dermatitis were recorded as having pellagra. In the course of the canvass, cases with manifestations more or less suggestive of the disease were from time to time encountered, but in the absence of a clearly marked bilaterally symmetrical eruption were recorded at most as "suspects."

The date of the first appearance of the eruption was assumed to mark the onset of the attack. This date could be fixed fairly accurately in most adults, but was frequently rather difficult of determination in children, for many times it happened that in these the existence of an eruption was not recognized until attention was called to it in the course of the canvass. In such instances the date could frequently be placed as within the period of the immediately preceding two weeks by the fact of the absence of the eruption at the date of the preceding examination, or, in the event of the individual not having been seen at the immediately preceding visit, the date could, as a rule, be placed as falling within the preceding four weeks. A definite date, however, so far as possible, was always assigned even in such instances. In selecting it, the appearance and stage of the eruption, with such other circumstances as the history of the case might bring out, were used as a guide. In general, it may be said that in the vast majority of our cases the date of "onset" is probably correct within less than a week, and in practically all cases it may be said that the eruption appeared not later than this date. It is possible that some of the cases recorded as occurring late in the year were really relapses, the eruption in the early part of the year having escaped our observation.

It is recognized that in assuming that the appearance of the eruption marks the onset of the attack of pellagra a certain error is involved. In many of our cases a definite history of symptoms antedating the eruption was obtained; in a much greater proportion (children for the most part), however, such history either could not be elicited or it was so vague as to be of no value in fixing the date of onset. In the latter event the assumption that the first appearance of the eruption marks the onset of the disease was, therefore, practically unavoidable; hence, for the sake of uniformity and in order to eliminate any possible bias, this rule was adopted and applied in all cases. It follows, therefore, that our "date of onset" should be interpreted as indicating that the attack began "not later than" that date.

In computing the incidence of pellagra among the total population studied, as well as the general incidence according to sex, age, occupation, and month of onset, all cases as defined above were considered without regard to the locality in which the onset of the 1916 attack occurred and without regard to the question of whether the 1916 attack was the initial or a recurrent attack.

The data relating to population were secured by a census of the villages made during May and June, 1916. The population is as nearly as possible that which was observed for pellagra prevalence. In some of the tabulations which are presented care has been taken to consider only those households which were under biweekly observation for specified periods.

The population of the several villages used in computing incidence according to sex, age, and occupation is slightly less than the total population, for the reason that data for some of the households and for some individuals were incomplete in these and some other respects, and hence could not be used. The total population of the seven villages enumerated in May and June, 1916, and used for the computation of pellagra incidence was 4,399, while the population used in computing sex, age, and occupation incidence aggregated 4,161.

Total Incidence

A total of 115 definite cases was recorded in the seven villages during the period April 16–December 31, 1916, representing a rate of 26.1 per 1,000 of population. These cases occurred in 77 households, so that on the basis of a total of 798 white mill workers' households, it appears that 9.6 per cent of these included some one or more members with a definite attack of pellagra in 1916.

There were recorded also 73 cases in which the eruption did not conform fully with the criteria we had adopted. These are some of the "suspects" to which previous reference has been made. We are satisfied that all of these may properly be classed as pellagra. If this were done, we would have a total of 188 cases and an incidence rate of 42.7 per 1,000 of population, a rate which is probably more closely representative of the actual condition than is that for our definite cases alone. As it has seemed wiser, however, to adhere strictly to our definition of pellagra, we have segregated these from our definite cases and have not considered them in relation to any of the factors that we have attempted to study. [Tabulation of these statistics deleted. ED.]

It may here be noted that the number of cases recorded by us is believed to represent pretty closely, though perhaps not quite fully, the total incidence for the year, even though the search for cases did not begin until about the middle of April or the first of May. Subsequent experience has shown that but few cases develop during the first three months of the year in the locality studied; and as it is highly probable that a considerable proportion of the few developing earlier in the year would have continued active into the period when our canvass for cases began, the number missed was probably too small to affect the general rate very materially.

Incidence According to Sex and Age

The incidence of the disease during 1916 among persons of different sexes and of various age periods is shown in Table 30. The ages in

TABLE 30—*Pellagra incidence by sex and age in seven cotton-mill villages of South Carolina during 1916.*
(Definite cases in white population.)

Age periods.	Males.			Females.			Total.		
	Number.	Pellagrins.		Number.	Pellagrins.		Number.	Pellagrins.	
		Number.	Per 1,000.		Number.	Per 1,000.		Number.	Per 1,000.
Under 1 year........	65	0	0.0	63	0	0.0	128	0	0.0
1 year..............	57	0	.0	56	0	.0	113	0	.0
2 years.............	59	0	.0	54	5	92.6	113	5	44.2
3 years.............	82	2	24.4	74	5	67.6	156	7	44.9
4 years.............	76	1	13.2	62	3	48.4	138	4	29.0
Under 5.............	339	3	8.8	309	13	42.1	648	16	24.7
5-9.................	313	20	63.9	296	15	50.7	609	35	57.5
10-14...............	279	5	17.9	258	4	15.5	537	9	16.8
15-19...............	242	2	8.3	279	3	10.8	521	5	9.6
20-24...............	221	1	4.5	234	12	51.3	455	13	28.6
25-29...............	156	0	.0	180	5	27.8	336	5	14.9
30-34...............	131	1	7.6	139	8	57.6	270	9	33.3
35-39...............	119	1	8.3	116	5	43.1	235	6	25.5
40-44...............	81	1	12.3	76	5	65.8	157	6	38.2
45-49...............	63	0	.0	59	3	50.9	122	3	24.6
50-54...............	46	1	21.7	45	1	22.2	91	2	22.0
55-59...............	32	1	31.2	40	0	.0	72	1	13.9
60-64..............	16	2	125.0	19	0	.0	35	2	57.1
65 years and over...	33	2	60.6	39	1	25.6	72	3	41.7
All ages........	2,071	40	19.3	2,089	75	35.9	4,160	115	27.6
Under 15 years......	931	28	30.1	863	32	37.1	1,794	60	33.4
15 years and over...	1,140	12	10.5	1,226	43	35.1	2,366	55	23.2

this table are grouped according to the conventional divisions—by single years up to 5, and by 5-year periods up to 65 years.

This tabulation suggests that certain age periods may be further grouped according to the incidence curves for the two sexes. This has been done in Table 31. [Graphic representation deleted. ED.]

If the population of the pellagrous households alone—that is, of only those households in which definite cases of pellagra occurred in 1916—is considered, the variations in incidence (per cent) according to sex and age in this population appear to be similar to the variations indicated by the rate per 1,000 of the entire population censused, as may be seen by comparing Tables 31 and 32.

Table 32, showing the number and per cent of members of differ-

TABLE 31—*Pellagra incidence by sex and age in seven cotton-mill villages of South Carolina during 1916.*

(Definite cases in white population, the ages being classified into such periods as indicate the greatest variations.)

Age periods.	Males.			Females.			Total.		
	Pellagrins.			Pellagrins.			Pellagrins.		
	Num-ber.	Num-ber.	Per 1,000.	Num-ber.	Num-ber.	Per 1,000.	Num-ber.	Num-ber.	Per 1,000.
Under 2............	122	0	.0	119	0	.0	241	0	.0
2- 4..............	217	3	13.8	190	13	68.5	407	16	39.3
5- 9..............	313	20	63.9	296	15	50.7	609	35	57.5
10-19.............	521	7	13.4	537	7	13.0	1,058	14	13.2
20-29.............	377	1	2.7	414	17	41.1	791	18	22.8
30-44.............	331	3	9.1	331	18	54.4	662	21	31.7
45-54.............	109	1	9.2	104	4	38.5	213	5	23.5
55 years and over.	81	5	61.7	98	1	10.2	179	6	33.5
All ages.....	2,071	40	19.3	2,089	75	35.9	4,160	115	27.6

TABLE 32—*Pellagra incidence by sex and age among members of white pellagrous households in seven cotton-mill villages of South Carolina during 1916.*

Age.	Total.			Males.			Females.		
	Num-ber of per-sons.	Num-ber of pella-grins.*	Per cent pella-grins.	Num-ber of per-sons.	Num-ber of pella-grins.*	Per cent pella-grins.	Num-ber of per-sons.	Num-ber of pella-grins.*	Per cent pella-grins.
Under 5......	67	14	21.0	24	3	12.5	43	11	25.6
5- 9........	79	31	39.2	41	16	39.0	38	15	39.5
10-19.......	114	13	11.4	65	6	9.2	49	7	14.3
20-29.......	46	13	28.3	22	0	.0	24	13	54.2
30-44.......	70	20	28.6	37	3	8.1	33	17	51.5
45-54.......	16	3	18.8	12	1	8.3	4	2	50.0
55 and over..	12	3	25.0	6	2	33.3	6	1	16.7
All ages...	404	97	24.0	207	31	15.0	197	66	33.5

*Only those pellagrins are considered who had been members of the household regularly (i.e., exclusive of transient persons and of pellagrins the onset of whose 1916 attacks occurred in other households).

ent sexes and ages in pellagrous households who were affected with pellagra, is significant because it indicates pellagra incidence according to sex and age among persons living under generally closely similar household conditions. It will be observed that the ratio of female to male pellagrins among persons of all ages is about 2 to 1; this ratio varies considerably at different age periods, as is shown in the table below.

Before attaching significance to these variations, consideration should be given to the possibility of their being due entirely or in part to irregularities arising from the relatively slight amount of data. Furthermore, since pellagra incidence is closely related to the household diet and tends to occur by households rather than by individuals in a considerable proportion of instances, the age and sex composition of the households affected may influence materially the rate in a given age period. In those age periods when the distribution of the sexes tends to be very nearly equal, as in the adult periods up to old age, the possible effect of such a condition is slight. But among children, especially young children, and among old persons, the effect of this condition upon the rate per 1,000 may be considerable. The number of our pellagrous families actually is small, and individual families may "run to" boys or to girls; and among old persons in households affected there may chance to be a predominance of widowed or deserted men or women.

A scrutiny of our family schedules indicates that at least one of the variations in incidence according to sex is due to irregularities of this

Ratio of female to male pellagrins in population of white pellagrous households.

Age.	Per cent of members of pellagrous households who were affected with pellagra.		Ratio of female to male pellagra rate.
	Male.	Female.	
Under 5.......	12.5	25.6	2.0
5-9............	39.0	39.5	1.0
10-19.........	9.2	14.3	1.6
20-44.........	6.9	27.4	4.0
45-54.........	8.3	50.0	6.0
55 and over...	33.3	16.7	.5
All ages....	15.0	33.5	2.2

type. In the age period "under 5 years" the rate for females, as indicated in Table 30, is 42.1 per 1,000, as against only 8.8 for males. The pellagrins in this group were in 16 households, for 14 of which detailed data are available. The following are the statistics for these 14 households:

	Male	Female
(A) Total population "under 5 years"	5	15
(B) Number of pellagrins "under 5 years"	3	11
Per cent (B) of (A)	60	73

It appears, therefore, that the ratio of total males to male pellagrins and the ratio of total females to female pellagrins in the households affected by pellagra-causing conditions (allowing for the small numbers) was much the same and that there was, therefore, no real indication of a significant difference in incidence in the two sexes in this age period.

With these limitations in mind, the data appear to indicate that (1) the disease is rare at the age of 2 and under—no case in this age period was observed in the population studied during 1916; (2) among both males and females up to 20 years the incidence is similar, being higher among children between 2 and 10 years than in persons of the ages of 10 to 19, inclusive; and (3) among adults 20–54 years old the incidence is many times higher in females than in males.

These indications are in harmony with the results of other previous studies (Boudin 1861; Siler, Garrison, and MacNeal 1915). A discussion of their significance is reserved for a later communication.

Monthly (or Seasonal) Incidence

In computing the incidence of 1916 attacks according to month (or season) of onset for all persons affected with pellagra, and in relation to their sex and age, each case of pellagra has been credited to the month in which the eruption appeared. In order to determine the monthly incidence as accurately as possible, the number of cases credited to each month has been adjusted to a 31-day month basis, and the monthly indices have been computed with the monthly average for the year as the basis.

Table 33 shows the actual number of cases the onset of which occurred in each month, as well as the relative number after adjustment is made to a 31-day month, for males and females and for both sexes. [Graph plotting the relative number of cases deleted. ED.]

There was a sharp rise in incidence during April and May, reaching a well-defined peak in June. This was followed by an abrupt decline during July and August which was halted during September,

TABLE 33—*Monthly incidence of pellagra during 1916 in seven cotton-mill villages of South Carolina, actual number of definite cases for each sex, with onset in specified months, and the monthly percentage of cases after adjustment to a thirty-one-day month.*

Month.	Males.			Females.			Total.		
	Number of cases.	Number of cases adjusted to 31-day month.	Monthly percentage of cases.	Number of cases.	Number of cases adjusted to 31-day month.	Monthly percentage of cases.	Number of cases.	Number of cases adjusted to 31-day month.	Monthly percentage of cases.
January....	0	0	0	0	0	0	0	0	0
February...	0	0	0	1	1.1	1.4	1	1.1	0.9
March......	3	3	7.4	1	1.0	1.3	4	4.0	3.4
April......	6	6.2	15.3	7	7.2	9.5	13	13.4	11.5
May........	7	7.0	17.1	13	13.0	17.1	20	20.0	17.1
June.......	12	12.4	30.3	25	25.8	33.9	37	38.2	32.7
July.......	3	3.0	7.4	15	15.0	19.7	18	18.0	15.4
August.....	1	1.0	2.4	7	7.0	9.2	8	8.0	6.8
September..	6	6.2	15.3	4	4.1	5.4	10	10.3	8.8
October....	1	1.0	2.4	2	2.0	2.6	3	3.0	2.6
November...	1	1.0	2.4	0	0	0	1	1.0	.9
December...	0	0	0	0'	0	0	0	0	0
Total...	40	40.8	100	75	76.2	100	115	117	100
Monthly average...	....	3.4	....	....	6.4	....	....	9.8	....

but was resumed quite sharply during October. The season of onset appeared to be confined almost entirely to the six months, April to September, inclusive, and the period of greatest incidence clearly within the four months, April to July, inclusive. This agrees fairly well with the observations reported by other workers.

It should be observed that the data refer to monthly incidence ("onset") of attack and not to prevalence, since the duration of the attacks was not noted.

The monthly incidence of attacks among males and females appeared to be similar, with the exception of a secondary peak for males in September. The number of cases is too small, however, to warrant attaching significance to this irregularity. An examination of the detailed data shows that this was due to a predominance of males of the ages of 5 to 9 in two households affected with pellagra, and it may thus be regarded as accidental in a small group of individuals.

The possibility that seasonal incidence might vary among persons of different ages and of different family incomes was suggested by some tabulations made for experimental purposes, but, because of the necessity of subdivisions of the population into quite small groups, the results were not believed to be based on sufficient experience to warrant their presentation. The much larger experience afforded by our 1917 studies will, it is hoped, yield more satisfactory indications.

Incidence According to Occupation

On the basis of occupation the population of the villages naturally falls into two classes, namely, mill workers and non-mill workers. Persons classified as mill workers were those who had been employed in the cotton mills during 1916 up to the date of the census, or, in the case of persons incapacitated by pellagra or other causes, up to the time of the incapacitation. With few exceptions, mill workers had been so employed prior to January 1, 1916, for periods varying in length, some as long as 10 or 15 years. The inclusion of all persons employed in the mills in a single group rather than in groups for specific occupations within the mill is made because (1) the occupations within the mill are for the great majority of persons similar in character and (2) because a considerable proportion of the operatives frequently change from one kind of work to another.

Persons classified as non-mill workers included all not classified as mill workers. In the case of children, these included those at home or at school, a few having been employed in millwork in 1915 during school vacation. In the case of adults, the females were housewives, with negligible exceptions; the males included those unable to engage in millwork or who were idle for some unascertained reason, and a very small number employed at other miscellaneous occupations.

In order to compare the incidence of the disease in these two classes, the members of which lived under the same general household and community conditions, Table 34 was prepared. This, it may be seen, indicates that the pellagra rate among both males and females of all ages was considerably higher for the non-mill workers than for the mill workers. Since mill workers are all above the age of 10 years, the pellagra rates for the mill-working and the non-mill-working groups "10 years and over" afford a better basis of comparison. On this basis, the same condition is clearly indicated (Table 34). [Graphic representation deleted. ED.] As between the sexes the incidence among mill workers seems to follow pretty closely the corresponding general curves; that is, in the age group 10–19 years the rate for males is essentially the same as that for females; for the age groups 20–44 the rate for females is much higher than that for males. A comparison of the rates for the sexes, of those 10 years and over, of the non-mill-working group can hardly be made because of the small numbers among the males in all age groups save that between 10 and 19 years. For this age group the incidence was the same for both sexes.

TABLE 34—*Pellagra incidence according to occupation among white persons of different sex and age in seven cotton-mill villages of South Carolina during 1916.*

Age period.	Mill working.			Non-mill working.		
	Number of persons.	Pellagrins.		Number of persons.	Pellagrins.	
		Number.	Per 1,000		Number.	Per 1,000.
Males.						
All ages............	1,186	8	6.7	885	33	37.3
10 years and over...	1,186	8	6.7	233	10	42.9
Under 10............	0	0	.0	652	23	35.3
10-19...............	358	3	8.4	165	4	24.2
20-29...............	362	1	2.8	13	1	76.9
30-44...............	321	3	9.3	10	0	.0
45-54...............	93	0	.0	15	1	6.7
55 years and over...	52	1	19.2	30	4	13.3
Females.						
All ages............	639	8	12.5	1,450	66	45.5
10 years and over...	639	8	12.5	845	38	44.9
Under 10............	0	0	.0	605	28	46.3
10-19...............	332	2	6.0	205	5	24.4
20-29...............	198	4	20.2	216	12	55.6
30-44...............	95	2	21.1	236	16	67.8
45-54...............	9	0	.0	95	4	42.1
55 years and over...	5	0	.0	93	1	107.5
Total.						
All ages............	1,825	16	8.8	2,335	99	42.4
10 years and over...	1,825	16	8.8	1,078	48	44.5
Under 10............	0	0	.0	1,257	51	40.6
10-19...............	690	5	7.3	370	9	24.3
20-29...............	560	5	8.9	229	13	56.8
30-44...............	416	5	12.0	246	16	65.0
45-54...............	102	0	.0	110	5	45.5
55 years and over...	57	1	17.5	123	5	40.6

The Relation of "Disabling Sickness" to Pellagra Incidence[2]

In connection with the inquiry relating to occupation, it seemed of interest to determine the relation of disabling sickness to pellagra

2 Persons classified as "sick" were those who were "unable to work" on account of sickness or nonindustrial accident. See also Sydenstricker, Wheeler, and Goldberger, 1918, where the definition of "disabling sickness" is given and more fully discussed.

208

Community Studies

TABLE 35—*Cases of disabling sickness of less than three months' duration (exclusive of confinements), as ascertained by a census in May and June, 1916, and of pellagra during 1916, among non-mill-working and millworking females between the ages of ten and forty-five in seven cotton-mill villages of South Carolina.**

	Non-millworking.			Millworking.		
	Number of persons.	Cases.		Number of persons.	Cases.	
		Number.	Rate per 1,000.		Number.	Rate per 1,000.
Disabling sickness at date of census......	664	26	39.2	619	28	45.2
Pellagra during 1916...	657	33	50.2	625	8	12.8

*The actual rate of pellagra incidence during 1916 can not, of course, be compared with the rate of disabling illness as found for one day. The relative differences in rates according to occupation, however, are comparable, especially when the fact is taken into consideration that the majority of the pellagra cases had their onsets in May and June, the same months in which the census of disabling sickness was made.

incidence, and, accordingly, Table 35 was prepared. This shows that while the pellagra rate among non-mill-working females was approximately four times as high as that among mill-working females, the rate for disabling sickness appears distinctly higher in mill-working than in non-mill-working females. Pellagra would seem, therefore, to have been a relatively unimportant element in the higher sickness rate among mill-working females, and, conversely, the disability indicated by the higher sickness rate among mill-working females appeared not to influence materially the pellagra rate in this group. This does not seem to afford any support for the view entertained by many observers that general debility is an essential predisposing factor in the production of pellagra.

Summary

1. During 1916 the incidence of pellagra among the members of the families of white mill-operatives of seven representative cotton-mill villages of South Carolina was included in our study.

2. In a population of 4,399, a total of 115 definite cases, representing a rate of 26.1 per 1,000, was recorded. If 73 cases with ill-defined eruption recorded as "suspects" are included, there were

in all 188 cases and an incidence rate of fully 42.7 per 1,000 in this population.

3. The data appear to indicate that the disease is rare in children at the age of 2 and under; that among both males and females up to 20 years the incidence is similar, being higher among children between 2 and 10 years than in persons of the ages of 10 to 19, inclusive; and that among adults 20–54 years old the incidence is many times higher in females than in males.

4. There was a sharp rise in incidence during April and May, reaching a well-defined peak in June. The season of onset appeared to be confined almost entirely to the six months, April to September, inclusive.

5. The pellagra rate among both males and females was considerably higher for the non-mill workers than for the mill workers.

6. While the pellagra rate among non-mill-working females was approximately four times as high as that among mill-working females, the rate for disabling sickness appeared distinctly higher in mill-working than in non-mill-working females. The disability indicated by the higher sickness rate among mill-working females appeared not to influence materially the pellagra rate in this group.

References

Boudin, J. C. M. *Annal. d'Hyg.* (Paris), Vol. 15, 2nd S. (January, 1861), p. 17.

Goldberger, J., Wheeler, G. A., and Sydenstricker, E. "A Study of the Diet of Nonpellagrous and of Pellagrous Households," *J. Am. Med. Assn.*, Vol. 71 (September 21, 1918), pp. 944–49.

———. "A Study of the Relation of Diet to Pellagra Incidence in Seven Textile-Mill Communities of South Carolina in 1916," *Public Health Rep.* (Washington, D.C.), Vol. 35 (March 19, 1920), pp. 648–713.

Siler, J., Garrison, P. E., and MacNeal, W. J. "Statistics of Pellagra in Spartanburg County, etc.," *Arch. Int. Med.*, Vol. 15 (January, 1915), p. 98.

Sydenstricker, E., Wheeler, G. A., and Goldberger, J. "Disabling Sickness Among the Population of Seven Cotton-Mill Villages of South Carolina in Relation to Family Income," *Public Health Rep.* (Washington, D.C.), Vol. 33 (November 22, 1918), pp. 2038–51.

10. A Study of the Relation of Factors of a Sanitary Character to Pellagra Incidence in Seven Cotton-Mill Villages of South Carolina in 1916[1]

JOSEPH GOLDBERGER
G. A. WHEELER
EDGAR SYDENSTRICKER
R. E. TARBETT

Introduction

In the spring of 1916 a study was begun of the relation of various factors to pellagra incidence in some representative textile-mill communities in South Carolina. On a varying scale the study was continued through 1917 and 1918. The results of the first year's (1916) study with respect to diet (Goldberger, Wheeler, and Sydenstricker, 1918; also Mar. 19, 1920) have already been reported as have also the data relating to the general incidence (Goldberger, Wheeler, and Sydenstricker, July 9, 1920) of the disease in the population of the selected mill villages. In the present paper we wish to record the results of the part of this study dealing with the relation of sanitation to the incidence of the disease.

Locality and Population

Locality.—The study was made in seven representative cotton-mill villages in the northwestern part of South Carolina. Four (*At., In., Sn.,* and *Wy.*) are in Spartanburg County, two (*Sa.* and *Ny.*) in Oconee County and one (*Rc.*) in Chester County. All had previously been studied more or less intensively by the Thompson-McFadden Commission.

Population.—The villages were of about average size; none had over 800 or less than 500 inhabitants. Each constituted a distinct, more or less isolated community in close proximity to a cotton-cloth manufacturing plant and was composed practically exclusively of the mill employees and their families.

But few Negroes are employed in or about a cotton mill; these

1 *Public Health Rep.,* Vol. 35, No. 29 (July 16, 1920), 1701–14.

with their families usually live in a quarter somewhat apart from that of the white families. Contact between the two races in the mill is very slight; it is more frequent at the stores, which are patronized in common, and in the houses of some of the white operatives in which colored women are at times employed as laundresses or cooks, or to nurse the very young children while both parents are at work in the mill.

The families of only the white mill operatives were included in the study; those of the mill officials, store managers, and of Negro employees were not considered. There was, therefore, no significant difference in race or occupation (other than that of employment or nonemployment in the cotton mills) in the population studied. In evaluating the sanitary factors considered in determining the sanitary rating of a village, conditions in the Negro quarter were taken into account, but the pellagra rates represent the incidence in the white population as above defined.

The general data relating to population were secured by a census of the villages, made during May and June, 1916, in connection with the general study of which the present paper is a part.

Methods of Study

Pellagra incidence.—The method of determining the incidence of the disease has been described at length in previous papers (Goldberger, Wheeler, and Sydenstricker, Mar. 19, 1920; July 9, 1920). Briefly, in order to ascertain the incidence of the disease as completely as possible, the expedient of a systematic biweekly house-to-house search for cases was employed and almost exclusively depended on. A few cases, relatively negligible in number, came to our attention through the courtesy of the local physicians. In no instance, however, was a case recorded by us as pellagra until seen and the diagnosis confirmed by one of us (G. A. W. or J. G.).

Criteria of pellagra.—Only cases with a clearly defined, bilaterally symmetrical dermatitis were recorded as pellagra, and the date of the appearance of the eruption was assumed to mark the onset of the attack. It is recognized that in this assumption a certain error is involved. The fact, however, that in a very large proportion of our cases a history of symptoms antedating the eruption could either not be obtained or was so vague that a definite date of onset could not be fixed, made such assumption practically unavoidable; therefore, for the sake of uniformity and in order to eliminate any possible bias, this rule was adopted and applied in all cases.

Initial and recurrent attacks.—In recording our cases, inquiry was always made as to any previous attack, and the statement of the patient or responsible member of the family was recorded. The accuracy of the information thus secured is, however, open to doubt in many instances. It is highly probable, if not quite certain, that some of our recorded first attacks were really recurrences, and also that some of the cases recorded as recurrent were really initial. As there is no reason to believe that the trend of the error would vary materially in different villages, a comparison of villages on the basis of rates for initial attacks would seem permissible.

Comparison of Village Incidence of Pellagra

In Table 36 is presented the gross rate for all definite cases, without distinction as to whether initial or recurrent, recorded in each of the villages studied during the year. Quite marked variations in rates are shown, the extremes being 1.3 and 67.6 per 1,000 of population. The household incidence rate of the respective villages likewise shows considerable variation, the extremes being 0.8 and 25.4 per cent.

For the purpose of comparing villages with respect to incidence it would appear that these gross rates might be subject to inaccuracies arising from two circumstances; namely, (1) the inclusion of imported cases and (2) the possible differences in the degree of shifting in the populations of the several villages during the period of observation,

TABLE 36—*Incidence of all definite attacks of pellagra recorded in specified mill villages of South Carolina in 1916.*

(Rate based on population ascertained by census made in May and June, 1916.)

Mill village.	Number of persons considered.	Number of definite cases.	Cases per 1,000.
All villages..............	4,399	115	26.2
At.....................	579	14	24.2
In.....................	681	46	67.6
Ny....................	750	1	1.3
Rc....................	603	19*	31.5
Sn....................	642	8	12.5
Sa....................	504	15	29.7
Wy....................	640	12	18.7

*Includes one case the onset of whose attack occurred in 1915 and continued into 1916. Died, June, 1916.

and therefore in the degree of their "exposure" so far as length of residence during the 1916 "pellagra season" is concerned.

It is manifestly desirable to exclude, as far as possible, those cases that might have originated in localities other than those in which they happened to be recorded. Thus it was found that several cases were unmistakably active before coming to the village in which they were first observed; and several others might properly be classed as imported, since they could reasonably be associated with conditions possibly existing at previous places of residence. On the assumption of an unknown etiology and unknown period of development or incubation, it was necessary, for our present purpose, to assume some period which might be used to differentiate between imported and local cases. Accordingly, it was decided to discard as possibly imported all cases the onset of whose 1916 attack occurred within less than 30 days after the individual came to the village to reside. The resulting village rates are shown in Table 37. Comparing these rates with those in Table 36, it is seen that while the individual rates are slightly reduced, the relative standing of the villages is not affected. The corresponding comparison of household rates shows much the same insignificant effect on the rates. [Tabulation deleted. ED.]

In order to ascertain the comparability of the populations of the several villages with respect to exposure as affected by length of residence, records were kept of the moving in and out of families

TABLE 37—*Incidence of definite attacks of pellagra with onset after residence of not less than thirty days in a specified mill village of South Carolina in 1916.*

(Rate based on population ascertained by census made in May and June, 1916.)

Mill village.	Number of persons considered.	Number of definite cases.	Cases per 1,000.
All villages.................	4,399	103	23.4
At......................	579	12	20.7
In......................	681	44	64.6
Ny......................	750	0	0.0
Rc......................	603	15*	24.9
Sn......................	642	7	10.9
Sa......................	504	13	25.8
Wy......................	640	12	18.7

*Includes one case the onset of whose attack occurred in 1915 and continued into 1916. Died in June, 1916.

TABLE 38—*Population resident during various periods between March 1 and October 31, 1916, in specified mill villages of South Carolina.*
(Population as ascertained by census of white mill workers' households at various times between May 1 and October 1.)

NUMBER RESIDING THE SPECIFIED NUMBER OF MONTHS OR LONGER *

Mill village.	1 month.	2 months.	3 months.	4 months.	5 months.	6 months.	7 months.	8 months.
At.......	691	672	621	591	578	559	516	450
In.......	827	779	735	717	682	667	620	595
Ny.......	986	916	852	811	731	680	646	593
Rc.......	730	730	694	647	613	508	465	447
Sn.......	836	806	745	693	647	560	525	489
Sa.......	608	576	536	461	448	442	420	392
Wy.......	786	739	701	672	649	615	589	523
Total..	5,464	5,218	4,884	4,592	4,348	4,031	3,781	3,489

PER CENT RESIDING THE SPECIFIED NUMBER OF MONTHS OR LONGER

At.......	100	97	90	85	84	81	75	65
In.......	100	94	89	87	83	81	75	72
Ny.......	100	93	86	82	74	69	66	60
Rc.......	100	100	95	89	84	70	64	61
Sn.......	100	96	89	83	77	67	63	59
Sa.......	100	95	88	76	74	73	69	64
Wy.......	100	93	89	85	83	78	75	67
Total..	100	96	89	83	80	74	69	64

*Persons in households residing in the village less than one month have been omitted.

in each village subsequent to the May and June enumeration, and a census was taken of each family whose residence in the village began subsequent to this enumeration. On the basis of the data thus secured, Table 38 was prepared. This presents statistics of the total population which resided in each village for periods of one month or longer between March 1 and October 31, 1916. The period from March 1 to October 31 was selected because practically all of the 1916 attacks of pellagra had their onsets between these dates, the large majority being between May 1 and August 1.[2] Examination of

2   Since only one census was made of each household, a certain degree of inaccuracy in the statistics of population residing during any given period is probable. This arises from the fact that records were kept of the household

this table reveals evidence of different degrees of shifting in villages, which, while not very great, is yet sufficient to be kept in mind as a possible source of error. It suggests that small differences in rates based on the census population are not to be closely regarded.

In order to determine the effect on the rates of eliminating the possible error arising from different degrees of shifting among the populations of the different villages, we have computed a rate on the basis of the population resident throughout the period March 1– October 31, considering only those cases occurring in that population during this period. The resulting rates are shown in Table 39. A comparison of these rates with the gross, and what may be desig-

TABLE 39—*Incidence of all definite cases of pellagra with onset between March 1 and October 31, 1916, in persons of households all or part of the members of which resided continuously in the specified mill villages of South Carolina between those dates.**

(Only those cases considered having onset after a residence of not less than thirty days in specified village.)

Mill village.	Number of persons considered.	Number of definite cases.	Cases per 1,000.
All villages....	3,489	100	28.7
At..........	450	10	22.2
In..........	595	44	73.9
Ny..........	593	0	0.0
Rc..........	447	14	31.3
Sn..........	489	7	14.3
Sa..........	392	13	33.2
Wy..........	523	12	22.9

*Tabulation showing a comparison of relative pellagra incidence according to different methods of computation deleted. ED.

units with respect to their moving. It was impracticable to record the coming and going of every individual member of the household units. The moving in and out of individuals separately from their households, however, was relatively slight in any village and the error arising from this cause may be regarded as negligible. There was no reason to believe, moreover, that the shifting of individuals of a given sex or age was relatively greater in one village than in another.

nated as the refined rate, based on the census populations, shown in Tables 36 and 37, respectively, reveals on the whole remarkably little difference, a difference which in no way affects the relative standing of the villages. It would follow, therefore, that either of the rates based on the census population is satisfactory for comparative purposes. But it may be worth recalling that, for the reasons already mentioned, and also because of the fact that a single household with two or more cases of pellagra may appreciably affect the rate of a village of the size of those under consideration, but little if any significance, as reflecting community conditions, can be attached to any but quite well-marked differences in rates. With these considerations in mind, our villages would seem to fall into three groups: (1) *In.*, with an extremely high rate; (2) *Ny.* and *Sn.*, with markedly low rates; and (3) *Wy.*, *At.*, *Rc.*, and *Sa.* with moderate rates.[3]

In the foregoing comparisons of pellagra incidence, no distinction was made between initial and recurrent cases. Reference has already been made to the limitations attaching to such classification. Furthermore, in computing rates for these classes a serious source of possible error with respect to that for recurrent cases, if conventional practice is followed, should be noted. If, as some workers seem to believe, an essential etiological difference between an initial and a recurrent

TABLE 40—*Incidence of initial and of recurrent-attack cases of pellagra after a residence of not less than thirty days in specified mill villages of South Carolina in 1916.*

(Population ascertained by census made in May and June, 1916.)

Mill village.	Number of persons considered.	All cases.		Initial cases.		Recurrent cases.	
		Number.	Rate per 1,000.	Number.	Rate per 1,000.	Number.	Rate per 1,000.
All villages....	4,399	103	23.4	63	14.3	40	9.1
At............	579	12	20.7	4	6.9	8	13.8
In............	681	44	64.6	29	42.6	15	22.0
Ny............	750	0	0.0	0	0.0	0	0.0
Rc............	603	15*	24.9	6*	10.0	9	14.9
Sn............	642	7	10.9	4	6.2	3	4.7
Sa............	504	13	25.8	12	23.8	1	2.0
Wy............	640	12	18.7	8	12.5	4	6.2

*Includes one case the onset of whose attack occurred in 1915 and continued until 1916. Died in June, 1916.

3 The differences in the rates are so marked that it has not seemed worthwhile to compute them to a standard population.

attack exists, it would necessarily follow that the rate for recurrent attacks should be based not as is that for first attacks, on the population as a whole,[4] but on the number of individuals in that population having a history of a previous attack of the disease.[5] For this purpose a record of all resident pellagrins would be necessary. Such we found it impracticable to secure, and so we are not in a position to make a comparison of the villages on the basis of rates for recurrent attacks determined in this way.

With the reservations suggested by the foregoing consideration in mind, we present Tables 40 and 41, in which are shown the incidence rates for initial and for recurrent attacks recorded in 1916. In the former table the incidence is computed for the population as censused in May and June; in the latter for the population residing continuously between March 1 and October 31. It will be observed in each of these tables that although the rate for initial attacks is in general decidedly lower than that for all cases, the relative position

TABLE 41—*Incidence of initial and of recurrent-attack cases of pellagra with onset between March 1 and October 31, 1916, in persons of households, all or part of the members of which resided continuously in the specified mill villages of South Carolina between those dates.*

(Only those definite cases considered having the onset after a residence of not less than thirty days in specified villages.)

Mill village.	Number of persons considered.	All cases.		Initial cases.		Recurrent cases.	
		Number.	Rate per 1,000.	Number.	Rate per 1,000.	Number.	Rate per 1,000.
All villages......	3,489	100	28.7	54	15.5	46	13.2
At.............	450	10	22.2	3	6.7	7	15.5
In.............	595	44	73.9	26	43.7	18	30.3
Ny.............	593	0	0.0	0	0.0	0	0.0
Rc.............	447	14	31.3	5	11.2	9	20.1
Sn.............	489	7	14.3	4	8.2	3	6.1
Sa.............	392	13	33.2	8	20.4	5	12.8
Wy.............	523	12	22.9	8	15.3	4	7.6

4 Strictly speaking the rate for initial attacks should be based on that portion of the population never previously affected. The possible error arising from using the entire population as a base may, even in these relatively small units, be regarded as negligible because of the relatively small number of that part previously affected.

5 This would be unnecessary if the number of such present in the several villages formed a fairly uniform proportion of the population. There is reason to believe, however, that this ratio varies considerably.

of the villages is not materially affected. Furthermore, a comparison of the rates for initial cases obtained by the methods of computation represented in these two tables shows but slight and unimportant differences, so that a comparison of villages on the basis of either of the rates for initial cases would seem to be permissible. It may be noted also that the relative incidence for recurrent cases differs distinctly from that for first attacks.

Taking into account the small size of the population units, the small number of cases, and the previously mentioned sources of error affecting the rates, especially the rates for recurrent cases, it would seem that a comparison of villages on the basis of the rates for cases, without distinction as to whether initial or recurrent, would be the most significant; that on the basis of rates for initial cases next; and that on the basis of rates for recurrent cases least.

Sanitation

An examination of the various factors, which, taken together, constituted the sanitary character of each of the several villages studied, showed rather marked differences in certain respects. Characterizing these factors singly or as a whole, broadly, as good, bad, or indifferent, while possibly satisfactory for some purposes, did not seem to lend itself very well to an intensive study of the relation of these factors to the incidence of pellagra, particularly as such general characterizations were open to the influence of personal bias. As Surg. W. H. Frost had developed a method for a survey of sanitary conditions with a definite system of weighted ratings for each of the several constituent factors in connection with his stream-pollution investigations, a request was made of Surg. Gen. Rupert Blue for the detail of a sanitary engineer, trained in Surg. Frost's procedure, to make an independent survey of the mill villages in which we were carrying on our study and to furnish us with a report of his findings, including a sanitary rating of each village.

In response to this request, Mr. R. E. Tarbett, Sanitary Engineer, United States Public Health Service, was detailed and made such a survey of the villages in November, 1916. From his detailed report are taken the ratings summarized in Table 42. [Tabulation of data with respect to extent to which various types of water supply and conservancy were used deleted. ED.] The general sanitary rating being the sum of the individual ratings after weighting, and as the weighting will naturally vary somewhat with the varying judgment of the importance to be attached to the individual factors, this gen-

TABLE 42—*Summary of ratings of sanitary factors in specified mill villages of South Carolina in 1916.*
(By R. E. Tarbett, Sanitary Engineer.)

			Ratings.			
Mill village.	Water supply.	Disposal of human excrement.	Sanitary control (flies, food-stuffs, and milk).	Control of communicable diseases.	Domestic environment and habits of population.	All factors.*
	Per cent.	Per cent.	Per cent.	Per cent.	Per cent.	Per cent.
At............	65.60	45.00	44.00	17.50	33.33	49.33
In............	49.30	2.00	39.50	17.50	33.33	28.49
Ny............	60.00	66.00	36.00	20.00	33.33	53.12
Rc............	90.00	100.00	66.50	70.00	66.66	87.06
Sn............	77.53	35.84	39.50	17.50	41.60	44.46
Sa⁺...........	25.00	4.00	36.50	15.00	33.33	18.72
Sa#...........	60.00	75.00	36.50	15.00	33.33	55.43
Wy............	47.51	0.00	36.50	15.00	33.33	26.43

*This represents the sum of the ratings of all factors after due weighting. The weights assigned being as follows: Water supply, 40; disposal of human excrement, 32; general sanitary control, 12.5; control of communicable diseases, 12.5; and domestic environment, etc., 3.
⁺For period January-July, 1916.
#For period July-November, 1916. "Sanitary" privies replaced surface closets in July.

eral rating will be affected accordingly. The relative standing of the villages, however, will not be affected.

Typhoid incidence being justly regarded as a good index of sanitary conditions, we made a record of all cases of typhoid fever encountered in the course of the canvass for pellagra. It was impracticable for us to apply laboratory diagnostic tests to these cases, so that, with the exception of a few concerning which information was secured from the medical attendant, our diagnoses are based on the history and brief clinical observation of the case. It was likewise impracticable for us to attempt to trace the source of infection. We deemed it expedient, therefore, to credit the cases to the village in which recorded. As there seems no reason to believe that the trend of the errors involved in this would vary materially in the different villages, we are disposed to regard the relative incidence of these cases as not without value as an auxiliary, though, because of the small number of cases, necessarily a subordinate index of sanitary conditions. In all, 38 cases, representing a rate of 8.6 per 1,000 of the aggregate population, were recorded. [Tabulation of distribution of cases among the villages deleted. ED.]

Relation of Sanitary Factors to Pellagra Incidence

Thus far we have considered the rates of incidence of pellagra in the several villages and have seen that these might properly be compared on the basis of certain of those rates. As a measure of the sanitary conditions in the villages, we have the ratings assigned by Sanitary Engineer Tarbett after an independent survey, and as an auxiliary but subordinate index, we have the typhoid incidence recorded in connection with the canvass for pellagra. We are in position, therefore, to proceed with a study of the relation of factors of a sanitary character to the incidence of the disease.

In order more readily to ascertain any existing correlation between sanitary conditions and pellagra incidence, we have prepared Tables 43, 44, and 45. It may here be observed that the pellagra incidence rates presented in these tables are based on the populations as censused by us in May and June, 1916, for cases with onset after a residence of not less than 30 days in the specified village. Of the rates

TABLE 43—*Relation of pellagra and typhoid incidence to sanitary character of water supply of specified mill villages of South Carolina in 1916.*

(Pellagra cases with onset after a residence of not less than thirty days in specified village; typhoid cases credited to village in which recorded. Rates based on population as censused in May and June. Villages in order of increasing water-supply ratings. Water-supply ratings by Sanitary Engineer R. E. Tarbett.)

Mill village.	Water supply rating.	Typhoid.	Pellagra.	
		All cases, rate per 1,000.	All defi- nite cases, rate per 1,000.	First at- tack, rate per 1,000.
	Per cent.			
Sa..............	25.00*	19.8	25.8	23.8
Wy..............	47.51	17.2	18.7	12.5
In..............	49.30	8.8	64.6	42.6
Ny..............	60.00	1.3	0.0	0.0
At..............	65.60	3.5	20.7	6.9
Sn..............	77.53	12.5	10.9	6.2
Rc..............	90.00	0.0	24.9	10.0

*The rating for this village is for the period anterior to and coincident with the pellagra season. In the other villages no changes occurred during the year.

examined and, as has been seen, found equally suitable as a basis for the comparison of villages, we have chosen these because the method of computing them conforms most closely to conventional practice.

In Table 43 we present the pellagra incidence data in relation to the sanitary character of the water supply as rated by San. Engr. Tarbett. [Graphic representation deleted. ED.] No significant correlation is perceptible; the two villages representing the extremes of pellagra incidence (*In.* and *Ny.*) have water supplies with a difference in rating of little or no significance. Likewise, no consistent correlation between the incidence of pellagra and that of typhoid is here discernible. In contrast, however, a suggestive tendency to inverse correlation between typhoid incidence and water-supply rating is perceptible.

In Table 44 is presented the pellagra incidence data in relation to the rating of the efficiency of disposal of human excreta in the several villages. [Graphic representation deleted. ED.] Although the

TABLE 44—*Relation of pellagra and typhoid incidence to efficiency of methods of disposal of human excrement in specified mill villages of South Carolina in 1916.*

(Pellagra cases with onset after a residence of not less than thirty days in specified village; typhoid cases credited to village in which recorded. Rates based on population as censused in May and June. Villages in order of increasing excreta disposal rating. Excreta disposal ratings by Sanitary Engineer R. E. Tarbett.)

| | | Typhoid. | Pellagra. | |
Mill village.	Excreta disposal rating.	All cases, rate per 1,000.	All definite cases, rate per 1,000.	First attack, rate per 1,000.
	Per cent.			
Wy.............	0.00	17.2	18.7	12.5
In.............	2.00	8.8	64.6	42.6
Sa.............	*4.00	19.8	25.8	23.8
Sn.............	15.84	12.5	10.9	6.2
At.............	45.00	3.5	20.7	6.9
Ny.............	66.00	1.3	0.0	0.0
Rc.............	100.00	0.0	24.9	10.0

*The rating for this village is for the period anterior to and coincident with the pellagra season. In the other villages no change occurred during the year.

villages representing the extremes of pellagra incidence recorded by us are close to the respective extremes of excreta disposal rating, this suggestion of an inverse correlation is not borne out when the data are further examined: Of the two villages representing the extremes of efficiency of excreta disposal, the one (*Rc.*) with the highest rating (a water carriage system) had a pellagra incidence rate that differed in but negligible degree from that of the village (*Wy.*) with the lowest rating (surface privies), the incidence rate for "all definite cases" being slightly but not very significantly higher in the former and for "first attack cases" slightly but insignificantly higher in the latter village. Similarly we fail to find any consistent correlation between pellagra incidence and the typhoid rate, although a distinct tendency to inverse correlation between the latter and the ratings for excreta disposal is perceptible.

As may be seen by reference to Table 42, the variations among the villages in rating for efficiency of "sanitary control" (control of fly prevalence, protection of foodstuffs and of milk) are with one

TABLE 45—*Relation of pellagra and typhoid incidence to general sanitary rating of specified mill villages of South Carolina in 1916.*
(Pellagra cases with onset after a residence of not less than thirty days in specified village; typhoid cases credited to village in which recorded. Rates being based on population as censused in May and June. Villages in order of increasing sanitary rating. Sanitary ratings by Sanitary Engineer R. E. Tarbett.)

Mill village.	General sanitary rating.*	Typhoid.	Pellagra.	
		All cases, rate per 1,000.	All defi- nite cases, rate per 1,000.	First cases, rate per 1,000.
	Per cent.			
Sa.......................	+18.72	19.8	25.8	23.8
Wy.......................	26.43	17.2	18.7	12.5
In.......................	28.49	8.8	64.6	42.6
Sn.......................	44.46	12.5	10.9	6.2
At.......................	49.33	3.5	20.7	6.9
Ny.......................	53.12	1.3	0.0	0.0
Rc.......................	87.06	0.0	24.9	10.0

*Represents the sum of the ratings of all factors after due weighting.
+Rating for this village is for the period anterior to and coincident with the pellagra season. In the other villages no changes of sanitary significance were observed during the year.

exception, very slight. This is likewise true of the ratings for efficiency of "control of communicable diseases" and of those for
"domestic environment." In the case of the ratings for all three of
these groups of factors, it is the same village (*Rc.*) that stands out
conspicuously above the others. As this village is one of those having
an intermediate pellagra incidence rate it is clear that no consistent
correlation between any of these three groups of factors and the
incidence of the disease is indicated.

Having thus examined the relation of each of the important sanitary factors or groups of factors in their relation to the incidence of
pellagra, it will be of interest next to study the relation of the incidence of the disease to the general quality of the sanitation of the
several villages as indicated by the rating representing the sum of
the weighted ratings of the individual factors or groups of factors.
For this purpose Table 45 has been prepared. [Graphic representation deleted. ED.] Study of this fails to reveal any consistent correlation between the quality of sanitary conditions and the incidence of
the disease; nor, as we have previously seen, does there seem to be
revealed any consistent correlation between pellagra and typhoid
incidence. On the other hand, an inverse correlation between typhoid
incidence and sanitary conditions is, as might have been expected,
quite clearly suggested.

Conclusions

This study of the relation of factors of sanitary importance to the
incidence of pellagra in seven representative mill villages has failed
to reveal any consistent correlation between them. Although based
on a rather small mass of data and, in itself, not warranting any conclusions, it may, nevertheless, be noted as not without significance
that this result, at any rate, affords no support for the view until
recently, at least, quite widely entertained in this country, that
pellagra is "an intestinal infection transmitted in much the same
way as typhoid fever"; nor does the evidence adduced in favor of
this view by other workers, when rightly considered, afford it any real
support.[6]

It may be of interest to add that the results of the very much more
extensive study of this subject carried on by us during 1917 and 1918,

6 See Goldberger and Wheeler, 1920, and Goldberger, Wheeler, and Sydenstricker, March 19, 1920, for a discussion of this evidence. The explanation
of the very marked difference in incidence recorded for some of the villages
will be considered in a forthcoming paper.

to be presented in a later communication, are in harmony with and
confirm those here recorded.

References

Goldberger, J., and Wheeler, G. A. "The Experimental Production of
Pellagra in Human Subjects by Means of Diet," *Hyg. Lab. Bull.* (Washington, D.C.), No. 120 (February, 1920).

————, and Sydenstricker, E. "A Study of the Diet of Nonpellagrous and
of Pellagrous Households, etc.," *J. Am. Med. Assn.*, Vol. 71 (September
21, 1918), pp. 944–49.

————. "A Study of the Relation of Diet to Pellagra Incidence, etc.,"
Public Health Rep. (Washington, D.C.), Vol. 35, No. 12 (March 19,
1920), pp. 648–713.

————. "Pellagra Incidence in Relation to Sex, Age, Season, Occupation,
etc.," *Public Health Rep.* (Washington, D.C.), Vol. 35, No. 28 (July 9,
1920), pp. 1650–64.

11. A Study of the Relation of Family Income and Other Economic Factors to Pellagra Incidence in Seven Cotton-Mill Villages of South Carolina in *1916*[1]

JOSEPH GOLDBERGER
G. A. WHEELER
EDGAR SYDENSTRICKER

In the spring of 1916 we began a study of the relation of various factors to pellagra incidence in certain representative textile-mill communities of South Carolina. On a varying scale the study was continued through 1917 and 1918. The results of the first year's (1916) study with respect to diet (Goldberger, Wheeler, and Sydenstricker, 1918 and Mar. 19, 1920), to age, sex, occupation, disabling sickness,[2] and to sanitation (Goldberger, Wheeler, and Sydenstricker, July 16, 1920) have already been reported. At the present time we wish to record the results of the part of the study dealing with the relation of conditions of an economic nature to the incidence of the disease.

Review of Literature

A close association of pellagra with poverty has been repeatedly remarked upon since the time of the first recognition of the disease. In the earliest account, Casal (1870, p. 93), discussing the diet of those persons attacked by the disease, remarks that "they eat meat very rarely since most pellagrins are poor field laborers, and this circumstance does not permit them to eat meat daily nor even from time to time." Continuing, he says: "Their only beverage is water. Their clothes, beds, habitations, etc., are strictly in keeping with their extreme poverty." Further along, discussing the treatment of the disease, Casal states that "milk, thanks to the butter it contains, is certainly capable of supplying the nutritive lack of the other foods; they use it but rarely without having first removed the butter, since

---

1   *Public Health Rep.*, Vol. 35, No. 46 (November 12, 1920), 2673–2714.
2   Goldberger, Wheeler, and Sydenstricker, July 9, 1920; Sydenstricker, Wheeler, and Goldberger, 1919.

these poor people sell the butter in order that they may be able to buy other necessaries, thus using in their own diet what remains in the milk after having thus treated it."

Much more definite and direct is Strambio (1796) who states that "thus much is certain, that pellagra is most at home where poverty and misery reign and increases as they increase."

Very interesting and significant is Marzari's observation (cited by Russell, 1845, p. 167). "I have several times observed," he states, "that if a villager falls into poverty, as happens so often as a result of a storm, drought, or other calamity, pellagra does not fail to crown his misfortune and put an end to his miserable existence."

Holland (1820), in introducing his discussion of the cause and symptoms of pellagra in a paper read in 1817, based on observations of his own and on information secured from Italian physicians in the course of a journey to Italy, remarks: "The pellagra is a malady confined almost exclusively to the lower classes of the people, and chiefly to the peasants and those occupied in the labors of agriculture." He repeats this two or three times in other connections. In his discussion of the etiology of the disease (p. 322) we find the following highly suggestive statements: "Though I have spoken of Lombardy as one of the most fertile portions of Europe, yet to those who consider the little certain relation between mere productiveness of soil and the prosperity or comforts of the population dwelling upon it, it will not appear very extraordinary that the peasants of this district should be subject to various physical privations unknown to the people of countries which are much less favored by nature. The fact unquestionably is, whatever be our speculations as to the cause, that the peasants of Lombardy do for the most part live in much wretchedness, both as regards the quantity and quality of their diet and the other various comforts of life. It further seems probable, if not certain, that this evil has been progressively augmenting within the last 50 years; partly, perhaps, an effect of the wars which have so often devastated the country by marches and military contributions; partly a consequence of the frequent changes of political state; together with the insecurity, the variable system of government, and the heavy taxes and imposts attending such changes. To these causes may be added a decaying state of commerce and a faulty system of arrangement between landlords and the cultivators of the soil, all tending to depress agriculture and to reduce the peasantry at large to a state of much misery and privation." Continuing this discussion, Holland remarks further (p. 333): "Animal food rarely forms a part of their diet, and although living on a soil which produces wine their poverty almost precludes the use of it, even when sickness and debility render it most needful. The same condition of poverty is evident in their clothing, in their habitations, and in the want of all the minor necessaries and comforts of life. The immediate effect of these privations is obvious in the aspect of squalid wretchedness and emaciation which forms so striking a spectacle at the present time throughout the greater part of Lombardy. I say particularly *at the present time* [italics in original], because whatever may have been the progress of misery among the peasants of this country during the last half century it appears to have increased in a tenfold ratio during the last two years, the effect of bad harvests added to the preceding wars and political changes which have distressed this part of Italy."

Hameau (1829), in the first recorded observations of pellagra in France, reported that "this disease attacks individuals of both sexes and all ages, but I have not yet seen it in any but the poor and uncleanly who subsist on coarse food."

Lalesque (1846), in his account of pellagra of the Landes, cites a number of instances illustrating the conditions of misery under which pellagra occurred, finally exclaiming (p. 421): "These are the individuals attacked by pellagra, for it attaches itself to poverty as the shadow to the body."

In a discussion of pellagra in Gorz-Gradisca, Berger (1890) very significantly observes: "The appearance during the last decennium of diseases of the vine, the reduction in value of the product of the soil because of foreign competition, crop failures, increase in taxes, increasing living costs, all operated to undermine economic conditions, particularly of the poorer country folk, and thus prepared favorable conditions for the spread of the disease."

Discussing the therapy and prophylaxis of pellagra in Bessarabia, V. Rosen (1894) bewails the attendant difficulties "in that, on the one hand, the alimentation with cornmeal porridge is a deeply rooted national custom, and, on the other, that the disease attacks the poorest class of the population; 'N'am vaca, n'am lapte a casa' ('I have no cow and no milk in the house') is uniformly the reply of the patient to questions in relation to this subject," and Sofer (1909, p. 219), discussing the economic status of pellagrins (in Austria), remarks that "89.9 per cent haven't even a cow."

The extremely unfavorable economic conditions of those subject to pellagra (in Austria-Hungary, at least), is further strikingly suggested by the character of some of the recommendations for its control. Thus Von Probizer (1899, p. 141) urged, as a necessary measure, "pecuniary aid by the Government in view of the deplorable condition of the peasantry in the affected localities."

V. Babes (1903), writing on pellagra in Roumania, remarks (p. 1187) that "practically all pellagrins are very poor"; and goes into some detail in describing the unfavorable economic condition of the Roumanian peasant, which leaves him in debt to the landowner and the tax collector.

In modern Spain we have Calmarza (1870) remarking (p. 66) that although he had seen cases in well-to-do individuals, the disease only exceptionally occurred in those of this class. He adds (p. 67) also that in his experience, unlike the reported observations of others (Roussel, 1866, p. 431), pellagra is quite common in beggars. In discussing the etiological role of widowhood, this keen observer expresses the opinion (p. 68) that this plays a part only in proportion as it tends to bring about a depression in economic well-being and a consequent insufficient alimentation. Huertas (1903) describes the disease as occurring among the most miserable class of the population of Madrid, who live on the food picked from the city's garbage.

In Egypt Sandwith (1903) found the disease highly prevalent among the poorer peasants of Lower Egypt. "In one village," he reports, "where the inhabitants are especially well to do because they get regular pay throughout the year from the Domains administration, there were only 15 per cent of pellagrous men, while among the men of the village, which has the reputation of being the poorest, the percentage rose as high as 62."

Gaumer (1910), discussing pellagra in Yucatan, states that the disease did not become epidemic in that state until 1884, two years after a destructive invasion by locusts or grasshoppers. "Among the better classes the disease seldom made its appearance. . . . It was the middle and lower classes who, from reduced circumstances, were obliged to purchase the cheapest corn in the market that suffered most from the ravages of the disease.

"From 1891 to 1901 Yucatan produced sufficient corn for home consumption, and new cases of pellagra were no longer to be found. . . .

"From 1901 to 1907 the corn crops were almost total failures and corn was again imported in greater quantities than ever before. . . .

"Pellagra again became epidemic, but was not then confined to the middle and lower classes, as in the former invasion. The wealthy hemp owners, on account of the exorbitant prices paid for hemp, found it was more profitable to import than to raise corn for home consumption, thus compelling even well-to-do people to consume the imported article," which was believed to have been spoiled in transport from the United States. "Pellagra then spread alike among the rich and poor, until by the close of 1907 about 10 per cent of the inhabitants were victims of the disease. . . ."

In Barbados, B. W. I., the disease, according to Manning (1907), is "confined to the laboring classes and is most prevalent among those who are badly off or poverty stricken. It is very seldom found among the whites, but cases do occur among those in straitened circumstances." In the pioneer reports on pellagra in the United States such references as are made to the relation of economic status to the disease are of a very general character and appear for the most part to be echoes of European opinion. So far as we are aware credit for the first study of this relationship is due to Siler and Garrison (1913). This study was made in South Carolina in 1912 and relates to pellagrins alone. In recording their data relating to the economic conditions under which the patients lived, Siler and Garrison adopted five classes, namely, squalor, poverty, necessities, comfort, and affluence. Of the 277 cases so classified, the economic conditions were reported as poor (squalor, poverty, necessities) in 83 per cent, within the average (comfort) in 15 per cent, and well above the average (affluence) in 2 per cent.

Jobling and Petersen (1917) in their second year's study of the epidemiology of pellagra in Nashville, Tenn., "endeavored to make a most accurate study of the economic condition of pellagrous patients. In order to do this," they state that their examiners "ascertained the average rentals for the entire city, the weekly income of the pellagrin when a wage earner, and the total income of the pellagrous family." From these data the amount of money available for each pellagrin per week was computed by dividing the total income by the number of individuals, children being accorded the same value as adults.

They found that 70 per cent of their white adult male pellagrins were wage earners, more than 60 per cent of whom earned $10 or more per week. Of the white adult females, 22 per cent were wage earners, and of these, 56 per cent earned less than $10 per week. Of the colored wage earners, 66 per cent of the males earned less than $10 per week, while a similar per cent of the females earned under $8 per week.

When the amount of money available for each pellagrin per week was estimated, Jobling and Petersen found that of the whites 56.5 per cent and of the colored 24 per cent had an available income of $2.50 or more per week.

These workers also made an estimate of the economic status of the pellagrous class on the basis of rentals, which they considered a "fairly reliable basis" for this purpose. They found that of the whites 11 per cent and of the colored 16 per cent owned their own homes or were buying them on the installment plan. "The rentals paid by the balance were practically all under $15 per month, only 3 per cent of the cases occurring in families paying more than this amount. Of the colored families few pay more than $8 per month."

It will be observed that the study of Jobling and Petersen, like that of Siler and Garrison, concerns itself exclusively with the pellagrin. Neither study affords any basis for a comparison with the economic distribution of the general population so that neither these nor, so far as we are aware, any previous observations give us any means of measuring in a definite objective manner the degree of association between economic status and pellagra incidence. This deficiency we have endeavored to repair by the study that we shall now proceed to detail.

Plan and Methods of Present Study

Locality

The study was made in seven representative cotton-mill villages situated in the northwestern part of South Carolina.

Population

The villages were of about average size; none had over 800 or less than 500 inhabitants. Each constituted a distinct, more or less isolated community in close proximity to a cotton-cloth manufacturing plant and was composed practically exclusively of the mill employees and their families. The few Negro families present and living somewhat apart were not considered, so that our study deals with an exclusively white population, which, with hardly a single exception, was of Anglo-Saxon stock born in this country of American-born parents. Besides the Negroes, there were also excluded from this study the mill executives, store managers, clerks, and their households, so that we had left for study an exceptionally homogeneous group with respect to racial stock, occupation, and general standard of living, including dietary custom. An enumeration of the population was made in May and June in connection with the collection of our dietary and economic data, and totaled about 4,160 people, included in about 750 households.

Pellagra Incidence

The procedure adopted for determining the incidence of pellagra in this population has been described at length in a previous paper of this series (Goldberger, Wheeler, and Sydenstricker, Mar. 19, 1920).

Briefly, in order to ascertain the incidence of the disease as completely as possible, the expedient of a systematic biweekly house-to-house search for cases was employed and practically exclusively depended on.

Only cases with a clearly defined, bilaterally symmetrical dermatitis were recorded as pellagra; cases with poorly defined eruptions, or those with more or less suggestive manifestations but without clearly marked eruption, were recorded at most as "suspects" and are excluded from present consideration.

Just as in our study of pellagra incidence in relation to diet, so here, in relating pellagra incidence to economic conditions, no distinction is made between first and recurrent attacks, but all active cases as above defined are considered. So-called inactive or quiescent cases, that is, individuals who had had the disease in a previous year but during 1916 presented no definite eruption or evidence sufficient to be classed as "suspects," are considered as nonpellagrous.

As a considerable proportion of the population of any village is of transient character (see in this connection Goldberger, Wheeler, and Sydenstricker, July 9, 1920) and as much of the pellagra occurs in this class [tabulation deleted. ED.], some assumption was necessary on the basis of which cases might be assigned to households and villages. Accordingly the rule was adopted that a case was to be charged to a household or village only if the affected individual had been a member of that household or had resided in the village not less than 30 days immediately preceding the beginning of the attack (as above defined).

Season

It would seem reasonable to expect, if diet, economic status, or other factor has any influence in relation to the seasonal rise in incidence of the disease, that this influence is most effective during a period immediately anterior to the sharp rise and peak of incidence. Such statistics of pellagra morbidity as were available to us at the beginning of our study indicated that the rise of the seasonal curve of pellagra incidence in the southern states began in the late spring and reached its peak in June. It was assumed, therefore, that the factors favoring the production of pellagra were most effective during the season beginning some time in the late winter or early spring and continuing up to or possibly somewhat into June. The period actually selected by us as representative of this season extended from April 16 to June 15, 1916. Information relating to family income, household food supply, and the composition of the households, etc., for sample sections of this period was secured by trained enumerators who canvassed the village in successive 15-day periods under the immediate direction and supervision of one of us (E. S.).

Dietary Data

The methods adopted for securing data relating to diet have been described fully in a previous communication (Goldberger, Wheeler, and Sydenstricker, Mar. 19, 1920). It will suffice in the present connection to recall that these data relate to the food supply of the household, not to that of the individual, and so do not indicate the differences that may have existed in the diets of the individual members. It being impracticable to secure our dietary data simultaneously in all villages, the record of household food supply secured in the several villages was for successive 15-day periods between April 16 and June 15. It was assumed that an accurate record for a 15-day period would be a sufficiently representative sample of the supply of the season immediately anterior to the peak of seasonal incidence of the disease, that is, of what may be considered as the pellagra-producing season.

Data Relating to Economic Conditions

Since nearly 90 per cent of the individuals composing the population studied were found to be dependent upon the income of family groups composed of more than one person, family income was adopted as the basis for classifying the population according to economic status.

Family income.—The data relating to family income were secured by inquiries of the housewife or of some other responsible member or members of each family, supplemented by data from the mill payrolls. For the latter we are greatly indebted to the willing cooperation of the administrative officials of the mills.

The information obtained from the families covered (*a*) the rate of daily earnings of each member earning wages during the half month preceding the week of the canvass and the various rates of daily earnings of all members who had been employed during the 12 preceding months; (*b*) the days not at work for all members who had worked for wages during the 12 preceding months; (*c*) the income from all other sources during the preceding half month as well as during the preceding 12 months, this information being secured in detail for each source of income. On the basis of this information it was possible to approximate the total income of each family for the half month preceding the visit of the enumerator, and, roughly, for any part or all of the preceding year.

Finding that approximately 90 per cent of the total income of the families studied came from the earnings of wage-earning members, the family statements of earnings during this half-month period were compared with the records on the mill payrolls, and, in the great majority of instances, were found to agree closely with them; but in order to reduce the error arising from even slightly inaccurate statements as to wages, the payroll records instead of the family statements have been used to supply the earnings data. For that small proportion of family income made up of wages earned in employment outside of the mills and of the amounts derived from other miscellaneous sources, the family statement was necessarily accepted.

On the basis of the results of some preliminary tabulations it was decided that the family income during the half month preceding the week of the enumerator's canvass would be a fairly accurate indication of family income during the season selected as most significant in relation to the occurrence of pellagra. The basis for classifying families with respect to income was, therefore, the total cash income of each during a 15-day period between April 16 and June 15, 1916. A half-month sample period was used, partly because it corresponded to the sample period for which dietary data were secured and partly because a majority of the mills in the villages paid at semimonthly intervals. The payroll data from other mills were adjusted to a half-month basis.

In the course of the canvass of the homes of the mill workers' families other data affecting the economic status of the families were also collected. These related principally to length of experience in mill work, occupational status of wage earners, and the amount and incidence of disabling sickness (see Sydenstricker, Wheeler, and Goldberger, 1918) among wage-earning and other members of households.

Availability of food supply.—With the view of studying the relation of food availability to pellagra incidence, information was collected under the immediate direction of one of us (E. S.), relating to conditions that might affect the supply of a given food or foods. In collecting and recording this information a uniform method was followed as closely as possible except where specific points suggested the advisability of special inquiry. The principal sources of information and the nature of the information sought were as follows:

(1) Statements were obtained from households as to the immediate source of every article of food entering into their half-month's supplies. Thus it was ascertained, for example, whether the fresh milk used by the household was produced at home, purchased from another mill worker's household in the village, or from some specific farmer, dairy, or store, or donated by a relative, neighbor, or other person. In the event that a household had a source of supply not common generally to households in the village, inquiries were directed with a view of ascertaining the length of time the household had had such a supply, particularly, with respect to the period after January 1, 1916.

(2) From farmers, hucksters, or "peddlers" selling from house to house, statements were secured relating to the quantities sold, prices, frequency of selling, and character of produce sold since January 1, 1916.

(3) From managers and clerks in the stores, markets, and other retail establishments at which mill workers' households largely dealt, data were secured relating to (a) prices during the 15-day period and price changes during 1916; (b) sources of each food sold, whether direct from near-by farms or through middlemen from local agricultural territory or from other sections of the United States; (c) names of brands and quantities of the foods sold; (d) practices with respect to credit to mill workers' households, especially as affected by the amount of earnings by the mill workers.

Economic Classification

Method of classification according to economic status.—As has already been mentioned, the great majority of the individuals composing the population studied were members of families who subsisted on the income of families composed of several persons; the small proportion not subsisting on such family income were boarders living under substantially the same conditions as the families with which they boarded. It would seem permissible, therefore, to classify these economically with the members of the family with which they boarded, although it is fully recognized that in so doing a certain, though, for the present purpose, unimportant, error is involved.

In classifying this population according to economic status on the basis of family income the conventional method of using total family income for a given period was found to be so inaccurate in many instances as to be misleading. The average total annual cash income of all of the families for which income data were secured was about $700, and relatively few had annual incomes of over $1,000. Thus the range of total income was relatively small and the families were, from this point of view, fairly homogeneous. They differed, however, very markedly in size and with respect to the age and sex of their members. Manifestly it was improper to classify, for example, a family whose half-month's income was $40, and was composed of only a man and his wife, with one whose half-month's income was also $40, but was composed of a man, his wife, and several dependent children. Since family income, for the purpose of this study, was used as an index of the economic status of individuals who composed the family group, it was necessary to take into consideration the number of such individuals in comparing one family with another. A per capita statement of income, however, while more accurate than the statement of total income, was subject to the inaccuracy arising from differences in the age and sex of members of the families to be compared. It appeared advisable, therefore, to employ a common denominator to which the individuals of both sexes and of all ages could be reduced in order to obtain a more accurately representative method of expressing the relative size of the families to be compared.

In the absence of a better common denominator for this purpose, the Atwater (1915) scale of food requirements was employed, and the size of each family was computed according to this scale and expressed in terms of "adult male units." The scale used appears below. The assumption in the use of this scale was that the expenditures for total maintenance for individuals varied according to sex and age in the same proportion as did their food requirements. The assumption is by no means as accurate as could be desired; in its favor, however, it may be said that since family

Age.	Equivalent adult male unit.	
	Male.	Female.
Adult (over 16)...	1.0	0.8
15 to 16..........	.9	.8
13 to 14..........	.8	.7
12................	.7	.6
10 to 11..........	.6	.6
6 to 9............	.5	.5
2 to 5............	.4	.4
Under 2..........	.3	.3

expenditures in the great majority of cases equaled total family income, and since food expenditures were nearly half (among poorer families considerably more than half) of total expenditures, a scale based on food requirements alone is obviously very much more accurate than one omitting any consideration whatsoever of the number, sex, and age of the individuals composing the families to be compared with respect to income.[3] For the present purpose,

TABLE 46—*Number of families and members of families and their equivalents in adult male units in seven cotton-mill villages of South Carolina, classified according to family income during a fifteen-day period between April 15 and June 16, 1916.*

Half-month family income per adult male unit.	Families.	Persons.*	Equivalent adult male units.+
	Number.	Number.	Number.
Less than $6.00	217	1,289	866.2
$6.00-$7.99.....................	183	972	675.9
$8.09-$9.99.....................	139	704	529.2
$10.00 and over.................	208	800	607.1
All incomes.................	747	3,765	2,678.2
	Per cent.	Per cent.	Per cent.
All incomes.................	100.0	100.0	100.0
Less than $6.00.................	29.1	34.2	32.4
$6.00-$7.99.....................	24.5	25.8	25.2
$8.00-$9.99.....................	18.6	18.7	19.8
$10.00 and over.................	27.9	21.3	22.6

*Exclusive of persons paying board and including only those dependent upon family income.
+According to the Atwater scale for food requirements.

3   In order to establish a more accurate basis for computing the size of families in comparing their incomes, a detailed study of expenditures for individuals in a number of representative families in cotton-mill villages was undertaken during 1917. While the tabulations of these data were not completed in time for use in the study of the data collected in 1916, it appears that the Atwater scale is roughly indicative of the variations, according to sex and age, in the consumption of all articles for which there are individual expenditures. It should be noted that before using the Atwater scale in the preliminary computations of family income, several published estimates of the cost of maintenance for individuals of various ages were examined. These estimates were based, in several instances, upon the results of investigation

therefore, the total income of each family as defined above, has been divided by the number of "adult male units" subsisting on the family income, and the resulting figure has been termed the "family income per adult male unit."

Results of classification.—The 747 families for which income data were sufficiently accurate and complete for consideration have been classified by this method and grouped into four convenient classes, each containing a fair proportion of the total number. Table 46 presents this classification and also the resulting distribution of individuals and their equivalent "adult male units."

The differences in income are also indicated in Table 47, which permits of a comparison of the results of classification on the basis of the average income during the half-month period per family, per person, and per "adult male unit." It will be noted that the same *general* differences in *average* incomes for the four groups are indicated by any of the three methods of classification. For reasons already stated, however, the "adult male unit" method is believed

TABLE 47—*Average half-month family income, computed in terms of "per family," "per person," and "per adult male unit,"* for various income classes of the population in seven cotton-mill villages in South Carolina.*

Half-month family income per adult male unit.	All family income during a half month.	Average income during a half month.		
		Per family.	Per person.	Per adult male unit.+
Less than $6.00..............	$3,990.45	$18.38	$3.09	$4.61
$6.00–$7.99..................	4,780.85	26.12	4.92	7.07
$8.00–$9.99..................	4,642.29	33.40	6.55	8.77
$10.00 and over..............	7,777.99	37.39	9.72	12.81
All incomes..............	21,191.58	28.36	5.63	7.92

*According to the Atwater scale for food requirements.
+Exclusive of persons paying board and including only those dependent upon family income.

of actual expenditures of individual members of families. Using the estimated expenditures for an adult male as 100, the estimates for individuals of other ages of either sex were expressed relatively and compared with the Atwater scale. It appeared that, in most instances, the scales were fairly similar. [Tabulation of data deleted. ED.]

to be more accurately representative of actual conditions than either of the others and, therefore, to be preferred for the classification of individual families; it is the method hereinafter employed.

Before entering upon a consideration of the relation of family income to pellagra incidence it will be desirable to make brief reference to the factors affecting family income. An analysis of our data with a view of determining, so far as practicable, what these were, showed the principal ones to be as follows: (a) Supplemental income, chiefly from boarders; (b) the number of dependent persons, principally children, in proportion to the number of wage-earning persons in the family; and (c) the earning capacity of the wage earners, including chiefly the factors of natural ability, length of training, and state of health. In the classification of this population according to "family income per adult male unit," those persons in the higher income classes appeared distinctly to have the advantage in each of these respects over those in the lower income classes.

Pellegra Incidence According to Economic Status

Having considered the methods employed for securing the basic data relating to the occurrence of the disease and for securing those relating to the classification of the population with respect to economic status, we may now proceed to determine the relationship existing between the economic status of the family and the degree of incidence of the disease.

We have in all 747 households for which our data are sufficiently complete and accurate to permit of classification according to income. There were recorded among the members of these households 97 definite cases of pellagra. In Table 48 we have distributed these households in accordance with the family income per "adult male unit" during the sample half-month period and have indicated therein also the number and per cent of the households in each of the resulting five income classes that were affected with pellagra to the extent of (a) one or more cases, (b) two or more cases, and (c) three or more cases.

It will be observed that the proportion of families affected with pellagra declines with a marked degree of regularity as income increases. This inverse correlation is even more clearly shown when weight is given to households with more than one case of the disease,[4]

4   Upon the basis of the average half-month income per adult male unit for each of the income classes and the corresponding pellagra rate per 1,000 persons, the Pearsonian coefficient of correlation is -0.91 ± 0.05. While the small number of classes considered must, of course, be taken into account,

TABLE 48—*Number and per cent of households of different income classes affected with pellagra in seven cotton-mill villages of South Carolina in 1916.*

Half-month family income per adult male unit.	All households.	Pellagrous households in which were--		
		One or more cases of pellagra.	Two or more cases of pellagra.	Three or more cases of pellagra.
		NUMBER.		
Less than $6.00........	217	28	17	7
$6.00-7.99.............	183	21	3	1
$8.00-$9.99............	139	8	4	0
$10.00-$13.99..........	144	3	0	0
$14.00 and over........	64	1	0	0
All incomes........	747	61	24	8
		PER CENT.		
Less than $6.00........	100.0	12.9	7.8	3.2
$6.00-$7.99............	100.0	11.5	1.6	.5
$8.00-$9.99............	100.0	5.8	2.9	0.0
$10.00-$13.99..........	100.0	2.1	0.0	0.0
$14.00 and over........	100.0	1.5	0.0	0.0
All incomes........	100.0	8.2	3.2	1.1

as is done in Table 49, in which the incidence of pellagra is expressed as a rate per 1,000 persons in each income class.

The occurrence of multiple-case families, especially from the point of view of difference in income, invites special comment. The 97 cases of pellagra occurred in 61 families. In each of 24 of these families, two or more cases occurred, while in each of 8, three or more cases developed. Taking into consideration the size of the families and assuming that all individuals were equally susceptible to the disease,[5] a computation of the probability of the occurrence of multiple-case families according to purely chance distribution indicated that in the 747 families we should expect about 90 families

---

the expression indicates high degree of correlation (—1.0 being perfect inverse correlation).

5 So far as sex and age are concerned, all families (with but few exceptions) contained fairly comparable proportions of "susceptible" individuals.

TABLE 49—*Number of definite cases of pellagra and rate per 1,000* among persons of different income classes in seven cotton-mill villages of South Carolina in 1916.*

Half-month family income per adult male unit.	Total.			Males.			Females.		
	Number of persons.	Number of cases.	Rate* per 1,000.	Number of persons.	Number of cases.	Rate per 1,000.	Number of persons.	Number of cases.	Rate per 1,000.
Less than $6.00.....	1,312	56	42.7	650	20	30.8	662	36	54.4
$6.00–$7.99.........	1,037	27	26.0	521	6	11.5	516	21	40.7
$8.00–$9.99.........	784	10	12.8	376	4	10.7	408	6	14.7
$10.00–$13.99.......	736	3	4.1	363	0	0.0	373	3	8.0
$14.00 and over.....	291	1	3.4	161	1	6.2	130	0	0.0
All incomes.....	4,160	97	23.3	2,071	31	14.9	2,089	66	31.6

Comparison of crude pellagra rates and of rates after adjustment for age to a standard population for each income class.
(Standard population=total population, all incomes.)

Family income per adult male unit.	Case rate per 1,000.	
	Crude.	Adjusted.
Less than $6.00................	42.7	41.0
$6.00–$7.99....................	26.0	24.8
$8.00–$9.99....................	12.8	14.2
$10.00–$13.99.................	4.1	5.2
$14.00 and over...............	3.4	2.5

*Since a marked variation in the pellagra rate according to age and sex was found for the population studied (Goldberger, Wheeler, and Sydenstricker, 1920 b), and since, ordinarily, differences in the distribution of persons according to age occur in different economic groups, computation of rates adjusted to a standard population was made. The influence of differences in the sex distribution in any age group was insignificant, and practically the same incidence rates were obtained after making adjustments to a standard age distribution, as is shown in the above table:

with one case each, about 8 families with two or more cases, while the probability of households each with three or more cases would be less than 2 in 10,000. The actual occurrence of 24 families with two cases each and of 8 families with three or more cases would thus seem to be far in excess of the result of chance.[6] The fact that multiple-case families occurred only in the lower-income classes and that families with three or more cases occurred practically only in the lowest-income class plainly shows that the tendency toward concentration of cases in certain families increases as income diminishes. Pellagra incidence in the population studied therefore not only varied inversely according to family income, but with

6 Acknowledgment is made to Associate Statistician F. M. Phillips, United States Public Health Service, for assistance in this computation.

decreasing income it seemed to show an increasing tendency to affect members of the same family.

Discussion

The very marked inverse correlation between low income and pellagra incidence naturally calls for explanation. Under the conditions of the study the following possibilities in this regard suggested themselves for consideration:

(a) Bad hygiene and sanitation;

(b) Difference in sex and age composition of the population in the several income classes; and

(c) Difference in diet.

(a) *Bad hygiene and sanitation* are in general closely associated with poverty so that the incidence of a disease, the dissemination of which is favored by such conditions, may be expected to be unusually high in the lower economic strata. Consequently it is natural to suspect that a disease found to be highly prevalent in an environment of poverty is dependent on the almost inevitably attendant unhygienic and insanitary conditions for its propagation, and to assume that it is of microbial origin. The possibility of an essential infective etiological factor in this disease has therefore been given careful consideration, and in a previous paper (Goldberger, Wheeler, and Sydenstricker, July 16, 1920) we reported the results of our study of the relation of certain factors of a sanitary character to the incidence of pellagra in these villages. No consistent correlation was found.[7] This, coupled with the results of the other of our own studies (see discussion by Goldberger and Wheeler, 1920, pp. 36–41) and of the studies of other investigators (White, 1919; and Boyd and Lelean, 1919), and with the fact of the complete absence of any unequivocal evidence in support of an essential infective etiological factor in this disease, not only renders discussion of hygienic and sanitary factors in the present connection unnecessary but, we believe, permits of their dismissal from further serious consideration.

(b) *Differences in sex and age composition of the population in the several income classes.—*We have shown in a previous communication (Goldberger, Wheeler, and Sydenstricker, July 9, 1920) that

7 The data collected during 1916 were not in a form to permit the study of the relation of crowding in the home to pellagra incidence. We may state, however, that a preliminary analysis of a considerable mass of data bearing on this point, collected during 1917, shows very little, if any, correlation between them when the effect of income is minimized.

the incidence of the disease in the population of these villages differs markedly in the sexes and at certain age periods; it is conceivable, therefore, that differences in the sex and the age distribution in the different income classes might give rise to the phenomenon under discussion. That this is not the case, however, is evident (1) when it is recalled that we are dealing with a population composed of family units and (2) when we compare the indications afforded by Tables 49 and 50, showing, respectively, the sex and the age distribution of the population of each economic class, and note the agreement in the indications afforded by the crude rates and by the rates after adjustment to a standard population (footnote to Table 49).

(c) *Differences in diet.*—The results of budgetary investigations have repeatedly demonstrated the association of marked variations in diet with variation in family income. (In this connection see Sydenstricker, 1915.) It seemed doubly pertinent, therefore, to inquire what, if any, variations in diet were associated with variations in income among the families of our cotton-mill villages. Accordingly, we prepared Table 51, showing the average food supply of the households of the several income classes. To facilitate comparison between the averages thus presented, indices have been computed, the figures for the households with the highest income being used as the base. It will be noted that, from the point of view of income, the following general tendencies are suggested:

1. The smaller the income the smaller were the supplies purchased of all meats (except salt pork), green vegetables, fresh fruits, eggs, butter, cheese, preserved milk, lard, sugar (including sirup), and canned foods.

2. The smaller the income the larger were the supplies purchased of salt pork and corn meal.

3. In the households of the various income classes the quantities of the purchased supplies[8] of dried peas and beans, potatoes, dried fruits, wheat flour and bread, fresh milk, and rice appeared without any consistent trend.

Thus it appears that there were associated with differences in family income quite definite differences in household food supplies. In order to determine the outstanding differences more clearly, the

8 Practically all food supplies, with the exception of fresh milk, were purchased (i.e., not home-produced) during the season (the late spring) of the year under consideration. Households securing supplies of milk from home-owned cows have not been included in Table 51, since supplies of food from this source constitute a factor affecting the diet of the population apart from the factor of family income. They are considered in another connection.

households with intermediate incomes were disregarded and comparison was made of the food supplies in households presenting the greatest contrast from an economic standpoint (i.e., those households representing the respective extremes of family income), with the result that not only did the differences already noted stand out more clearly, but, in addition, it appeared that the supplies of wheat flour and bread and of fresh milk were appreciably smaller in the poorest households.

In that part of our study dealing with the relation of household food supply to pellagra incidence (Goldberger, Wheeler, and Sydenstricker, Mar. 19, 1920) a very definite significant relationship between the character of the diet and the incidence of the disease was demonstrated, and since, as we have seen above, a marked inverse correlation exists between the amount of family income and the degree of incidence of the disease, it follows that the character of the diet of the population under consideration may be expected to vary with the amount of family income, in the sense at least that

TABLE 50—*Number and per cent of persons in each income class, classified according to age, in seven cotton-mill villages of South Carolina in 1916.*

(The classes being divided from each other at those ages at which the pellagra incidence rate for the whole population varies most sharply.*)

Half-month family income per adult male unit.	Age group.							
	All ages.	Under 5 years.	5-9	10-19	20-29	30-44	45-54	55 years and over.
NUMBER.								
Less than $6.00.........	1,312	260	251	317	162	217	49	56
$6.00-$7.99.............	1,037	162	166	270	172	166	60	41
$8.00-$9.99.............	784	104	108	229	149	114	48	32
$10.00-$13.99...........	736	95	69	173	215	102	46	36
$14.00 and over.........	291	27	15	71	91	63	9	15
All incomes..........	4,160	648	609	1,060	789	662	212	180
PER CENT.								
Less than $6.00.........	100	19.8	19.1	24.2	12.4	16.5	3.7	4.3
$6.00-$7.99.............	100	15.7	16.0	26.0	16.6	16.0	5.8	3.9
$8.00-$9.99.............	100	13.3	13.8	29.2	19.0	14.5	6.1	4.1
$10.00-$13.99...........	100	12.9	9.4	23.5	29.2	13.9	6.2	4.9
$14.00 and over.........	100	9.3	5.2	24.4	31.3	21.6	3.1	5.2
All incomes..........	100	15.6	14.6	25.5	19.0	15.9	5.1	4.3

*See Goldberger, Wheeler, and Sydenstricker, March 19, 1920.

the lower the income the more the character of the diet will tend
to approach that associated with pellagra. This is confirmed by
the quite definite differences in food supply above actually shown
to be associated with differences in family income, and further by
the fact that when comparison is made, such as Table 51 permits,
it is found that in a general, but quite definite, way the food supply
of the households of the lowest-income class tends to be similar to
that of the group of pellagrous households in each of which at
least two cases of pellagra occurred prior to August 1, 1916; that is,
similar to that of the group whose food supply more closely approximates a representative sample of a pellagra-producing diet than does
any other afforded by our study. [Graphic comparison deleted. ED.]

Differences in Incidence Among Households

From the foregoing considerations the conclusion would seem to
be suggested that the inverse correlation between pellagra incidence
and family income depended in large measure, if not entirely, on the
unfavorable effect of a low income on the character of the diet. In
this connection, however, it must be noted and consideration must
be given to the fact that a large proportion of households with low
incomes were not affected with the disease.

(Similarly, a large proportion of the members of pellagrous households were apparently unaffected by the disease. As has already been
stated, the present study deals with the household, not with the
individual, excepting only as to pellagra incidence. We have, therefore, no special data on which an explanation of the exemption
of the unaffected members of a household might be based. Nevertheless, in the light of (a) certain general observations and (b) of
analogies to such food deficiency diseases as scurvy and beriberi,
together with (c) the knowledge gained as the result of the newer
work of many students in the field of diet and nutrition, the following suggestions may properly be submitted for consideration
in this connection:

1. *Differences in diet consumed among individuals of the household.*—Although all members of a household presumably have the
same diet available, as the result of individual likes and dislikes,
observable at almost any table, slight differences in diet actually
consumed are common and marked differences, amounting in some
instances to outstanding individual eccentricities, are not rare.
Furthermore, differences in diet actually consumed may arise from,
or be accentuated by, food eaten between meals and by supplemental
foods of one kind or another in respect to which individuals of

TABLE 51—Average supply (per adult male unit) during a fifteen-day period between April 15 and June 16, 1916, of various purchased articles of food* in households of different income classes and in the group of households in each of which two or more cases of pellagra occurred prior to August 1, 1916.

GRAMS PER ADULT MALE UNIT PER DAY.

Half-month family income per adult male unit.	Salt pork	Corn meal and grits	Dried peas and beans	Potatoes	Dried fruits	Wheat flour, bread	Fresh milk (bought)	Sugar sirup	Butter	Rice	Canned vegetables	Preserved milk	Lard and lard substitutes	Canned meats	Cheese	Eggs	Green vegetables +	Fresh fruits	Canned corn	Canned fruits	Jellies and jams	Fresh meats	Canned peas and beans	Cured lean meats
$14.00 and more..	39	126	31	71	10	447	319	59	30	8	58	4	63	20	3	59	105	41	9	27	11	47	9	53
$10.00–$13.99....	49	152	31	107	9	434	302	61	35	6	36	4	54	12	2	57	63	33	10	26	10	32	6	28
$8.00–$9.99......	54	151	35	97	9	410	342	67	14	5	37	3	49	16	3	44	60	31	8	24	8	30	4	24
$6.00–$7.99......	56	174	33	88	9	460	317	55	19	4	46	1	49	14	2	38	61	30	6	14	9	21	5	20
Less than $6.00..	54	169	31	73	10	399	282	50	19	5	35	2	37	12	2	33	49	19	4	12	5	19	2	12
Pellagrous households......	65	150	34	60	10	361	127	48	11	6	20	2	35	16	#	31	61	10	6	16	6	16	2	8

RELATIVE NUMBERS. BASE: SUPPLY PER ADULT MALE UNIT PER DAY IN HOUSEHOLDS WITH HIGHEST INCOMES.

	Salt pork	Corn meal and grits	Dried peas and beans	Potatoes	Dried fruits	Wheat flour, bread	Fresh milk (bought)	Sugar sirup	Butter	Rice	Canned vegetables	Preserved milk	Lard and lard substitutes	Canned meats	Cheese	Eggs	Green vegetables +	Fresh fruits	Canned corn	Canned fruits	Jellies and jams	Fresh meats	Canned peas and beans	Cured lean meats
$14.00 and more..	100	100	100	100	100	100	100	100	100	100	100	100	100	100	100	100	100	100	100	100	100	100	100	100
$10.00–$13.99....	126	121	100	151	90	97	95	103	117	75	62	100	86	60	67	97	60	81	111	96	91	68	67	53
$8.00–$9.99......	138	120	113	137	90	92	107	114	47	63	64	75	78	80	100	75	57	76	89	89	73	64	44	45
$6.00–$7.99......	144	138	107	124	90	103	99	93	63	50	79	25	78	70	67	64	58	73	67	52	82	45	56	38
Less than $6.00..	138	134	100	103	100	89	88	85	63	63	60	50	59	60	67	56	47	46	44	44	45	40	22	23
Pellagrous households......	167	119	110	85	100	81	40	81	37	75	34	50	55	80	..	53	58	24	67	59	55	34	22	15

*For explanation of terms, see Goldberger, Wheeler, and Sydenstricker 1920a, appendix.
+ Includes string beans.
# Less than 0.5 of a gram.

the same household may differ considerably. Clearly, then, a knowledge of the exact composition of the diet of a household or other dietary group does not necessarily justify the assumption of a knowledge of the composition of the diet consumed by an individual member of such household or group. Failure to appreciate this, it may be noted, has been a frequent cause of serious error and consequent confusion in connection with studies of food-deficiency diseases.

2. *Differences in individual susceptibility or resistance.*—Assuming identity of diet actually consumed, differences in incidence among individuals of the same household or other dietary group may result from individual variation in resistance or susceptibility, which may conceivably be related to (*a*) an inherent individual characteristic, (*b*) the age or sex of the individual, (*c*) the existence of some exhausting underlying disease or condition (hookworm, dysentery, duodenal fistula), or (*d*) to unlike physical strain or exertion.

3. *Combinations of factors 1 and 2.*)

Thus, in the village of *In*, where the highest of the incidence rates observed by us in 1916 occurred and where the rate among persons constituting the households with incomes under the average was 90 per 1,000, over 65 per cent of these poorer households appeared not to be affected, and, in varying degree, this was true of each of the seven villages studied. That the exemption of these families from pellagra was not due to a lack of subjects of "susceptible" sex is evident from what has already been said on this point; and that it could not be attributed to lack of human material of "susceptible" age appears very clearly when the distribution of the population according to age is compared for the pellagrous and for the poorer nonpellagrous households in a representative village, as is done in Table 52. Manifestly, therefore, the amount of family income—that is, money income (in the sense here used), such as wages, cash payments from boarders, cash receipts from sales of supplies, and other sources—was not the sole factor determining the character of the household diet.

This is quite in accord with common experience, which teaches that there are many factors that, singly or in varying combinations, may have an important influence on the character of the diet and that may vary among and thus may distinguish different households of the same income. In illustration of this, reference may be made to the group of factors that tend to determine the amount and proportion of family income available for the purchase of food, an example of which is the occurrence of sickness or injury, making an

TABLE 52—*Age distribution of population constituting the non-pellagrous households with low family income* and the pellagrous households of the mill village of In.*

Households.	Age groups.							
	All ages.	Under 5.	5-9	10-14	20-29	30-44	45-54	55 and over.
	NUMBER OF PERSONS.							
Nonpellagrous.........	265	52	53	61	33	45	14	7
Pellagrous............	168	31	32	49	19	31	5	1
All households......	433	83	85	110	52	76	19	8
	PER CENT.							
Nonpellagrous.........	100.0	19.6	20.0	23.0	12.5	17.0	5.3	2.6
Pellagrous............	100.0	18.5	19.0	29.2	11.3	18.5	3.0	.6
All households......	100.0	19.2	19.6	25.4	12.0	17.5	4.4	1.8

*That is, under $8 per adult male unit during a half-month period in the late spring of 1916.

unusual draft on the family income. Related to such factors are the general spirit of the household with respect to thrift (which, when unwisely directed, may be harmful) and the intelligence and ability of the housewife in utilizing the available family income.

More tangible than these, and perhaps of more immediate practical importance in its effect on the household diet, is the difference among households with respect to the availability of food supplies. We found that, among households with similar incomes and of the same village and thus with access to the same markets, there were some more favorably situated in having sources of food supplies that others either did not possess or possessed in a lesser degree. Such sources frequently were gardens, home-owned cows, swine, poultry, and the like.

Differences in Incidence Among Villages

Besides differences among households with similar incomes and of the same village, quite marked differences in pellagra incidence were also observed, as has already been pointed out, among the villages themselves. We have sought to determine the explanation of this by considering in order the various possibilities that suggested themselves.

(*a*) The general environment (except as to condition of sanitation and food supply), the origin and type of the population, the character of work, and the general habits of living among these populations being, as we have already stated, strikingly similar, do not call for consideration in the present connection.

(b) Differences in sanitary conditions among villages were noted and their relation to differences in the incidence of the disease was studied without, however, discovering any consistent correlation among them. Reasons have been given why hygienic and sanitary factors might be dismissed from consideration in the attempt to explain the inverse correlation between family income and the incidence of pellagra (see p. 241). Further discussion of these factors in the present connection would therefore seem to be unnecessary.

(c) The marked association between low family income and pellagra incidence suggested the possibility that the difference in incidence among villages might be associated with a difference in the proportion of families of low incomes included in the populations of the several villages. But if the differences in the proportion of the population which had low incomes in the various villages be compared with the differences in pellagra incidence, as is done in Table 53, no consistent correlation is disclosed. Clearly the differences in pellagra incidence among these villages cannot be ac-

TABLE 53—*Comparison of the relation of rate of pellagra incidence to proportion of population of low family income in seven mill villages of South Carolina in 1916.*

Village.	Per cent of population whose half-month family income per adult male unit was less than—		Pellagra rate per 1,000 population (all incomes) in 1916.
	$6.00	$8.00	
All villages.........	31.5	56.5	23.4
At...................	37.0	64.3	20.7
In...................	40.9	66.6	64.6
Ny...................	26.2	45.7	0.0
Rc...................	13.2	23.7	24.9
Sn...................	38.3	58.1	10.9
Sa...................	28.3	57.4	25.7
Wy...................	31.0	64.0	18.7

Pearsonian coefficient of correlation: r=0.33± 0.23

counted for by differences in the economic status of the populations concerned.

(d) As family income is simply an index of the power to buy, and as this power is obviously limited by the cost of the thing desired (in this instance food), the thought naturally suggests itself that differences in prices in the different villages might be of importance in the present connection. That this was a negligible factor, however, is shown by the fact that we found no significant differences in food prices in the different villages.

(e) That individuals of "susceptible" ages may have been present in relatively insignificant numbers in the villages among whose poorer households few if any were affected by the disease, and that this may account for the differences, is an explanation that may be dismissed from consideration when the age distribution of the population is compared according to village, as may be seen by reference to Table 54.

(f) We thus come to a consideration, finally, of differences among villages with respect to availability of food supplies on the local markets or from home production. More or less marked differences in this respect were found to exist. In relating these to differences in pellagra incidence it should be borne in mind that the availability to a consumer of a supply of a given article or group of articles of food is often involved in a number of interrelated conditions, the influence of any one of which may be difficult to measure. Therefore, in analyzing community conditions affecting the supply of any article or articles of food, only the outstanding and clearcut differences between localities can be considered. Furthermore, since even considerable differences in pellagra incidence among localities of small population are not necessarily a reflection of community conditions, it seemed desirable to select for the study of the relationship under consideration villages presenting the most marked contrast in the incidence of the disease, thereby avoiding the possibly confusing effects of irregularities likely to arise in attempts to relate community conditions of food availability to pellagra rates for which community conditions were possibly responsible only in part or not at all. There was, moreover, the compelling practical consideration to thus restrict ourselves in the fact that the amount of labor involved in a detailed study of conditions in each of our villages was beyond the physical capacity of the available personnel to perform. Accordingly we selected for study *Ny* village, with no pellagra, and *In* village, with a rate of not less than 64.6 per 1,000 during 1916. The facts, as we were able to determine them relating to the avail-

TABLE 54—*Comparison of the age distribution of the population constituting the households with low family incomes* of seven cotton-mill villages of South Carolina.*

Villages.	All ages.	Classified by age periods (years).						
		Under 5 years.	5-9	10-19	20-29	30-44	45-54	55 and over.
		NUMBER OF PERSONS.						
At...............	367	65	65	82	63	59	18	15
In...............	433	83	85	110	52	76	19	8
Ny...............	331	60	56	87	45	57	15	11
Rc...............	206	37	42	50	34	32	5	6
Sn...............	338	65	46	69	61	52	14	31
Sa...............	268	51	51	68	40	34	14	10
Wy...............	407	62	72	120	39	73	24	17
All villages....	2,350	423	417	586	334	383	109	98
		PER CENT.						
At...............	100.0	17.5	17.5	22.3	17.2	16.1	4.9	4.1
In...............	100.0	19.2	19.6	25.4	12.0	17.5	4.4	1.8
Ny...............	100.0	18.1	16.9	26.3	13.6	17.2	4.5	3.3
Rc...............	100.0	18.0	20.4	24.3	16.5	15.5	2.4	2.9
Sn...............	100.0	19.2	13.6	20.4	18.0	15.4	4.1	9.2
Sa...............	100.0	19.0	19.0	25.4	14.9	12.7	5.2	3.7
Wy...............	100.0	15.2	17.4	29.5	9.6	17.9	5.9	4.2
All villages...	100.0	18.0	17.7	24.9	14.2	16.3	4.6	4.2

*That is under $8 per adult male unit during a half month in the late spring of 1916.

ability of supplies of various foods in these two villages, are briefly summarized in the following:

(1) *Retail grocery establishments.*—In both villages the mill workers' households purchased their supplies of all foods from the company stores and from grocery stores in adjacent communities, with the exception of fresh meats, fresh milk, and varying proportions of their supplies of eggs, butter, green vegetables, and fresh fruits. Exclusive of the articles named, the availability of supplies of all foods appeared to be the same in both villages for the reasons that (a) in both villages there existed company stores which carried in stock practically the same kinds of foods and were operated along

similar lines from the point of view of credit allowances to mill workers, and (b) within a mile of either village were general grocery stores carrying in stock the same kinds and varieties of foods as those sold at the company stores. The company stores at *Ny*, however, did not sell fresh vegetables, potatoes, and fresh fruits, there being an agreement with the lessee of the village market to the effect that the latter should have the exclusive store privilege of selling these articles. A much more regular and abundant supply of fresh vegetables and fruits was available at the *Ny* market than at the *In* company store.

It is of interest to note that the *In* households, whose incomes were less than the average income for the two villages, relied to a greater extent upon the company store than the *Ny* households with similar incomes. This is indicated by the purchase and food supply records during the 15-day period from May 16 to May 30, 1916, which show that 60 per cent of the *In* households purchased all of their groceries (exclusive of home produce and produce from near-by farms) from the company store as compared with only 13 per cent of the *Ny* households.

(2) *Fresh-meat markets.*—In *Ny* there was a fresh-meat market which had been open seven days in the week the year round for several years. This market, as already noted, also sold fresh fruit and vegetables. The nearest other market was 1 mile away, and this market operated a wagon which regularly had taken orders and delivered fresh meat in the village at the doors of the mill workers' households during the spring and the preceding fall and winter. At the town of Seneca, 4 miles away, there were two other fresh-meat markets which were occasionally patronized by *Ny* mill workers. In *In* village there was no fresh-meat market, and there had not been any since the last of February, 1916. In October, 1915, a privately operated market was opened in the basement of the company store building. This market was kept open every week day until about January 1, 1916, but, from all accounts, it was poorly managed. For this reason and for the reason that locally produced fresh meats became scarce after January 1, the market was open only one or two days a week during January and February and its credit trade was severely curtailed, being now limited to those households which had been prompt in settlements. In the latter part of February the market ceased to be operated. In the town of Inman, a mile or more from the mill village, there was a market selling fresh meat for cash only, which had a few regular customers among the mill

workers. No other market was accessible except in the city of Spartanburg, 13 miles away.

With the exception of a small amount of poultry purchased at home or purchased from near-by farmers, the sole sources of fresh meats in the two villages during the late spring of 1916 were these fresh-meat markets. The difference in availability of a fresh meat supply in the two villages is clearly reflected in the records of actual purchases during the 15-day period May 16–30, 1916, illustrated in Table 55, thereby suggesting a marked contrast in fresh-meat consumption between the two villages for households of similar incomes.

(3) *Produce from adjacent farm territory.*—The two villages presented a striking contrast with respect to the availability of food supplies from adjacent farm territory.

In the mill village of *In* there were no regular sellers of farm produce during the spring of 1916; farmers visited the village only occasionally and then practically solely in order to dispose of such goods as they had been unable to sell in the near-by town of Inman. The absence of hucksters was so marked that repeated and detailed inquiries were made of mill workers' households and of other persons living in or in close touch with the village, and the village was several times canvassed in order to secure as complete and accurate information as possible in relation thereto. *Ny*, on the other hand, appeared to be a center for marketing produce from near-by farms. In addition to a number of farmers who marketed their produce in

TABLE 55—*Comparison of availability of fresh meat as shown by the number of purchases and the average daily supply of this food during the period May 16–30, 1916, in households, with family incomes less than the average, of two mill villages of South Carolina.*

Number of purchases during 15-day period.	Village of Ny.(average daily supply per adult male unit, 31.2 grams.)		Village of In. (average daily supply per adult male unit, 7.0 grams.)	
	Number of households purchasing.	Per cent of total households.	Number of households purchasing.	Per cent of total households.
None....................	17	31.0	46	65.8
1........................	6	10.9	18	25.7
2........................	7	12.7	4	5.7
3........................	7	12.7	1	1.4
4........................	6	10.9	1	1.4
5........................	6	10.9	0	0.0
More than 5............	6	10.9	0	0.0

that village occasionally, not less than 22 farmers who habitually sold in the village at retail were found and interviewed in a single canvass of the adjacent territory. These regular hucksters came to the village once a week or oftener practically the year round. Of the 22 who were interviewed, 15 sold fresh milk and butter, 10 sold eggs, 7 sold poultry, 5 sold fresh pork, 2 sold fresh beef, and practically all of them sold potatoes and vegetables. Those selling milk and butter delivered regularly throughout the year and marketed other produce in different seasons. Thus, eggs were sold principally in the spring, poultry in the summer, autumn, and winter, fresh beef and pork in the autumn and winter, and green vegetables in the spring, summer, and autumn. On the basis of statements made by those selling produce regularly, not less than 41,000 quarts of fresh milk (about 790 quarts weekly), 12,000 pounds of butter (about 230 pounds weekly), 1,800 dozen eggs, and 4,200 pounds of live poultry, fresh beef, and fresh pork were sold during the 12 months ending May 30, 1916. These totals do not include quantities sold by other farmers or by stores and markets.

This contrast in available sources of farm produce is indicated also by the statements of actual purchases by the households in the respective villages, secured in the course of the dietary canvass. These statements have been summarized for households of similar incomes in Table 56. A striking difference is shown in the extent to which the households in *Ny* and *In* relied upon near-by farms for supplies of certain foods.

The difference between *Ny* and *In* in availability of food supplies from adjacent farm territory was so pronounced that further inquiries were made into some of the underlying conditions in order to discover, if possible, what other economic factors were responsible for bringing this about. From these inquiries it appeared that at least two conditions were important in causing the difference in availability of the supply of the foods in question: namely (*a*) differences in the kind of agriculture in the territory adjacent to the villages, and (*b*) differences in marketing conditions. The two are closely related, but for the sake of clearness it will be advantageous to discuss them separately.

(*a*) Contrast in the kinds of agriculture near the two villages.—A census of the farm products in the agricultural territory adjacent to the two villages was not undertaken, but from observation in the course of several trips and canvasses in the sections in question it was quite clear that a marked contrast existed in the kinds of agriculture pursued. The territory around *In* was planted principally in cotton, and relatively little diversification in crops existed. Truck farming on any considerable scale was not engaged in. Few beef cattle were raised and milch cows apparently were usually not more than sufficient to supply the household needs of the farmers. Many farmers had no cows or pigs or even poultry. The agriculture in the *In* section seemed rather typical of the cotton areas in South Carolina. Cotton was the predominant crop; all other products were incidental, none of them constituting the principal output of any farm, so far as was observed. The territory around *Ny*, on the other hand, was exceptional for South Carolina in that a considerable amount of diversified farming was carried on, although not fully comparable in this respect with the farming sections in states where one-crop agriculture has not been the rule. Cotton was a relatively less important crop, and beef cattle, swine, poultry, and milch cows seemed much more abundant than in the *In* section. Apparently greater emphasis was given to gardens, and the amount of truck produced was noticeably larger. The physical character of the section apparently was one cause of this difference in products. The land around *In* is almost level, lies well below the foothills of the Blue Ridge Mountains, and is well suited for the growing of cotton. The land around *Ny* is quite rolling and even hilly, being, in fact, in the foothills of the mountains and thus not so well suited to cotton

TABLE 56—*Comparison of availability of certain foods in two cotton-mill villages of South Carolina, as indicated by the proportion of the households with family incomes under the average of the contrasted villages purchasing the specified articles from nearby farms during the period May 16–30, 1916.*

Article purchased.	Ny.			In.		
	Average quantity per household purchasing.	Households purchasing.		Average quantity per household purchasing.	Households purchasing.	
		Number.	Per cent of total households.		Number.	Per cent of total households.
Fresh milk.......	22.5 qts.	24	51.0	29.3 qts.	3	4.5
Butter...........	3.4 lbs.	23	49.0	4.0 lbs.	1	1.5
Eggs.............	2.9 doz.	19	40.5	6.0 doz.	1	1.5
Fresh vegetables.	....	31	66.0	....	1	1.5
Fresh fruit......	....	8	17.0	....	0	0.0
Poultry..........	4.0 lbs.	1	2.1	3.0 lbs.	1	1.5
Any of the above articles.......	....	40	83.3	....	6	9.0
None.............	....	8	16.7	....	61	91.0

growing. Land not suitable for the cultivation of cotton and, hence, available and used for corn and truck products was consequently far more abundant near *Ny* than near *In*.

(*b*) Contrast in market conditions.—Conditions affecting the market for farm produce from the two sections were quite different in some important respects. The village of *Ny* is itself more isolated than the village of *In* and is not near any important community. The nearest railway station is a mile away and is surrounded by only about a dozen houses, including three small stores. Seneca, the nearest town of any size (population 1,313 in 1910), is some 4 miles from *Ny*, and Greenville, the nearest city (population 15,741 in 1910), is about 40 miles distant. Seneca exports comparatively little produce and hence its market is limited to local needs which are not sufficient to absorb all the miscellaneous farm products of the vicinity. *Ny* is thus a competitor for such produce as the adjacent farm territory affords. The village itself has been in existence without much change in size for about 25 years, and we found that some of the sellers of farm produce had been visiting it regularly for over 10 years. On the other hand, *In* mill village is almost on the outskirts of the town of Inman (population 474 in 1910), which is on the railroad connecting Spartanburg, S. C., with Asheville, N. C. The demands of the Inman market for farm products are far from being confined to securing sufficient supplies for the needs of its townspeople, since several resident buyers purchase the surplus produce of the adjacent territory and ship it to Spartanburg. Since Spartanburg (population 17,517 in 1910) is but 13 miles distant along a good highway, buyers from that city cover the territory around *In* village fairly thoroughly, and farmers having produce to market often take it to the city when they go there to avail themselves of Spartanburg's superior shopping advantages. The position of *In* village appears, therefore, to be distinctly disadvantageous with respect to farm produce since it must compete for this not only with the town of Inman but, more important, also with the city of Spartanburg. So far as could be ascertained in 1916, no regular trade with near-by farms had been established, and, as has been pointed out, such casual trade as existed was only that afforded by occasional visits of hucksters who, after making the rounds in the town of Inman, had unsold remnants of produce.

(4) *Home-provided foods.*—Specific inquiries were made of all mill workers' households regarding their possession of cows, poultry, and gardens and, as far as practicable, regarding their importance particularly during the spring of 1916. Different proportions of the

households in the two villages were found to have such sources of food supplies.

(a) Milch cows.—There was but little difference in the proportion of households in either village owning productive cows during the spring of 1916, the percentage being 17.2 for *Ny* and 23.3 for *In* among households having less than the average income. Such difference as existed in this respect was in favor of *In*. But it should be noted in this connection that 33.3 per cent of the *In* households had no fresh-milk supply at all during the 15-day period for which household supply records were kept, as against only 8 per cent of the *Ny* households (see Table 57). This difference in distribution was caused by the larger proportion of *Ny* households that purchased milk from hucksters, since, as shown in Table 56, 51 per cent of *Ny* households purchased fresh milk from hucksters as against 4.5 per cent of *In* households.

(b) Swine.—Slaughtering of hogs is done in autumn and winter. This is a general practice and prevailed in *Ny* as well as in *In*. Home-produced pork did not figure in the spring food supply of mill workers' households in either village, except in the form of cured and salt meat. Of the *Ny* households, 17 per cent slaughtered home-raised hogs as compared with 33.3 per cent of *In* households. All of these households slaughtered their hogs before February 1, 1916, the majority in either village slaughtering before Christmas, 1915. Of the *Ny* households, 11 per cent cured home-slaughtered meat, as compared with 29 per cent of *In* households; but very little of this meat was on hand for use in the late spring. Inquiries of households slaughtering swine revealed the fact that in less than 5 per cent of such households were there any supplies of home-cured pork on hand on May 16, 1916, these being principally salt pork. The home-produced pork, therefore, did not appear to enter in significant degree into the spring food supply of the households in either village.

(c) Poultry.—Inquiries of households having less than the average income showed that 40 per cent of the *Ny* households and 25 per cent of the *In* households either did own poultry during the winter and spring months ending May 30, 1916, or were owning poultry at the time of the canvass (from June 1 to June 10, 1916). The average number of poultry consumed per household during the preceding year was 22 in *Ny* and 8 in *In*. The per cent of *Ny* households reporting consumption of home-owned poultry during the spring of 1916 was 19, as against 3 per cent for *In*. Thirty-two per cent of *Ny* households reported a fairly regular supply of eggs from

TABLE 57—Percentages of cotton-mill operatives' households having supplies of various articles of food in different quantities per adult male unit per day, compared for the mill villages of Ny and In, South Carolina.*

(All households considered have incomes of less than the average for the two villages.)

Article of food	Village	Average daily supply per adult male unit.	None.	Per cent of households whose average daily supply per adult male unit was—		
				Some, but less than one-third of the average of all households.	One-third or more, but less than the average of all households.	The average or more than the average of all households.
		Grams.				
Fresh meats...........	Ny....	34	31.2	6.2	16.7	45.8
	In....	7	67.2	10.4	13.4	9.0
Cured lean meats......	Ny....	24	37.5	4.2	27.1	31.2
	In....	20	46.3	6.0	14.9	32.8
Canned meats..........	Ny....	19	22.9	10.4	37.5	29.2
	In....	17	35.8	3.0	31.3	29.9
Eggs..................	Ny....	34	31.2	4.2	31.2	33.3
	In....	50	7.5	6.0	26.9	59.7
Fresh milk............	Ny....	426	8.3	10.4	45.8	35.4
	In....	457	33.3	0.0	30.2	36.5
Preserved milk........	Ny....	1	87.5	2.1	2.1	8.3
	In....	3	73.6	1.5	1.5	22.4
Butter................	Ny....	26	16.7	10.4	33.3	39.6
	In....	30	14.9	16.4	21.4	46.3
Cheese................	Ny....	3	87.5	2.1	0.0	10.4
	In....	+	97.0	0.0	0.0	3.0
Dried peas and beans..	Ny....	32	25.0	14.6	29.8	39.6
	In....	25	32.8	7.5	29.9	29.9
Canned peas and beans.	Ny....	2	83.3	0.0	0.0	16.7
	In....	4	85.1	0.0	0.0	14.9
Wheat flour...........	Ny....	358	6.2	0.0	43.7	29.2
	In....	358	18.5	3.1	32.3	46.2
Wheat bread, cakes, and crackers........	Ny....	13	18.7	12.5	33.3	35.4
	In....	18	25.4	6.0	22.4	46.3
Cornmeal..............	Ny....	139	29.8	4.3	29.8	36.2
	In....	180	20.9	0.0	17.9	61.2
Grits.................	Ny....	4	87.5	0.0	0.0	12.5
	In....	2	95.6	0.0	0.0	4.5
Rice..................	Ny....	4	75.0	0.0	0.0	25.0
	In....	5	70.2	0.0	0.0	29.9
Salt pork.............	Ny....	54	4.3	4.3	57.2	34.0
	In....	53	10.4	0.0	41.8	47.8
Lard and lard substitutes........	Ny....	41	6.2	4.2	52.1.	37.5
	In....	40	10.4	3.0	37.3	49.3
Green string beans....	Ny....	11	68.7	0.0	0.0	31.2
	In....	1	100.0	0.0	0.0	0.0
Canned string beans...	Ny....	1	97.9	0.0	0.0	2.1
	In....	4	89.5	0.0	0.0	10.5
Green vegetables (bought)............	Ny....	88	14.6	12.5	39.6	33.3
	In....	46	22.7	16.7	37.9	22.7
Other canned vegetables..............	Ny....	36	29.2	2.1	22.9	45.8
	In....	36	26.9	7.5	28.4	37.3
Fresh fruits..........	Ny....	40	25.0	10.4	20.8	43.7
	In....	20	43.9	9.1	28.8	18.2
Dried fruits..........	Ny....	12	53.2	0.0	17.0	29.8
	In....	8	70.2	1.5	6.0	22.4
Canned fruits.........	Ny....	10	66.7	0.0	2.1	31.2
	In....	20	56.7	0.0	1.5	41.8
Irish potatoes........	Ny....	34	45.8	4.2	20.8	29.2
	In....	60	53.7	3.0	3.0	40.3
Fresh sweet potatoes..	Ny....	0	0.0	0.0	0.0	0.0
	In....	0	0.0	0.0	0.0	0.0
Canned sweet potatoes.	Ny....	5	81.2	0.0	0.0	18.7
	In....	3	88.1	0.0	0.0	11.9
Sugar.................	Ny....	46	10.4	4.2	45.8	39.6
	In....	39	9.0	9.0	43.3	38.8
Sirup.................	Ny....	17	68.7	0.0	2.1	29.2
	In....	17	64.2	0.0	0.0	35.8
Jellies and jams......	Ny....	3	70.2	0.0	4.3	25.5
	In....	9	40.3	1.5	0.0	58.2

*Tabulation of approximate average daily supply of various foods in these same households deleted. ED.
+Less than 0.5 gram.

home-owned hens as against 21 per cent of *In* households. It appears that the advantage in the supplies of home-produced poultry and eggs during the preceding winter and spring lay distinctly with *Ny* households.

(*d*) Gardens.—Home gardens were much more generally found in the village of *In* than in *Ny*. Nearly 92 per cent of the *In* households had gardens planted on June 1, 1916, as against less than 23 per cent of *Ny* households. The opportunity afforded by suitable garden space was decidedly better in *In* than in *Ny*; practically every home in *In* had a good-sized garden plot, whereas many of the *Ny* households had no suitable space at all.

It was quite evident, however, that home gardens contributed but very slightly, if at all, to the food supply of households in either village during the spring of 1916. With the exception of an occasional ("rare" is perhaps a more accurate term) "mess" or dish of greens, a very little lettuce, and a few young onions, the gardens had yielded no supplies during 1916 up to about June 1. Not until after June 15 did garden produce become abundant, a condition that was somewhat contrary to the expectation of the authors, who had anticipated finding considerably earlier garden production in this section. The principal reason for this tardiness appears to be the fact that gardens in mill villages are usually planted later than gardens elsewhere in this section. Difficulty in getting the ground prepared early enough, owing in part to the fact that the long hours of work in the mill leave no available daylight for gardening until well along in the spring, lack of initiative in making other preparations, and possibly other causes, apparently almost preclude good early spring gardens in most of the mill villages studied, including *Ny* and *In*, although climatic conditions ordinarily are such that gardens can be made to yield supplies of early varieties of vegetables during May and even in April. Aside from a half dozen households reporting that they had had radishes, lettuce, or English peas, only about one-third of the *In* households reported that they had had greens or young onions even occasionally and in small quantities before this date. In *Ny* the proportion was even less.

Summing up the principal differences in availability of food supplies during the spring of 1916 as between *Ny* and *In*, it may be said that (1) supplies of fresh milk, butter, green vegetables, and fresh fruit were available to a greater degree (better distributed among the households) in *Ny* than in *In*, because, in the farm territory adjacent to *Ny*, there was a larger production of these articles of food and because *Ny* occupied a more advantageous location as a market for such products, and (2) that a supply of fresh meat was available to a greater degree in *Ny* than in *In* because of the existence of a fresh-meat market in *Ny* all the year around. In practically all other respects the availability of food supplies appeared to be generally similar in the two villages.

The conditions outlined above are reflected in a comparison of the total food supplies during the 15-day period May 16–30, 1916, of households in *Ny* and *In*. In this comparison (Table 57) in order to eliminate as far as practicable the influence of differences in economic status, only those households with less than the average of incomes[9] have been considered.

In Table 57 is shown the average quantity of each article of food for all the households considered, as well as the percentages of the households in each village which had various quantities of each article of food, such quantities being expressed in terms of the average for all households in order to shorten the statistical presentation.

This comparison indicates that during the 15-day period, May 16–30, 1916, (1) supplies of fresh meat, fresh milk, green vegetables, and fresh fruit were more abundant (i.e., better distributed) in *Ny* than in *In* households; (2) supplies of cured and canned meats, salt pork, butter, flour, lard, and lard substitutes, and dried peas and beans in *Ny* households were quite similar to those in *In* households; and (3) supplies of eggs, corn meal, Irish potatoes, and most canned goods were more abundant in *In* than in *Ny* households. Other differences in the supplies of articles of food occurring either rarely or in small quantities are indicated.

From the foregoing considerations it clearly appears that the character of the household food supply in the two villages was considerably influenced by the availability of certain foods, notably fresh meats, fresh milk, green vegetables, and fresh fruits, all of which were relatively less abundant or less equally distributed in *In* than in *Ny*. It is clear also that these differences in the food supply of *Ny* and *In* households are quite similar to the differences which, as already reported, we found to exist in the food supply of nonpellagrous and of pellagrous households. (Goldberger, Wheeler, and Sydenstricker, 1918; also Mar. 19, 1920.)

We have here, therefore, a striking and significant correspondence between the differences in the availability of certain foods (and thus,

9   The average half-month family income per adult male unit for all households in *Ny* and *In* was $7.99. Hence, all households with such incomes under $8 were considered.

it is permissible to assume, in the character of the diet) in the two villages, on the one hand, and the difference with respect to the incidence of pellagra among their households on the other. Since between these two villages no other differences to which significance could properly be attached were disclosed by our study, the conclusion would seem to be warranted that the difference in the availability of food supplies above summarized was the outstanding determining factor in relation to the marked difference in the incidence of the disease.

Thus, of all the factors we have studied in relation to differences in pellagra incidence among our villages, the factor of food availability is the only one in connection with which significant evidence of such relationship was found. The conclusion would, therefore, seem to be warranted that in this factor we have the explanation for the differences among the villages studied in the incidence of the disease, so far as this incidence was a reflection of community conditions.[10]

Discussion

From the data presented in the foregoing pages it is evident that a variety of factors of an economic nature, through their effect on the character of the household diet, had an important influence on the incidence of pellagra in the communities studied. Among these factors family income and food availability stand out most conspicuously.

As has been seen, the data presented reveal a very marked inverse correlation between family income and the incidence of the disease. When it is recalled that the range of income enjoyed by our families

---

10 If such factor as food availability operated to affect the rate of pellagra incidence in our villages, then it may be reasonably expected that in the locality with exceptionally unfavorable conditions of food availability, family income would be less efficient as a protective factor than in other similar localities with better conditions of food availability. With a view of testing this we compared the pellagra incidence rate for each of our income classes of *In* village in which we believed food availability conditions were least favorable with that of a group of five villages in which conditions in respect to food availability are believed to have been better. It was seen that (1) the incidence rate in those income groups in which a significant number of cases occurred was decidedly higher in *In* village; and (2) that the curve of incidence showed a highly suggestive tendency to extend to a higher plane of income in *In* village than in the group of five villages. The indications thus afforded would, therefore, appear to be consistent with and to bear out the assumption which was tested. [Tabulation deleted. ED.]

was small (see p. 237), that the amount of income of even the highest of our income classes was actually quite low (but few had annual incomes of over $1,000), the reduction of incidence to the point of practical disappearance of the disease in this income class is all the more striking and significant. It would seem quite impressively to indicate that the occasional occurrence of the disease in well-to-do individuals must be regarded as a relatively quite exceptional occurrence, and that the explanation of such occurrence must be sought in circumstances of a special or exceptional character.

Cases in the well-to-do, instances of which have been observed repeatedly since the time of Strambio (1796), are of more than ordinary interest because of the perplexity and confusion to which they tend to give rise with respect to the etiology of the disease. Favorable economic status of the individual tends to create the presumption that diet can have little or no etiological significance, since there can be no question of the ability of such individual to provide himself with a liberal diet. Natural as this presumption may be under the circumstances, it nevertheless involves danger of serious error. This results from the implied assumptions that because of financial ability, not only was a satisfactory diet available, but that such was also consumed. Even granting what is not necessarily the case, that financial ability to provide may be assumed to be invariably synonymous with the actual provision of a good diet[11] and that a liberal diet was actually available to the individual, it by no means follows that such diet was in fact consumed. For such assumption would totally ignore the existence of individual likes and dislikes, more or less marked examples of which may be observed at almost any family table.

A great variety of causes may operate to bring about individual peculiarities of taste with respect to food. They may have their origin in the seemingly inherent human prejudice against the new and untried food or dish; they may date from some disagreeable experience associated with a particular food; they may arise as the result of ill-advised, self-imposed, or professionally directed dietary restrictions in the treatment of digestive disturbances, kidney disease,

11 In this connection the following from Roussel (1866, pp. 430–431) is of interest: "Almost all the individual histories, found in the literature of pellagra in the well-to-do, are remarkable because of this constant fact . . . namely, that because of some misfortune or by reason of some unwholesome trait (mauvaises habitudes), such as avarice, these well-to-do or wealthy pellagrins subsisted exactly as did the poor pellagrins about them."

etc.; they may originate as a fad; and in the insane they may arise because of some delusion such as the fear of poisoning, etc.

The individual peculiarities of taste which may thus arise have a significance in relation to pellagra that has been but little appreciated until recently (Goldberger, 1914 and 1916). In much the greater proportion of a moderate number of cases in well-to-do individuals with a good diet presumably available, coming under our observation, a significant eccentricity in diet could readily be determined (unpublished observations). Vedder (1916, pp. 157–160) and Roberts (1920) have reported observations of a similar character. It is of interest to note also that analogous facts have been recorded in connection with beriberi (see Vedder, 1913, pp. 154, 156, 171, 180, 184). Therefore, in seeking to explain cases of pellagra in individuals believed to have a good diet available, this factor must be given due consideration.

With conditions (including labor supply) in the cotton-milling industry substantially stable, family income may, in general, be expected to fluctuate but little from year to year. With conditions unsettled, family income may either fall or rise very considerably; a depression, accompanied by increasing unemployment and, possibly, reductions in wage rates will be reflected in a reduced family income, while industrial prosperity, with a diminution of unemployment and, possibly, increased wage rates, will be reflected in larger family income. In the former event we may have a diminution in family income to the point of inability to provide the family with a proper diet, with a consequent danger of the development of pellagra and thus with a more or less marked rise in the incidence rate of the disease. In the latter event we have the opposite effects, with a tendency to a reduction in or practical disappearance of the disease. In this we have, we believe, an illustration of the manner of operation of one of the most powerful factors in relation to the endemic and epidemic prevalence of the disease. Through its effect on diet, economic status is also an important element in, if not the entire explanation of, the oft repeated observation of the occurrence of a marked increase in the incidence or the development of an epidemic of the disease following on crop failure[12] (Weiss, 1914, p. 327) or other cause of "hard times," as was actually observed in the United States in 1915, following depression consequent on the outbreak of the World War in 1914, and as there is some reason to fear may

12 It should not be forgotten that overproduction, by glutting the market, may affect family income (of the farmer) as disastrously as may crop failure.

again be observed in the spring of 1921 if the present depression, especially in the price of cotton and cotton-textile manufacturing, continues.

At this juncture it may be well to point out that family income should always be considered in connection with living (food) costs if confusion and error are to be avoided. It is the purchasing power of family income that is significant and not necessarily its absolute amount.

Although economic status (as typified by family income) is, ordinarily, perhaps the most important factor (particularly in industrial communities) in relation to fluctuation in incidence of pellagra in different years,[13] marked changes in food availability conceivably play a similar rôle (particularly in agricultural communities). The reported occurrence, in some localities, of a sharp increase in the prevalence of the disease following an epizootic among swine or cattle (Niederman, Konrad, and Farkas, 1898) or after the loss of these through floods, we believe, is to be explained, in part, at least, in this manner.

The very great importance of food availability in relation to pellagra prevalence seems heretofore not to have been very clearly recognized. Under some circumstances, as we have shown, this factor may operate notably to affect the character of the diet and thus the incidence of the disease. Our data dealt with differences in availability between localities of relatively small area, but it is readily conceivable that analogous differences may exist between areas of great extent such as there is reason to believe actually is the case between the northern and southern parts of the United States. This difference is probably an important factor (together with the well-known difference in dietary habit, Sydenstricker, 1915) in the notable inequality in the incidence of the disease in these two sections of the country.

The results of the present study clearly suggest fundamental lines along which efforts looking to the eradication of the disease should be directed, namely, (1) economic, by improvement of economic status (income), and (2) food availability, by improvement in availability of food supplies.

Measures for improving the economic status of those people most subject to the disease, are in the main, outside of the sanitarian's sphere and but little subject to his influence. While much the same

13 We hope to consider the relation of economic status to the course of the disease from year to year in a separate paper.

may be said to apply to the conditions of food availability, this field is more easily accessible, both directly and indirectly, to his activities and influence. Thus, for instance, by avoiding ill-considered regulations governing milk production he can, negatively at least, favor an adequate supply of this invaluable food. Furthermore, he can and should aid in improving the conditions of food availability by lending his powerful influence in support of and, by cooperating with, the agencies at work in this field, in their efforts to stimulate milk production (particularly through cow ownership) and to induce the farmer to adopt a suitable system of crop diversification.

And in this connection it may perhaps be remarked that certain preliminary observations have created in our minds a rather strong suspicion that the single-crop system as practiced in at least some parts of our southern states, by reason of apparently unfavorable conditions of food supply and of other conditions of an economic character bound up therein, will be found indirectly responsible for much of the pellagra morbidity and mortality with which local agricultural labor is annually afflicted.

Although considerable study will be required to determine definitely the factors responsible for the high incidence of the disease in the rural areas in question, it would, nevertheless, seem to be the part of wisdom to make an earnest effort to improve conditions in the ways suggested above.

Summary and Conclusions

1. In the present paper are reported the results of the part of the pellagra study of cotton-mill villages, during 1916, dealing with the relation of conditions of an economic nature to the incidence of pellagra. It is the first reported study in which the degree of the long-recognized association between poverty and pellagra incidence is measured in a definite, purely objective manner.

2. The study was made among the white mill operatives' households in seven typical cotton-mill villages of South Carolina. Pellagra incidence was determined by a systematic, biweekly, house-to-house canvass and search for cases, only active cases being considered. Information relating to household food supply, family income, etc., was secured by enumerators for a sample section of the period April 16 to June 15, assumed to be representative of the season during which the factors favoring the production of pellagra were assumed to be most effective.

3. Family income was made the basis of classification according to economic status, the Atwater scale for food requirements being

used for computing the size of families in comparing their incomes.

4. In general, pellagra incidence was found to vary inversely according to family income. As the income fell, the incidence of the disease rose and showed an increasing tendency to affect members of the same family; as the income rose, incidence fell, being reduced almost to the point of practical disappearance in the highest of our income classes, although the income enjoyed by this class was comparatively quite low.

5. The inverse correlation between pellagra incidence and family income depended on the unfavorable effect of low income on the character of the diet; but family income was not the sole factor determining the character of the household diet.

6. Differences in incidence among households of the same income class are attributable to the operation of such factors as tend to determine the amount and proportion of family income available for the purchase of food, the intelligence and ability of the housewife in utilizing the available family income, and to the differences among households with respect to availability of food supplies from such sources as home-owned cows, poultry, gardens, etc.

7. Differences in incidence among villages whose constituent households are economically similar, are attributable to differences among them in availability of food supplies resulting from differences (a) in the character of the local markets, (b) in the produce from adjacent farm territory, and (c) in marketing conditions.

8. The most potent factors influencing pellagra incidence in the villages studied were: (a) low family income, and (b) unfavorable conditions regarding the availability of food supplies, suggesting that under the conditions obtaining in some of these villages in the spring of 1916 many families were without sufficient income to enable them to procure an adequate diet, and that improvement in food availability (particularly of milk and fresh meat) is urgently needed in such localities.

References

Atwater, W. O. "Principles of Nutrition and Nutritive Value of Food," *Farmers' Bull.* (U. S. Dept. of Agric., No. 142), 1915, p. 33.

Babes, V. "Ueber Pellagra in Rumanien," *Wien Med. Presse,* Vol. 44 (1903), pp. 1184, 1239.

Berger, L. "Pellagra," *Wiener Klinik Wien,* Vol. 16 (1890), pp. 161–79.

Boyd, F. D., and Lelean, P. S. *Report of a Committee of Enquiry Regarding the Prevalence of Pellagra Among Turkish Prisoners of War* (Alexandria, Egypt, 1919). Also *J. Roy. Army Med. Corps,* Vol. 33 (1919), p. 426 et al.

Calmarza, J. B. *Memoria Sobre La Pelagra* (Madrid, 1870).

Casal, G. "Obra Postuma del Dr. Casal Publicada en 1762," *Corresp. Med.* (Madrid), Vol. 5 (1870), p. 78.

Gaumer, G. F. "Pellagra in Yucatan," *Trans. Nat'l Conf. on Pellagra* (Columbia, S. C., 1910), pp. 101–107.

Goldberger, J. "The Cause and Prevention of Pellagra," *Public Health Rep.* (Washington, D.C.), Vol. 29 (September 11, 1914), pp. 2354–57.

————. "Pellagra—Causation and a Method of Prevention," *J. Am. Med. Assn.*, Vol. 66 (February 12, 1916), pp. 471–76.

————, Wheeler, G. A., and Sydenstricker, E. "A Study of the Diet of Nonpellagrous and of Pellagrous Households, etc.," *J. Am. Med. Assn.*, Vol. 71 (September 21, 1918), pp. 944–49.

————. "A Study of the Relation of Diet to Pellagra Incidence in Seven Textile-Mill Communities of South Carolina in 1916," *Public Health Rep.* (Washington, D.C.), Vol. 35 (March 19, 1920), pp. 648–713.

————. "Pellagra Incidence in Relation to Sex, Age, Season, Occupation, and 'Disabling Sickness' in Seven Cotton-Mill Villages of South Carolina during 1916," *Public Health Rep.* (Washington, D.C.), Vol. 35 (July 9, 1920), pp. 1650–64.

————. "A Study of the Relation of Factors of a Sanitary Character to Pellagra Incidence in Seven Cotton-Mill Villages of South Carolina in 1916," *Public Health Rep.* (Washington, D.C.), Vol. 35 (July 16, 1920), pp. 1701–14.

Hameau. "Note sur une maladie peu connue observée dans les environs de la teste (Gironde)," *Jour. de Med. Prat. (etc.) de la Soc. Roy. de Med. de Bordeaux*, Vol. 1 (1829), pp. 310–14.

Holland, H. "On the Pellagra, A Disease Prevailing in Lombardy," *Med. Chir. Trans.* (London), Vol. 8 (1820), pp. 313–46.

Huertas, F. "La Pelagra en España," *Arch. Latin. de Med. y de Biol.* (Madrid), Vol. 1 (October 20, 1903), pp. 9–15.

Jobling, J. W., and Petersen, W. "The Epidemiology of Pellagra in Nashville, Tennessee, II," *J. Infec. Dis.*, Vol. 21 (August, 1917), pp. 109–31.

Lalesque, fils. *Actes de l'Acad. Roy. d. Sc. (etc.) de Bordeaux* (1846), p. 421.

Manning, C. J. *Report on Certain Cases of Psilosis Pigmentosa Which Have Recently Occurred at the Lunatic Asylum* (Barbados, 1907).

Niederman, J., Konrad, E., and Farkas, E. "A Report on Pellagra in Transylvania" (abstract), *Lancet* (London), Vol. 2 (July 16, 1898), p. 164.

Probizer, von. "Die Pellagra," *Die Heilkunde* (Wien), Vol. 4 (December, 1899), pp. 139–42.

Roberts, S. R. "Types and Treatment of Pellagra," *J. Am. Med. Assn.*, Vol. 75 (July 3, 1920), pp. 21–25.

Rosen, H. V. "Ueber die Pellagra in Russland, Petersburg," *Med. Wchnschrft.*, n. F. Vol. 11 (1894), pp. 21–23.

Roussel, T. *La Pellagre* (Paris, 1845).

————. *Traité de la Pellagre, . . .* (Paris, 1866).

Sandwith, F. M. "How to Prevent the Spread of Pellagra in Egypt," *Lancet* (London), Vol. 1 (March 14, 1903), p. 723.

Siler, J., and Garrison, P. E. "An Intensive Study of the Epidemiology of Pellagra," *Am. J. Med. Sci.* (Philadelphia), Vol. 146 (July and August, 1913).

Sofer, T. "Die Pellagra in Oesterreich und ihre Bekampfung als Volks-krankheit," *Therap. Monatshefte*, Vol. 23 (April, 1909), pp. 216, 219.

Strambio, G. *Abhandlungen ueber das Pellagra* (Leipzig, 1796).

Sydenstricker, E. "The Prevalence of Pellagra—Its Possible Relation to the Rise in the Cost of Food," *Public Health Rep.* (Washington, D.C.), October 22, 1915.

————, Wheeler, G. A., and Goldberger, J. "Disabling Sickness Among the Population of Seven Cotton-Mill Villages of South Carolina in Relation to Family Income," *Public Health. Rep.* (Washington, D.C.), Vol. 33 (November 22, 1918), pp. 2038–51.

Vedder, E. B. *Beriberi* (New York, 1913).

————. "Dietary Deficiency as the Etiological Factor in Pellagra," *Arch. Int. Med.*, Vol. 18 (August, 1916), pp. 137–72.

Weiss, E. "Die Pellagra in Sudtirol und Die staatliche Bekampfungsaktion," *Das Osterreichische Sanitätswesen* (Wien), Vol. 26 (May 7, 1914), pp. 309–31.

White, R. G. *Report on an Outbreak of Pellagra Among Armenian Refugees at Port Said, 1916–17* (Cairo, Egypt, 1919).

12. A Study of Endemic Pellagra in Some Cotton-Mill Villages of South Carolina.[1] An Abstract

JOSEPH GOLDBERGER   G. A. WHEELER
EDGAR SYDENSTRICKER   WILFORD I. KING

As a part of the field investigations of pellagra conducted by the Public Health Service there was begun in the spring of 1916 a study of the relation of certain social, hygienic, sanitary, and economic factors to pellagra incidence in some representative South Carolina textile-mill communities, so-called cotton-mill villages, in which the disease was believed to be endemic. On a varying scale, but without interruption, this study was continued until the fall of 1921; that is, during a period of about five and a half years.

During 1916 this study was carried on in 7 villages. As it progressed it was more and more felt that the mass of data being collected would prove to be too small to afford entirely convincing indications with respect to certain important phases of the investigation. For this reason and because it seemed desirable to observe the possible fluctuations in the incidence of the disease from year to year and to study some of the factors possibly related to such fluctuations, it was arranged to continue the study, and for at least one year to carry it out on a much larger scale. Accordingly, early in January, 1917, a considerable number of additional villages were taken under observation, and by the end of February, 17 villages in addition to the 7 of 1916 were settled upon for study. These 24 villages were kept under surveillance for pellagra throughout the year 1917.

With the beginning of 1918 the scale of the investigation was reduced to about that of 1916, surveillance of 18 of the 24 villages studied during 1917 being discontinued. Of the 6 continued under observation during 1918, 2 had been among the 7 studied in 1916. At the beginning of 1919 the scale of the investigation was further reduced by discontinuing observation of all but 1 of the villages. This 1 village (*In*) was 1 of the original 7 and was continued under

1 *Public Health Rep.*, Vol. 43, No. 41 (October 12, 1928), 2645–47. The complete report appeared as, "A Study of Endemic Pellagra in Some Cotton-mill Villages of South Carolina," *Hyg. Lab. Bull.*, No. 153 (January, 1929), 1–85.

surveillance throughout 1919, 1920, and up to October 15, 1921—or, in all, for about five and a half years.

The results of the first year's study have already been published.[2] In the present communication, much delayed by, among other reasons, the pressure of other continuing studies, we desire to record certain of the results of that phase of the subsequent study concerned with the incidence of the disease and the relation of this incidence to certain social, climatic, sanitary, economic, and dietary factors.

During 1917 in an aggregate population of 22,653 individuals, 1,147 cases of pellagra (an incidence rate of 50.6 per 1,000) were observed. Of the 4,104 households among which that population was distributed, 18.5 per cent had at least one member affected by the disease in that year.

Pellagra (in an endemic locality) is very much (two to six times) more prevalent than the experience of the physicians of the locality would seem to indicate.

The fatality rate of the endemic disease, when definitely marked cases of all grades of severity are considered, would appear not to exceed 3 per cent.

Striking peculiarities of age and sex distribution of the disease were observed.

The observations of age incidence appear to indicate, what seems not to have been recognized heretofore, that endemic pellagra is preponderatingly a disease of children of from 2 to 15 years of age.

Explanations of the peculiarities of age and of sex incidence are suggested.

The single woman, as compared with the married, widowed, or divorced, is relatively exempt from the disease. In the population group under consideration, the single woman is usually a wage earner, which may place her in a somewhat more advantageous position with respect to diet than her married or widowed sister.

The incidence of the disease was found to be markedly seasonal; 80 to 90 per cent of all cases had their "onset" within the period April to July, inclusive. One explanation suggested, in view of the proved dietary relation of the disease, is the variation in diet brought about by the seasonal modification of the food supply.

The seasonal incidence of cases distinguished by their occurrence singly or otherwise in a household, and as initial and recurrent attacks, was studied.

The disease was found to have a marked and very sharply limited

2 See Chapters 8, 9, 10, and 11.

season of prevalence the curve of which, with a slight lag, paralleled that of incidence.

The study failed to disclose any consistent correlation between sanitary conditions and pellagra incidence. Such association as may at times be observed is regarded as accidental and to be explained by the intimate relation of the endemic disease to economic status, of which the sanitary condition may be an index.

The study reveals the existence of a striking inverse correlation between the incidence of the endemic disease and family income.

The continuous study of a selected village during a period of nearly six years appears to demonstrate that income shortage was a fundamental, though indirect, controlling factor in relation to the year-to-year fluctuation in the incidence of the disease. It is therefore inferred that the year-to-year fluctuations in the incidence of the endemic disease are bound up with fluctuations in economic conditions that influence the ability of a certain section of the population to procure an adequate diet.

Marked seasonal variations in the food supply of a selected village are demonstrated. A relation of this variation in food supply to the striking seasonal incidence and prevalence of the disease is suggested.

13. *Pellagra in the Mississippi Flood Area.*

REPORT OF AN INQUIRY RELATING TO THE PREVALENCE OF
PELLAGRA IN THE AREA AFFECTED BY THE OVERFLOW OF THE
MISSISSIPPI AND ITS TRIBUTARIES IN TENNESSEE, ARKANSAS,
MISSISSIPPI, AND LOUISIANA IN THE SPRING OF 1927.[1]

JOSEPH GOLDBERGER
EDGAR SYDENSTRICKER

The following report deals with an inquiry relating to pellagra prevalence and conditions related thereto in the area recently overflowed by the Mississippi River and its tributaries in the states of Tennessee, Arkansas, Mississippi, and Louisiana.

In the course of this survey the writers visited Dyersburg and vicinity in Tennessee; Little Rock, Pine Bluff and vicinity, England and vicinity, and Marked Tree and vicinity in Arkansas; Jackson, Greenwood, and Indianola in Mississippi; and New Orleans, Baton Rouge, Alexandria, and Monroe in Louisiana. These localities were visited because of their accessibility and in the belief that at these places information concerning representative samples of the affected area could most satisfactorily be secured. As will appear, the information available frequently related to the respective states as a whole, so that whatever may be stated as to the conditions in the overflow area must not be taken as without applicability to some of the other parts of the states affected.

Pellagra Prevalence

With respect to pellagra prevalence, an endeavor was made to secure all available pertinent information from the state health departments concerned, from county health officers or directors of health units where there were such, and from practicing physicians in the localities visited. In only one of the four states visited, namely, Mississippi, are there normally anything like complete official morbidity reports of pellagra. In the present instance, however, by reason of the disorganization caused by the overflow, even in that state the morbidity reports for the counties affected by the overflow were very incomplete or altogether lacking, so that such information as

1 *Public Health Rep.*, Vol. 42, No. 44 (November 4, 1927), 2706–25.

could be secured relative to the prevalence of pellagra this year in the overflowed area of Mississippi cannot properly be compared with official records for preceding years.

At Dyersburg, Tenn., at a conference called in anticipation of our visit by Dr. E. L. Bishop, commissioner of public health of Tennessee, the director of the health unit of that town and of Dyer County, the county health officers of the neighboring counties Lauderdale and Lake, and several practicing physicians from these counties, were interviewed and statements of their experience with pellagra this year as compared with preceding years were secured.

At Little Rock, Ark., conference was had with Dr. C. W. Garrison, state health officer. At Pine Bluff, Ark., the director of the county health unit had canvassed the physicians practicing in his county in anticipation of our visit, and from them had secured statements relative to pellagra incidence in 1927 as compared with preceding years. This information was furnished us and, in addition, in company with one of the physicians having an extensive plantation practice in the vicinity of Pine Bluff, we visited some of his patients at their homes. Through the kind offices of Doctor Garrison, we were enabled to meet the physicians of England, Ark., who took us to see some of their patients on near-by plantations and gave us their opinions regarding the prevalence of the disease in this and preceding years. Similarly, at Marked Tree, Ark., we conferred with several of the physicians practicing there and in the surrounding country, and were shown some of their patients. Here, too, we secured valuable incidence data from a field representative of the National Red Cross, who had canvassed the practicing physicians in this region.

In anticipation of our visit to Mississippi, Dr. F. J. Underwood, executive officer of the Mississippi State Board of Health, had arranged for a conference with the director of the health unit and the local practicing physicians at Greenwood, Miss., and for one with the county health officers of the delta counties at Indianola, Miss. At each of these conferences statements of pellagra incidence were secured from the health officials and practicing physicians.

At New Orleans, Dr. Oscar Dowling, president of the Louisiana State Board of Health, furnished us with what information he had of pellagra morbidity in his state. As pellagra morbidity is but very imperfectly reported in Louisiana, as in nearly all states except Mississippi, the most definite evidence at hand was a statement from the superintendent of the state asylum at Pineville, La., indicating a very definite increase in pellagra admissions for 1927. This institution serves the northern part of the state and thus reflects the conditions obtaining in that portion of the state. In addition, we visited Baton Rouge, where we met the superintendent of the other of the two state asylums for insane, that at Jackson, La., who stated that there had been no appreciable increase in admissions to his institution. This asylum is for patients from the southern parishes of the state, and the incidence found there may thus be considered as an index of conditions in the area served by it. At Alexandria, La., the director of the health unit was consulted with regard to pellagra in that locality. Similarly, at Monroe, La., the director of the health unit and the city and county health officers were visited, and statements were obtained regarding pellagra in that locality.

The information secured from all these sources was, for the most part, of a very general character. As already noted, no satisfactory official morbidity records were available in any of the states. Such information as the local health officers could give was based, with few exceptions, on canvasses of the physicians practicing in their jurisdiction. Very few of the physicians, however, keep their records in such a form as to enable them to make a numerical statement of cases treated. About all they could say was that they were or were not seeing more cases of pellagra, as the case might be, this year than last year, or, in some instances, more cases than they had seen altogether in the preceding period of, say, five or six years. The physicians in one of the localities visited were of the opinion that 25 per cent of the plantation population of that locality was affected with pellagra this year.

In evaluating the available information indicating an increased incidence, some allowance must be made for the effect of the abnormal conditions prevailing which probably tended to bring to the attention of physicians and health workers a larger proportion of existing pellagrins than would normally have been the case.

With all foregoing considerations in mind we submit the following summarized statement as our judgment with respect to pellagra incidence in the areas specified:

Tennessee.—All information obtainable indicates that there has been a notable increase in pellagra incidence in the overflow area of western Tennessee this year. Some evidence was also secured suggesting that there may be an increase of pellagra incidence also in some, at least, of the upland areas of the western counties of Tennessee.

Arkansas.—There is a considerable general increase in pellagra incidence in Arkansas this year as compared with 1926. This increase is particularly marked in the counties affected by the overflow, but these counties constitute the area in which pellagra is normally highly prevalent.

Mississippi.—There is probably an increased general incidence of pellagra in Mississippi this year. There are indications of a very high incidence in the delta counties. This is normally the case in this state. Some of the information obtained points to a much more marked increase in the overflow than in the upland areas of the delta counties.

Louisiana.—There is probably some increase of pellagra in Louisiana this year as compared with the corresponding period of 1926, this increase coming apparently principally from the northern portion of the state. No information was secured suggesting the existence of any abnormal incidence in the overflow area.

Notwithstanding the very general character of most of the information obtainable, we are satisfied that in the localities visited in Tennessee, Arkansas, and Mississippi the incidence of pellagra is abnormally high. The only available objective index of this that seems worthy of presentation was obtained from Doctor Leach, director of the health unit of Sunflower County, at Indianola, Miss. Under Doctor Leach's direction a house-to-house canvass in the vicinity of Indianola was made between June 20 and July 22, 1927, covering an unselected population of 4,179, among whom 102 cases of pellagra were recorded, an incidence rate of approximately 24.4 per 1,000. It is, of course, impossible to state definitely whether the incidence disclosed by this special canvass in Sunflower County is representative of all the delta counties or of the localities in the overflow areas in Tennessee and Arkansas. We are inclined to believe, however, that the incidence of the disease in the delta counties as a whole and in some, at least, of the localities visited in Tennessee and Arkansas, was not notably unlike that disclosed by the sample canvass in Sunflower County. Indeed, we think it possible that in some localities it may have markedly exceeded this rate.

While it is manifestly impossible, on the basis of the available data, to determine the actual pellagra incidence rate in the overflow area of Tennessee, Arkansas, and Mississippi, it may be permissible, on the basis of the results of the sample canvass in Sunflower County, Miss., and in the light of our experience, to suggest that this rate is probably of the order of 10 to 20 per 1,000 of the rural (tenant farm) population of that area. It should be kept clearly in mind, however, that this suggestion is essentially little better than a guess and is offered only in order to convey some concrete idea, however crude, of the magnitude of the problem we are considering.

Another way of visualizing the magnitude of the pellagra problem is to estimate the probable morbidity in the four states: Tennessee, Arkansas, Mississippi, and Louisiana on the basis of recorded deaths. The pellagra mortality records are approximately complete and may safely be used for such purposes. They are presented in the accompanying table (Table 58) for each state for the years 1924, 1925, and 1926. As may be seen, there has been a definite and more or less marked tendency to an increase in pellagra in these states during 1925 and 1926 as compared to 1924, the aggregate number of deaths in 1926 being fully 80 per cent larger than in 1924. We believe it conservative to expect that the number of deaths from pellagra during 1927 in these four states will be at least one-fourth to one-third larger than that for 1926. In other words, we think the number of deaths from pellagra that may conservatively be expected to occur during the present year, unless exceptionally potent measures intervene, will be little, if any, under 2,300 to 2,500. The studies of the Public Health Service workers indicate that the case fatality rate of pellagra, when all types of definitely recognizable cases are considered, does not exceed 5 per cent. On this basis, therefore, it may be expected that fully 45,000 to 50,000 individuals will have suffered a definitely recognizable attack of pellagra within the limits of these four states during 1927. It seems to us probable that about one-half of this number will be in the overflow area.

The overflow area of Tennessee, Arkansas, and Mississippi is normally an area in which pellagra has been quite prevalent ever since the disease was recognized in 1908 or 1909. Therefore, it seems to us highly probable, particularly in view of the depressed economic conditions in this area, associated with the low price of cotton in

TABLE 58—*Number of deaths and estimated number of cases of pellagra in specified states for 1924, 1925, and 1926, and estimated number of deaths and of cases of pellagra for 1927.*

State.	1924		1925		1926		1927	
	Deaths	Cases*	Deaths	Cases*	Deaths	Cases*	Deaths	Cases*
Tennessee.....	263[+]	.....	375[#]	.....	528[#]	.....	.....	.....
Arkansas......	164[#]	.....	313[#]	.....	491[#]	.....	.....	.....
Mississippi...	413[#]	.....	561[#]	.....	564[#]	.....	.....	.....
Louisiana.....	183[#]	.....	343[#]	.....	267[#]	.....	.....	.....
Totals......	1,020	20,000	1,592	32,000	1,850	37,000	2,300- 2,500	45,000- 50,000

*[+]Estimates. See text.
[#]From Mortality Statistics, Bureau of the Census.
[*]Direct from State health departments.

1926, that this area would have suffered an increased incidence even had no overflow taken place. Witness, for example, the well-known exceptionally high incidence of pellagra in 1915 following the depression in cotton values in 1914. However, the overflow (by causing a more than ordinary restriction (1) in the available supply of milk, through a decrease in the number of milch cows—from drowning or sale—and through the lowered milk yield of such cows as remained because of a period of low feeding; (2) in the supply of fresh meat and eggs, through loss of many of the home-owned poultry and swine; and (3) in the supply of fresh vegetables, through destruction of such gardens as were planted before the overflow and delayed planting because of the overflow) very probably accentuated the unfavorable dietary conditions that would have obtained in any event and thus may reasonably be presumed to have contributed to the existing increased prevalence. What portion of the existing increase is properly attributable to the factors resulting from the overflow it is impossible to say.

The lack of evidence of any increase in pellagra prevalence in the overflow area in Louisiana is of considerable interest, but with the meager information at present available it is difficult or impossible to explain. We shall not attempt to do so at this time.

Some Economic Factors Related to Pellagra Prevalence

With respect to the economic factors related to the prevalence of pellagra in the area under consideration, we made inquiries of physicians, health officers, tenants, planters, business and professional men, and of farm demonstration agents, county officials, and others in the localities visited. Without attempting to report in detail the statements made and the opinions expressed by the various individuals, the information so obtained is summarized in the following paragraphs:

1. The prevalence of pellagra at any given time in the lower Mississippi River area is involved in three sets of conditions, namely:

(a) The dietary habits of the inhabitants.

(b) The tenant farm system of cotton production, cotton being the chief crop throughout the lowlands along the lower Mississippi and tributary rivers.

(c) The availability of supplies of various foods which, in turn, is influenced by the one-crop type of agriculture, with the consequent lack of diversification, and by the dietary habits of the people.

2. Given certain dietary habits and conditions, the variants in the conditions affecting pellagra prevalence are essentially economic in

their character. In the past 12 years, when records of morbidity and mortality from the disease have become available, it has been plainly evident that an unprofitable year in cotton production in this area is followed by an increase in incidence and mortality, and, conversely, that an improvement in the economic situation is followed by a diminished prevalence.

3. In the present situation the outstanding fact, aside from the deprivation directly due to the recent overflow, is that the economic condition of the entire cotton-producing area is unfavorable. This is due principally, if not altogether, to the unprofitable cotton crops of 1925 and 1926. The financial resources of the cotton planters thus were already severely strained before 1927, and the economic status of the tenant population was already considerably below that of 1922 and 1923. The destruction of, or impossibility of planting, crops in certain sections and the serious delays in planting in other areas, resulting in only 25 per cent to 40 per cent of normal production, due to the overflow, undoubtedly has intensified a condition that already was distinctly unfavorable.

4. It was obviously impossible, in a rapid survey, to obtain anything more than the broad outlines of the situation. These, however, seem to be perfectly clear and not only were plain to anyone with an elementary understanding of the conditions ordinarily prevailing and those developing by reason of the flood, but were universally corroborated by all the evidence obtainable from those who were conversant with the situation. An estimate of the magnitude pellagra incidence will have attained by the end of 1927 has already been submitted. A forecast of what proportions pellagra will attain in prevalence during 1928 is extremely difficult or impossible to make, for the reason that it is so bound up with the economic factors already referred to. If the price of cotton continues to be relatively high, as present indications seem to promise, the financial condition of the planters obviously will be more favorable both for the remaining portion of the present year and for the ensuing year; but it must be remembered that since cotton is a highly speculative commodity, its price is subject to many indeterminable factors. Assuming, however, that the price of cotton will be favorable to the planters in 1927, those planters and the tenant population in the areas affected by the overflow obviously cannot benefit to any great extent from this favorable price, because of the fact that, in general, they will have little or no cotton to sell except such as was carried over from the high production year of 1926. All that it seems permissible to say is that since it has been observed that in the past an unfavorable cotton year is

followed by an increased incidence of pellagra, we may expect a high and possibly an increased prevalence in 1928 as compared with 1927, unless some important mitigating factor or factors intervene.

In order to clarify the foregoing summary, a brief statement may be made on the relation of economic conditions and of dietary habits and availability of food supplies to prevalence of pellagra in this cotton-growing area. The statement is based on information from the sources already mentioned in the light of the results of previous studies of the Public Health Service, and is expressed in general terms without attempting to include statistics, illustrations, or details. The particular economic factors involved which may be emphasized are the dietary habits of the rural population, the availability of food supplies, the prevailing practices of financing cotton production in this area, and the system of tenant farming.

The dietary habits of the tenants, in fact, of the population as a whole in this area, play an extremely important part, we believe, in the endemic prevalence of pellagra. The expression is common that the tenant families, both white and colored, subsist on the three "m's"—meat, meal, and molasses. The meat is salt pork, which includes very little lean; the meal is corn meal; the molasses is the sorghum, or cane. To these should be added wheat flour, used to some extent to supplement the corn meal, some rice, and dried beans. The customary ration supplied to tenants from stores and commissaries, whenever rations are prescribed, consists of these articles of food, and the tenant farmer, whether white or Negro, universally regards them as his staple diet. In this connection it may be remarked, as will be pointed out somewhat more fully later, that this makes a typical pellagra-producing diet.

It is important to bear in mind that the poorer the economic condition of the tenant, the more nearly exclusively will he tend to rely upon these articles of food for his diet. Thus, the factors that influence his ability to purchase or otherwise provide certain other necessary supplementary foods become factors that influence the prevalence of pellagra, and thus the incidence of the disease rises or falls in inverse association with them.

Supplementary to this staple or basic diet, a rather limited variety of foodstuffs is ordinarily available. These may be classified, for convenience of discussion, as home-produced, purchased, and wild.

The home-produced supplementary foods are milk (used almost altogether in the form of buttermilk), butter, poultry, and eggs, and a limited variety of vegetables, chiefly cabbage, collards, beans, peas, corn, okra, and tomatoes. To these may be added fresh pork. At first glance these constitute a rather impressive supply and diversity of foods, but as a matter of fact the diversity and quantity are not large. As to milk and butter supplies, our observation and the information obtained from farm demonstration agents and others lead us to estimate that, in ordinary times, only 30 to 40 per cent of the tenants own cows. The reasons for this lie partly in the fact that the tenants are too poor to purchase cows, partly in the fact that facilities for pasturage and feed are frequently not afforded by the plantation owners, and partly by the improvidence of the tenants themselves. The policy of some of the planters is responsible in some measure for the absence of cows for two reasons: (1) Because of the desire to use all the land for cotton, pasturage is not furnished and cows are then usually staked along the roadside during the cotton-growing season; and (2) because, as it is claimed by some planters, the tenants are prone to divert feed destined for mules and horses to feeding their cows. It may be observed also that seasonal variation in the ownership of cows as well as in milk production apparently takes place. Since the tenant farmer is usually at his lowest economic ebb during the late winter and early spring, he is sometimes forced to sell his cow for cash, especially when the purchase of feed becomes necessary. This tends to lessen somewhat the number of families owning cows at this season of the year. The supply of milk from the cows which are retained varies somewhat according to season, the supply being lowest in the winter and early spring, because of the scantiness of forage and feed.

While poultry is owned by 60 to 70 per cent of the tenants, the number of such poultry owned by a tenant is usually very small; the egg production is almost negligible and at best will not furnish more than a very occasional meal. Vegetable (garden) produce ordinarily is extremely limited in quantity. A well-informed farm demonstration agent in one of the counties gave us his observation that less than 2 per cent of the tenant population have gardens in the ordinary sense of the word and our own observation confirms the statement. Probably about 25 per cent have some form of garden, but most of these gardens contain usually only a few cabbages or collards, occasionally a few peas and beans, and still more rarely some tomatoes. The planting of gardens is not generally encouraged by the plantation owners for two reasons: (1) The fact that the gardens use space which otherwise might be planted in cotton; and (2) the making and maintenance of gardens entail labor on the part of the tenant and his family during the season when all the labor possible is required in the cotton fields. The result is that, although in the late winter or early spring, gardens may be planted, the opportunity for working them is lost later on at the time when cultivation is most necessary, so that the garden rarely contributes anything of importance to the food supply of the family. There seems to be a more or less general feeling among local observers that the scarcity of gardens is also due partly to the lack of energy and thrift on the part of tenants, partly to the fact that they are not in the habit of raising gardens, and partly to their ignorance of how to cultivate them. Probably other reasons may be suggested in the facts that the soil is not always well adapted for small garden cultivation and that the tenant farmer after he has finished his day's work in the field is without the needed energy to attempt to cultivate a garden entirely by hand. The ownership of swine is even more restricted than that of cows, and the fresh-meat supply from this source in the autumn and winter lasts but a comparatively short time.

A second source of supplementary food supply is wild vegetation and game. In the early spring a certain amount of greens of different varieties is to be had for the picking, and it is our information that they are used to a considerable extent at that season of the year. Fish are available at all seasons of the year to those who live near the streams or lakes, but here again it should be borne in mind that fishing is done only in those seasons and at times when work is not required in the fields. To a very limited extent wild game is available, especially during the autumn and winter.

A third source of supplementary foods, such as canned meats and, to a very limited extent, vegetables, such as potatoes, cabbage, and tomatoes, is available in the commissaries and stores. The favorite canned goods are salmon, corn, and tomatoes. Obviously, the availability of these foods to the tenant depends upon his ability to buy. In years when his income or credit from his crop is "good," he does not hesitate to purchase considerable quantities and a fair variety of all the articles of diet that the store supplies. In fact, he may be encouraged to do so by the plantation commissaries and other stores. In times of economic depression he is not only forced on his own account to limit his purchases of these kinds of food, but he is discouraged from purchasing by the merchant or storekeeper in order to keep him from getting too deeply into debt.

The method of financing cotton production bears an indirect but a definite and important relation to the economic status of the tenant class. In the first place, it must be kept in mind that while all agricultural production is more or less speculative, the speculative character of cotton production is even more pronounced than that of most other forms of agriculture, for three reasons: (1) Cotton in the section under consideration is almost the sole crop, and the chances of severe loss or considerable success to the entrepreneur fluctuates to a greater extent than in a section where the crops are diversified; (2) the product is a highly speculative one in that it is sold in a market which is very sensitive to many factors; (3) a considerable proportion of cotton planters apparently regard cotton production as a speculative activity rather than a regular or settled business.

From the point of view of the economic status of the tenant population, cotton plantations may be roughly divided into at least three types:

(1) There is the small, or relatively small, farm or plantation, chiefly in the "uplands," on which cotton is only one of the crops. This farm is usually owned by the resident planter or farmer. He may have a few acres in cotton, the other acreage being in hay, corn, possibly other grains, truck, and fruits. This type is not characteristic of the "delta" section, and it may be remarked that our information is to the effect that relatively little pellagra is incident in the section characterized by this diversification of crops. This is borne out by the peculiar distribution of the disease in Mississippi. The average yearly number of deaths for the three-year period 1924–1926 in that state was 513. Of this number, 280 deaths (a death rate of 38 per 100,000) occurred in the 17 counties[2] ordinarily considered as constituting the delta section, and 233 (or a death rate of 18 per 100,000) in the remainder of the state. In other words, the pellagra incidence (as indicated by the death rate) in Mississippi outside of the delta section was only about one-half that in the delta.

(2) The large plantation, owned either by an individual or by a corporation, ranging from two or three thousand acres to 30,000 acres or more. These plantations may be again classified into two subgroups: (a) Those owned and operated by resident planters, and (b) those operated by nonresident planters or corporations. Our information is to the effect that the tenants, on the whole, are usually better off economically here than on the small plantations of a type to be referred to later. The management of a plantation owned by a large corporation is usually more efficient. The resident owner is likely to devote his time and personal attention to the welfare of his plantation, and our information is that his tenants are likely to be composed of the more stable and efficient class. It is on these planta-

---

2 These are as follows: Bolivar, Coahoma, De Soto, Holmes, Humphreys, Issaquena, Leflore, Panola, Quitman, Sharkey, Sunflower, Tallahatchie, Tate, Tunica, Warren, Washington, and Yazoo.

tions, for example, that apparently the tenants are better equipped as to houses, gardens, and livestock, including cows.

(3) The plantations or tracts of land which are bought as a speculation by persons engaged in other business. A plantation is usually bought upon the payment of only a portion of the purchase price, a mortgage being carried for the remaining amount by a local bank, insurance company, or credit organization. The owner then obtains a supply of tenants and their families on the best terms possible and often secures a mortgage on his crop, although this is not in all cases necessary if he has sufficient working capital. If one or two unfavorable years are experienced, a speculative venture of this sort not infrequently comes to grief. For example, in 1926, when the cost of cotton production was some 2½ cents a pound higher than the average market price of cotton, the credit of such operators was severely strained, especially in view of the fact that they had not had a very successful year in 1925. The great deflation in land values is a further complicating factor in the present situation, bearing especially upon speculative ventures of this kind. Many of those individuals and companies that embarked upon cotton production in a speculative way without sufficient capital to weather unfavorable conditions were caught, and in a number of instances have been unable to meet the interest on their mortgages. In 1926 and 1927 the mortgage holders, in some instances, have attempted to operate these plantations themselves; in other instances the land has lain idle; in still others the mortgages have been reduced and the owner has been allowed to continue.

Now, the precise effects of these conditions upon tenant farmers are difficult to set forth in detail because of so many complicating factors that render the situation an extremely intricate one. But the major effect seems to be fairly clear, namely, that all planters, but particularly those who did not have and who do not now have adequate financial resources in the face of two or three years of unfavorable conditions, and in the face of such a catastrophe as the flood, are compelled to operate at the very least possible cost. This may be translated, according to our information, into a limitation of cash and credit advances to the tenant to the very least possible amount that can be arranged for. We have learned of some instances in which the amount of credit was cut from the usual $1 and $1.25 per acre per month to $0.75 and even $0.50. This condition bears most heavily upon the least fortunate class of tenants, for various reasons. In the first place, the tenants who contract with planters of this kind tend to be of the less efficient and more shiftless type;

they are largely the "moving" population of the cotton-growing area who have very few possessions, tend to be improvident, and perhaps invite less consideration from the planters themselves. Moreover, this type of plantation is not always operated by the most efficient managers, and these, in their turn, are likely to be rated more according to the cotton production per acre in the present rather than upon their ability to develop the future productivity of the land and the labor supply. It is perhaps not going too far to say that insofar as any lack of personal attention to the welfare of the tenants exists on the part of the manager or the planter, it is to be found on these plantations where the owner is nonresident.

This does not mean, however, that the pressure of unfavorable conditions in "poor" years is felt by plantations of this type only. We were informed of a number of instances of failures, in 1926 and 1927, of plantations owned and operated by large companies, and many of the smaller resident-owner plantations were severely hit by the succession of unprofitable years and the flood. The effect upon the tenant in all cases is much the same, except for the fact that the planter without considerable financial resources is obviously less able to "carry" his tenants without passing on to them some of the pressure to which he himself is subjected.

The economic status of the tenant may be understood more clearly if the system of share farming prevalent in the cotton-growing area of the Mississippi Valley is described briefly. Generally speaking, the system is similar throughout this area. The plantation owner enters into a contract about the first of the year with the tenant to plant, cultivate, and harvest cotton on a certain number of acres of land, varying from 15 to 40, the number of acres depending upon the richness and condition of the soil, its freedom from stumps, etc., and the number of individuals in the tenant's family who are capable of furnishing labor. Perhaps a fair average would be between 25 and 35 acres. The size of the tenant's share of the crop depends largely on whether or not mules or horses, implements, and seed are furnished by the plantation owner. The value of his crop obviously depends upon the production of the particular acreage and upon the price of cotton and cottonseed at the end of the season. The method by which the tenant is financed, since he is almost always without any ready funds and frequently already in debt, may be illustrated by the method obtaining in the delta section of the state of Mississippi, outlined below.

At Christmas the tenant receives what is generally known as "Christmas money," the amount ranging from $25 to $100, depending in large measure upon his efficiency, his indebtedness at the time, the prospects for a cotton crop, etc. This is paid to him in cash, and our information is that it is usually largely spent during the Christmas season. From about the first of the year until March 1 the only cash income which the tenant has is from odd jobs which he may be able to secure in lumbering, mending houses and barns, work on the roads and levees, etc. On the money thus earned, together with what he may have saved from the previous year's crop and the "Christmas money," the family must subsist until the crop season begins.

On March 1 the usual arrangement entered into is for the planter to make monthly advances in cash to the tenant of $1 to $1.25 per acre farmed. This ranges from $15 to $40 per month, averaging $25 or $30. During the period from March 1 to August 1 his family prepare the ground and plant and cultivate the cotton. The only other source of cash income during this period is from hoeing cotton for wages on other tracts of land, this being done chiefly by the women and the older children. The cash advances by the planter are made over a five-month period, beginning March 1, the last payment being made on July 1. After July 1 no further cash income is available until the crop is picked and ginned, except from very occasional odd jobs and from picking cotton on other tracts of land by members of the family capable of work. When the cotton is ginned in the fall, the tenant receives income from two sources: One is from the sale of cotton lint after the deduction of the cash advances made by the planter; the other is from the sale of the seed, all the money from the latter going to the tenant.

The money from the crop is the chief income of the family. Obviously, if the crop is of fair quantity and quality, the amount of income will depend upon the price of cotton at the time the cotton is sold. If conditions are unfavorable, as, for example, in a year when cotton prices are low (as in 1926), or when unfavorable growing conditions exist, as they did in certain areas in 1925 when heavy rains interfered with the quality and quantity of cotton, the tenant does not realize any great advantage from his crop. For the lint he may be, and in many instances actually is, in debt to the planter; the price of cottonseed, of course, varies closely with the price of cotton. In a "good" year the tenant tends to extravagance, to purchase beyond the limits of absolute need such things as clothing and cheap automobiles, and it is a very general observation that the Negroes and most of the white tenants in this section are rarely in possession of any surplus by the end of the year.

The method of cash advances to the tenant on his crop prevails generally throughout the delta section of Mississippi. It may be noted that this system marks a quite distinct change from that prevailing 10 years ago, when, instead of advances on the crop being made in cash, the advances were in the form of credit on the planter's commissary or store, or other stores when the planter himself did not operate one. The reason for this change, as stated by various planters and others, was that the scarcity of labor resulting from an exodus of Negroes since 1920 forced this change to conciliate and conserve the labor supply, the system of credit advances being objected to by the tenant and the cash advances preferred. The effect of this change has been a greater freedom on the part of the tenant to buy where and what he pleases, and a greater consumption of supplementary foods, automobiles, clothing, etc., in "good" years. Another possible effect is a tendency toward a restriction in the variety of diet on the part of some (improvident) tenants for the reason that too large a portion of the available money was spent for other (luxury) purposes than food.

While the system outlined above prevails generally throughout the Mississippi lowlands, certain variations are to be found. Thus, in Tennessee the older form of store credits instead of cash advances is prevalent. In Arkansas it was found that both of these systems existed, the tendency being toward a greater following of the practice of cash advances. Among the white tenants in Tennessee and Arkansas still another variation in method of financing the crop is to be found, whereby the tenant receives no cash advance or credit from the planter but mortgages his own crop to the commissary or store for supplies during the crop season.

Whatever particular form of this system prevails, the effect upon the economic status of the tenant farmer is practically the same. For the most part, except in unusually favorable years, the tenant is constantly in debt, or on the verge of debt, to the planter or the store. If he chooses to move, to change the plantation owner with whom he has a contract, care is taken by the next owner to ascertain how much the tenant is in debt to his former planter so that the new planter may take up this indebtedness for his new tenant.

The average tenant may thus be said to be chronically on the verge of deprivation, it being understood, of course, that some tenants never reach that border line, and that others are almost continuously under it. Even within the relatively narrow range of income in which all of these tenants must be classified by any ordinary standard, there are quite distinct gradations. The less energetic, less capable, and less efficient, "shiftless" class find themselves on or below the border line. Obviously, only a relatively small decrease in income is sufficient to force a considerable number of tenants who are on the border line into the class which actually suffers deprivation. This was true in 1915, again in 1921, and again in 1924 and 1926.

Now, the precise manner in which an unfavorable condition operates upon the tenant differs to some extent according to the individuals concerned, but in general it is somewhat as follows: If for any reason the tenant clears little, if anything, from his crop, the amount of his "seed money" is also limited, and he is thus at a distinct disadvantage during the winter and the following spring until, at least, a new crop is financed. If he is unable, for various reasons, to secure or to do other work, as has been described, he has no additional source of income. It may, therefore, happen that the tenant is so pressed during this period that if he owns a cow he is compelled to dispose of it, and to the extent that he thus deprives his family of milk he impoverishes the household diet. Furthermore, it is during this period that the annual movement of tenants occurs. Some, hoping to be more fortunate the following year, seek other plantations; some, disheartened by a bad year, may leave the section and either go to other cotton-growing areas in the lowlands or go to the uplands and the "hill country," leaving their debts behind them. On the other hand, after a favorable crop the proportion of such unfortunate tenants is reduced, although from every indication there is always a considerable proportion of tenants in this class.

In the present instance three unfavorable years have occurred, during the last of which (1926) the price of cotton fell on the average below the cost of production. The 1927 flood, obviously, has tended to intensify the severity of the resulting conditions, and it is reasonable to conclude that a larger proportion of tenants are this summer in a definitely unfavorable situation than has been the case for a number of years. This conclusion logically follows from the factual premises, but it may be remarked that throughout the flood area the information obtained was without exception corroborative of the accuracy of this inference.

The evidence of an unusually high incidence of pellagra this summer in the area under consideration is thus associated with factors of an economic character, the gravity of which has been accentuated by the overflow.

Recommendations

We may now turn to a consideration of practicable measures that may be applied in order (1) to mitigate or relieve the existing acute health situation, and (2) to influence the fundamental conditions responsible for that situation, with a view of minimizing their probable future effects.

In order to make clear the scientific basis for the recommendations which we shall presently outline for assisting those attacked with pellagra to regain their health, it seems desirable first of all to outline briefly the essentials of our knowledge of the cause and treatment of pellagra.

Broadly speaking, pellagra results from a deficiency in the diet of a specific pellagra-preventive dietary essential or vitamin which has been designated as factor, or vitamin, "P–P." In other words, it may be said that pellagra develops in those whose diet does not include enough of the foods which carry the vitamin P–P to supply the body's needs for this factor. This does not mean that the diet that leads to pellagra is entirely devoid of this essential factor; on the contrary, it is probable that a pellagra-producing diet practically always contains some of this vitamin, but the quantity is not enough for the nutritional needs of some or all of those subsisting on it.

The diet made up of the ingredients specified below in conventional quantities has been found associated with pellagra and, it is believed, will lead to the development of the disease in fully 40 or 50 per cent of those partaking of it within some three to six or eight months, *depending on the nutritional status of the individual when starting such diet.*

The components of a typical pellagra-producing diet may be the following: Corn meal (corn bread, boiled hominy, or mush), white wheat flour (biscuit), white rice, dried beans, "white meat" (salt pork), sorghum, or cane molasses, collards, or "greens." Such diet contains some vitamin P–P derived from the beans, collards, and corn meal, but too little to prevent pellagra. An increase in the ration of beans and collards or, better, the addition of some food or foods rich in this factor, would tend to diminish the incidence or altogether prevent the occurrence of the disease in those subsisting on this diet. In this connection it may be remarked that the diet made up as above specified is accurately representative of the main or basic portion (calorifically) of the diet of the rural population of the South, and, because of the three principal components, meal, meat, and molasses, to which in hard times it tends to be reduced, is designated in the vernacular as the "three m's" ration.

As has been remarked, when this diet is adequately supplemented with P–P-containing foods (such as milk, lean meat, and vegetables) pellagra does not occur. When the disease does appear, it is certain that, for some reason, the diet has not been adequately supplemented. This reason may be any one or some combination of the following: (1) Individual eccentricity of taste, especially where the variety of supplemental foods, and thus of choice, is restricted (exemplified by those who have a dislike for milk, for eggs, for fresh beef, etc.). (2) A shortage in supply of the supplemental P–P-containing foods, resulting, perhaps, from inaccessibility to markets, difficulties of transportation, particularly of the perishable foods, epizootic among the domestic animals (milch cows, poultry, swine); from fencing laws, which make it impracticable for many to keep milch cows or swine; from overflows, which may cause the drowning of milch cows, goats, poultry, or swine, or force the sale of such animals or, by leading to a shortage of stock feed, cause a reduced milk supply. (3) Insufficient cash or credit available for the purchase of an adequate diet.

Recent investigations having shown that the so-called vitamin B actually includes at least two distinct dietary essentials, namely, the antineuritic vitamin and the P–P factor, it has been inferred that all foods that are known to contain this so-called vitamin B contain the P–P factor. This inference has been borne out by the results of such tests of individual foods as have so far been made. It appears, however, that the different classes of foods, and, probably also, the foods of the different classes, vary considerably with respect to their richness in this P–P factor. This is of great practical importance, since it emphasizes the importance of quantity. Unfortunately, our knowledge of the quantity of factor P–P contained in the individual foods is extremely limited and, at best, of a very crude relative character, so that only a few very general statements can at present be made. Thus, when forming the principal supplemental source of factor P–P in connection with such basic diet as has been considered in the foregoing, there would be needed daily for fully preventive purposes in the adult, of lean beef (Hamburg steak) about (not over) one-half pound, of dried cowpeas fully one-half pound, of buttermilk about 1 quart, of canned tomatoes about 1 quart, of dried pure yeast about 1 ounce. If a combination of these or related foods is used, the quantities of each may or should, of course, be correspondingly reduced.

The foods that have preventive action have, of course, also curative value. In selecting the food or foods to be used in treating the sick, the physician must of necessity choose such as will most satisfactorily fit the tastes and digestive capacity of the patient. Such considerations and actual experience indicate that milk, fresh meat, eggs, and dried yeast are the foods of first choice. Unfortunately, it is frequently very difficult for the pellagrin to secure these foods, by reason of lack of means with which to purchase or because of a scant available local supply. As a consequence the patient all too frequently receives too little of the foods of which he is in greatest need, so that the course and progress of the attack are either altogether unfavorable, especially in the severe cases, or disappointingly tedious. This and other considerations which cannot here be discussed quite commonly tend to make the physician cling to the older ideas of drug treatment. There is no drug known that actually serves any useful purpose, unless it be to mitigate or relieve painful or disturbing symptoms or as a placebo. Almost always the money expended on drugs would be much more advantageously expended on the essential foods and the proper feeding of the patient.

With the foregoing elementary considerations relative to the cause and treatment of pellagra in mind, and in view of the difficult economic situation of nearly all pellagrins, we would recommend that the appropriate local relief agency or agencies furnish the local health officer with a supply of such nonperishable supplemental P–P rich foods, as dried pure yeast (preferably the killed culture), canned (chum) salmon, canned beef, and canned tomatoes, or adequate funds or credit with which to purchase such a supply, which he may then distribute on physicians' requisition or otherwise to those in need who are actually sick or present evidence of an impending attack of the disease. Since the vast majority of patients are able to be up, the question of hospitalization will arise only in a relatively small minority. In general, patients properly fed will regain their health and normal vigor in from 6 to 12 weeks. In the foregoing it is assumed that the patient has a sufficient supply of the basic staple foods.

It is believed that if the foregoing recommendation is promptly inaugurated and efficiently carried out, the acute pellagra situation will be mitigated if not altogether relieved. It must be noted, however, that this is not to be understood as solving the fundamental problem of pellagra. The solution of this, and thus the prevention of a recurrence of the disease next year and in the future, involves economic questions—income and food supply—the nature and complexity of which have already been outlined and which must be dealt with in other ways.

In any project or effort for the amelioration of conditions that are directly or indirectly responsible for the prevalence of pellagra among the agricultural tenant population of the cotton-growing area along the Mississippi and its tributaries, it is necessary to keep in mind two considerations of essential importance. The first is that the economic status of this population is bound up in the tenant system, which, in turn, is involved in single-crop agricultural production and the speculative character of agricultural finance as it is practiced in this area, the seasonal fluctuation in income of the tenant, the periodic or cyclical variation in profits, and other factors of an economic nature. The second consideration is that the dietary habits of the population in this section of the country are aggravated, if the term may be so used, by the peculiar limitations upon the supplies of foods, particularly foods of certain kinds, to which reference already has been made.

Thus it may appear at first glance that any attempt to remove the conditions which are fundamentally responsible for the prevalence of pellagra would involve a revolution of dietary habits and of the entire economic and financial system as it now exists. We are led, however, by our observations to believe that, regardless of changes that may be brought about or that may take place in these conditions, there seem to us to be some more direct and more immediately practicable approaches to the fundamental problem of pellagra which would be more specific in their effects.

We are fully aware that the extensive and valuable activities of the federal Department of Agriculture and of the state agricultural colleges and other agencies have been directed along at least some of the general lines which are suggested below; and our suggestions should not be taken as in any way implying that these activities are not fully commensurate with the demands of the situation. Since the aspect of the situation which concerns us here is primarily the public-health aspect, of which pellagra is only one index, we wish to invite consideration in a general way of certain measures which are either already under way or may, it seems to us, be undertaken for the improvement of specific conditions which are concerned more directly with the situation as a public-health problem.

In the first place, obviously any measure which will improve the economic condition of the tenant farm population, particularly of that portion of it which is liable to deprivation, will tend to lessen the prevalence of pellagra as well as of ill-health from most other causes. The stabilization of income of the tenant in such a way as to lessen the effect of seasonal and periodic limitations arising in part from the inability of the tenant at certain times to purchase such of those foods which are available would probably tend to operate in that way. It is generally recognized, we believe, that the diversification of agriculture in this area would be a measure for the stabilization of income, since the tenant's income would not then be so greatly subject to fluctuations as it is in the production and value of a single crop.

In the second place, there may be mentioned more specifically those efforts which do or may make food supplies available generally throughout the tenant population area and with less seasonal variation. Obviously, efforts looking toward crop diversification will have a direct bearing upon this objective, especially if the diversification includes truck, dairy, and cattle production. All efforts that will result in a greater increase in the milk supply may be regarded as definitely pellagra-preventive measures as well as measures for the improvement of health in general. From such information as has been furnished us in the areas concerned it is believed that a more general ownership of cows by the tenants themselves can be effected. Another suggestion which may be and has been made is for the establishment of plantation dairies operated by plantation owners or managers, the milk to be sold at a minimum price and to be included in the ordinary rations bought from the store or commissary. Another suggestion along this line is that of community dairies. In a similar way the efforts being made, by the Department of Agriculture and persons interested, toward more and better gardens among the tenants is a measure of great importance. It is believed that some practicable way can be found of providing for more convenient methods of the cultivation of gardens, such as the planting of garden produce in rows in the cotton fields themselves or the inauguration of plantation truck patches. In the latter case the produce may be sold, as in the case of the suggestion relating to milk, as are other goods in the plantation store or commissary. Again, an increase in cattle, swine, and poultry production, at least to the extent that will meet the local demand for fresh meat and eggs, is a matter which would have to be worked out in various ways to conform to local conditions. In short, the practicability and the economic and health advantage of promoting an increase in the production of food on the farm or plantation should be given the most earnest consideration.

The situation is manifestly one which calls for study with a view to working out practicable solutions of the economic and agricultural problems involved. In such study, however, the needs of health must be held in mind as of controlling importance.

PART FOUR

The Pellagra-Preventive Factor

14. Amino-Acid Deficiency Probably the Primary Etiological Factor in Pellagra[1]

JOSEPH GOLDBERGER
W. F. TANNER

Introduction

There is now at hand a considerable and convincing body of evidence in support of the view that diet is the primary controlling factor in the prevention and causation of pellagra. The more important part of this evidence may briefly be summarized as follows:

To begin with, account must be taken of the fact that no unequivocal evidence of the transmissibility of the disease has yet been adduced. Attempts to communicate the disease from the sick to the well by inoculation have failed in all reported instances.[2] The report of a successful inoculation of a monkey by Harris (1913) must be regarded, therefore, as in the highest degree doubtful; all the more as exhaustive efforts to confirm it, notably by Lavinder and Francis (1914) and by Harris himself, have failed.

In harmony with the negative results of experimental inoculation are the striking freedom from danger attaching to association and contact with cases in hospitals and the singular exemption of certain groups of residents in an endemic or epidemic institutional environment. It has repeatedly been observed, first, that at institutions (whether special or general hospitals) receiving cases of pellagra for treatment, physicians, nurses, attendants, etc., in frequent contact with the disease and directly or indirectly with the body discharges of persons sick with it, practically never develop the disease while so employed;[3] second, that employees (nurses, attendants, etc.) resident in institutions in which the disease has long been endemic or at times epidemic, many of whom also come in frequent association or intimate contact with cases of the disease or their body discharges or

---

1 *Public Health Rep.*, Vol. 37, No. 9 (March 3, 1922), 462–86.
2 Buniva, cited by Roussel; De Rolandis, cited by Roussel; Calmarza, 1870; McCafferty, 1909; Goldberger, 1916.
3 *La Pellagra in Italia*, 1880; Lavinder, 1911; Bouchard, 1862; Sambon, 1917. For an interesting account of medico-military observations in Rumania during the war, see Külz (*Arch. f. Schiffs u. trop. Hyg.* 1918, Vol. 22, pp. 401–403).

both, practically never contract it while so employed and so resident (Bouchard, 1862; Goldberger, 1914).

The striking exemption of certain groups residing in an endemic institutional environment has been found, in the instances studied by us, to be consistently associated with a significant difference in diet.

The controlling importance of diet is shown by the part it plays in the treatment, prevention, and production of the disease. Active cases of pellagra respond promptly and strikingly to an exclusively dietary treatment (Goldberger, 1916; Voegtlin, 1920). The relatively rare exceptions are no more than might be anticipated when the experience in scurvy and beriberi are kept in mind. The natural tendency to recovery without change of environment, and seemingly without therapeutic interference, is associated with a seasonal change in diet (Goldberger, et al., n.d.).

Of outstanding significance are, on the one hand, the demonstration that pellagra may be completely prevented by means of a suitable diet, without intervention of any other known factor, hygienic or sanitary,[4] and, on the other, the absence of any sound evidence that the disease is preventable by any other means (Nesbitt, 1916; Goldberger and Wheeler, 1920).

Although, as has already been stated, all attempts to transmit the disease from the sick to the well by inoculation have failed, an experiment to induce the disease in the human subject by feeding, carried out by Goldberger and Wheeler (1920) in 1915, was completely successful. At least 6 of 11 convicts who volunteered for the experiment and who subsisted on a diet consisting principally of the cereals, wheat, maize, and rice, with pork fat and some fresh vegetables (sweet potatoes, turnips, cabbage, greens), developed evidence which experienced observers recognized as that of pellagra; whereas, of a large number of controls, none presented any evidence justifying even a suspicion of the disease. In this connection it may be noted that symptoms and pathological changes resembling more or less markedly, but not certainly identical with, those occurring in pellagra have been reported in animals experimentally fed certain faulty diets.[5]

Finally, reference should perhaps also be made to the idea that in the causation of the disease there is, besides diet, also an essential

4 Goldberger, Waring, Willets, 1915; White, 1919; Stannus, 1920; Goldberger and Tanner, unpublished data.
5 Voegtlin, 1920; Chittenden and Underhill, 1917; Chick and Hume, 1920; McCarrison, 1921.

infective factor. According to this a faulty diet operates merely by lowering resistance to infection. This view has elsewhere already been discussed by Goldberger and Wheeler (1920), who have shown that it is untenable except in the form that a poor nutrition of a specific kind, the result of a faulty diet, is essential to enable the hypothetical infection to establish itself; that is, in the form calling for the concurrence of two specific extrinsic factors.

With respect to this more restricted conception it may be said, first, that it implicitly recognizes diet as the primary controlling factor; second, that unequivocal evidence of the existence of an essential infective factor has not yet been adduced; and, finally, that all the well-ascertained phenomena of the disease are either explicable by or at least not inconsistent with an exclusively dietary etiology, thus rendering superfluous the assumption of a second essential factor.

While it thus is clear that in the prevention and causation of pellagra, diet plays the dominating rôle, the question of the essential dietary factor or factors concerned is still undetermined.

In this paper we desire to record certain observations which bear directly on this question. First, however, we shall pass in review the literature more or less closely related thereto.

Review of Literature

A review of the older literature which, in the main, concerned itself with maize, particularly spoiled maize, although very interesting in retrospect, does not seem sufficiently pertinent in the present connection to warrant full presentation. It will suffice to recall the theory elaborated by Lussana and Frua and the closely related view advocated by Calmarza. Lussana and Frua (1856) contended that pellagra is due to an "insufficient neuromuscular repair" arising from "an alimentation of proteinaceous insufficiency in comparison with nondeficient respiratory quota" in a diet "fundamentally and almost exclusively composed of maize." This theory of relative protein insufficiency in pellagra may almost be considered the prototype of the theory advanced over a score of years later by Takaki (1885) in connection with beriberi and a rice diet.

Among other evidence adduced by Lussana and Frua in support of their contention was the markedly more favorable result of dietetic ("restorative nutritive") treatment based on their own theory than that obtained by treatment based on other hypotheses.

In this connection reference may be made to the fundamentally rather closely related theory suggested a few years ago by Deeks

(1912). Deeks seems to group pellagra with "hyperchlorhydria," "flatulent dyspepsias," "acute rheumatism and rheumatic affections," and "nephritis," as a "carbohydrate diathesis." He believes that it is not corn alone "but any cereal or starch food in conjunction with cane sugar, in a warm climate where there is lessened metabolic activity and consequent inadequate elaboration of digestive elements which initiates the autointoxication responsible for the symptom-complex known as pellagra. The proof thereof," he goes on to say, "lies not in the determination of the elusive complex physico-chemical substances, the result of fermentation or defective metabolic elaboration, but in the results obtained by physiological treatment based on the above-mentioned hypothesis." His treatment consists "(1) in limiting the nourishment absolutely to fresh fruit juice, preferably orange, meat broths, and milk, as long as there is nausea or vomiting, and the absolute avoidance of everything which contains sweet or starchy elements; (2) in the administration of from 15 to 30 drops of dilute nitric acid in three-fourths of a tumbler of water three times daily on an empty stomach. I have found by practical experience," he states, "that no substance will relieve as quickly or as satisfactorily gastric acidity as this mineral acid. When the stomach condition improves, which is generally in three or four days, a carbohydrate-free diet is ordered. This consists, in addition to the above, of eggs, meats of all kinds, fish, green vegetables, such as lettuce, celery, onions, tomatoes, beets, carrots, spinach, chayoti, vegetable marrow, okra, green peas, string beans, egg plant, etc., and fresh fruits of all kinds, there being no limitation." It may here be remarked, as has already been pointed out by Goldberger, Wheeler, and Sydenstricker (1920), that the idea that the production of pellagra is dependent on the excessive consumption of carbohydrates was suggested at least as far back as 1796 by Albera and by Strambio (1796). The essentials of Deeks's treatment are those of a long line of his predecessors, beginning with Casal himself.

Calmarza (1870) like many (if not most) Spanish students of the disease denied that maize had any necessary connection with pellagra and vigorously contended that the disease was due solely to an alimentation deficient in animal food, a diet too largely vegetable, providing, he claimed, too little nitrogen for human needs. Calmarza's contention did not receive the attention which it merited largely because of Costallat and Roussel (1866), who, being enthusiastic zeists, cast doubt upon the diagnosis of the cases of pellagra without maize reported by Calmarza and other Spanish observers.

The views relating to the nature of the dietary defect that may be considered as immediately pertinent to the present discussion date from 1912. In that year Funk (1912) included pellagra provisionally in a group of "deficiency diseases," all of which, he stated, could be prevented and cured by the addition of certain preventive substances called by him "vitamines."

Inspired by Funk's work and the other, then recent, developments in beriberi, Sandwith (1913, 1914) suggested that pellagra might be a "deficiency disease, waiting for a 'vitamin' to be discovered." At the same time, having in mind the work of Wilcock and Hopkins with zein, he vaguely suggested the possibility of a tryptophan deficiency on the basis, it would seem, of the mistaken impression that zein was the sole protein of maize, and in the belief that inferior or damaged maize was the cause of pellagra.

In 1914 Nightingale (1914) from his experience with a disease which he called "zeism," but which must be regarded as pellagra, concluded that the disease was due to the loss of some essential nutritive constituent during the process of grinding maize into meal, "probably of the nature of an organic salt." This recalls the suggestion made by Petrof (1907) in 1907 that pellagra is due to a deficiency in phosphorus. Petrof attempted to show that this deficiency arose as the result of a maize diet, of which the maize was poor in phosphorus, its poverty in phosphorus arising from being cultivated in a lime-poor soil.

In 1914, also, there was suggested by Voegtlin (1914) that in the study of the etiology of pellagra, serious consideration would have to be given to "(1) a deficiency or absence of certain vitamines in the diet; (2) the toxic effect of some substances, as aluminum, which occur in certain vegetable food; (3) a deficiency of the diet in certain amino-acids." Later, in a study of the influence of vitamins on the clinical course of pellagra, Voegtlin, in association with Neil and Hunter (1920), reported that the administration of extracts from yeast and rice polishings, which were highly efficient for the prevention of avian polyneuritis, in general failed to modify the course of the disease, but the administration to pellagrins of protein-free extracts obtained from liver and thymus gland presumed to contain both the antineuritic substance and the fat soluble vitamin "was followed by an improvement in their condition apparently comparable to that produced by the consumption of a diet rich in fresh animal proteins." The conclusion drawn was that "the dietary defect responsible for pellagra is distinctly (qualitatively) different

from and perhaps more complex than the one causing fowl polyneuritis and human beriberi."

McCollum, Simmonds, and Parsons, as a result of studies of faulty
diets in rats (1918) expressed the belief that pellagra is primarily
associated with the unsatisfactory character of three dietary factors,
namely, fat-soluble A, mineral elements, and protein mixture. A
year later these workers, after having attempted to produce in rats a
condition analogous to pellagra in man by feeding their animals
with diets similar to the diet employed by Goldberger and Wheeler
in their experiment on convicts, and observing in them only a
"generalized poor condition," concluded that pellagra is caused by
an infectious agent (1919). It may be remarked that this conclusion
appears in large measure to be based on the unwarranted assumption
that the distinctive symptoms observed in man, resulting from feeding a given diet, must necessarily be exactly reproduced in another
species, in this case the rat.

As a result of his experience with pellagra among Armenian
refugees, White (1919) has suggested that the causal factor may be a
deficiency of vitamin or of some other essential components of the
diet, such as tryptophan or an insufficiency or unsuitability of one of
the proximate principles in the dietary, such as the protein or fat.

On White's invitation, Wilson (1919) examined the diet concerned
in the outbreak among these refugees and as a result expressed the
opinion that the most probable cause of the outbreak was, first of all,
the low biological value of protein, next, the low total energy value,
and, finally, the low fat value. Wilson gave the results of his further
studies to the committee of enquiry which investigated the outbreak
of pellagra among Turkish prisoners of war. This committee (1919)
concluded that pellagra is due to deficiency in protein, as gauged by
its biological value.

Recently a full report of Wilson's important studies have appeared (1921). In this he makes comparisons of diets known to have
been connected with pellagra with those of known value in curing
and preventing the disease, from which he concludes that the etiological factor is a deficiency of protein in the food, best determined
by an estimation of its biological value by means of Thomas' figures.
He argues against a deficiency in vitamins, citing a markedly favorable effect in the reduction of pellagra observed among the inmates
of the Abassia Asylum for the Insane at Cairo, following the addition of 45 grams of meat and 50 of milk to a diet which already containing 100 grams of meat, 50 grams of milk, and 300 grams of fresh
vegetables, it was difficult for him "to suppose was lacking in either

vitamines, using the term generally, or in salts of lime, or that the additions made could have added anything of great importance in these respects." The deficiency of protein may, he considers, be "(a) primary, in which the supply is insufficient for the individual requirement or, when, owing to the indigestible character of the food, a somewhat restricted supply can not be utilized to the normal extent; (b) secondary, in which, owing to digestive disturbances or other causes, the supply of protein can not be assimilated." He looks upon indicanuria as an important indication of the loss of protein in the intestine, the amount present being, he estimates, sometimes sufficient to account for the loss to the body of a large proportion of the protein intake. He considers the indicanuria as closely related to the deficiency of gastric hydrochloric acid. Labor, by raising the level of protein requirement, especially when there is a deficient energy supply, is considered a factor in the causation of pellagra. He suggests that a deficiency of cholesterol may be related to some of the symptoms.

Wood (1920) from some experiments with fowls, and by reason of seemingly favorable results of treatment with maize germ and wheat bran, is disposed to suspect that a vitamin-B deficiency is involved in pellagra. However, he points out that there may be something else in the maize germ and the cortex of wheat that may account for the results observed. It may be remarked that there is nothing to show that other changes in the diet made at the same time could not explain the favorable results Wood attributes to maize germ and wheat bran.

In April, 1920, Chick and Hume (1920) reported symptoms resembling those of pellagra, produced in three monkeys by prolonged feeding on a low protein diet in which the proteins, almost exclusively those of maize, were at the same time of low biological value. Whether the condition of malnutrition produced in these animals may properly be regarded as corresponding to that of pellagra in man, depends, in the present state of our knowledge, on whether the eruption observed in one of the animals actually corresponded to the dermatitis of pellagra in man. So far as may be judged by the published description and colored drawing of the eruption, this is very doubtful. That some of the symptoms observed in these monkeys may have been due to an amino-acid deficiency in the experimental diet seems not improbable, and the improvement reported as having been observed in two of the three animals treated with tryptophan would suggest that a deficiency in at least this one

amino-acid was involved in the cause of the malnutrition observed
in these animals.

McCarrison (1921) has called attention to the parallelism of symptoms and pathological lesions of pellagra with those in the animals
(monkeys) experimentally fed by him on vitamin-deficient diets.
On the basis of these analogies he considers it probable "that deficiency of vitamines and the consequent disturbance of digestive
and endocrine functions play an important part in the production of
pellagra." Certain other considerations lead him to believe "that
pellagra may result either from deficient protein supply or from deficient protein assimilation consequent on vitamine insufficiency or
from a combination of both these causes." McCarrison does not
seem to have actually worked with the disease himself.

According to Hess (1921) "the experiences in the Central Empires
during the war render it improbable that pellagra is due merely to a
lack of adequate protein. Adequate protein was lacking to a marked
degree—milk, cheese, eggs, meat were all unavailable. Nevertheless
there was no prevalence of pellagra throughout these years." Evidently Hess assumes that the protein of milk, cheese, eggs, and meat
alone is "adequate" protein.

Impressed by certain striking epidemiological features and the
negative results of animal inoculation experiments, Goldberger
(1914) suggested in 1914 that pellagra is a disease essentially of
dietary origin caused either by a deficiency in the diet of some essential element or by the presence of some element in excessive
amounts; that is, by a diet faulty in some undetermined respect, but
the fault in which could be corrected by an increase in the fresh
animal food component (Goldberger, 1914 and 1916).

In 1918 Goldberger, Wheeler, and Sydenstricker (1918) reported
that the indications afforded by a study of the diet of nonpellagrous
and of pellagrous households clearly suggested that the pellagra-
producing dietary fault is the result of some one or, more probably, of a combination of two or more, of the following factors:
(1) A physiologically defective protein supply; (2) a low or inadequate supply of fat-soluble vitamin; (3) a low or inadequate supply
of water-soluble vitamin; and (4) a defective mineral supply.

In harmony with these indications are those afforded by the result
of Goldberger and Wheeler's (1920) feeding experiment in convicts.
The experimental diet, they state, was probably faulty in some degree with respect to the protein, mineral element, antineuritic, and,
possibly also, with respect to the fat-soluble vitamin. From this they
inferred that in relation to the production of pellagra their study

suggested that the dietary factors to be considered as possibly essential are an amino-acid deficiency, a deficient or faulty constitution of the mineral element, possibly, but doubtfully, a deficiency in the fat-soluble vitamin, and perhaps some as yet unknown factor.

In a more detailed report of the study of the diet of nonpellagrous and of pellagrous households, Goldberger, Wheeler, and Sydenstricker (1920) conclude that the indications of their study suggest that "the pellagra-producing dietary fault is the result of some one or of a combination or combinations of two or more of the following factors: (1) A physiologically defective protein (amino-acid) supply; (2) a defective or inadequate mineral supply; (3) a deficiency in an as yet unknown dietary essential (vitamine?)," none of the known vitamins being regarded as necessary factors.

Present Study of Preventive Dietary Factors

The following gives the details of some observations which were made in the course of studies of the prevention of pellagra at the Georgia State Sanitarium, one of the large southern asylums for the insane. We are deeply grateful to the trustees and officers of this institution for their sustained interest and cooperation.

I. *Mineral supplement.*—The high value which our experience at this asylum and the other service investigations had taught us to attach to milk, both as a prophylactic and therapeutic agent, suggested, among other things, the possibility that its value might be due to the inorganic elements of its ash. We therefore arranged to supplement the institution diet of a group of colored and one of white patients with an inorganic salt mixture, each daily dose of which contained the inorganic elements of the ash in a liter of whole milk (Sherman, 1918), this quantity of fresh whole milk as a supplement to the institution diet having shown itself to have decidedly beneficial effects in both prevention and treatment. We began with a single mixture of the following composition (quantities for one individual per day) prepared for us by Dr. Atherton Seidell, of the division of chemistry of the Hygienic Laboratory:

	Grams
$CaH PO_42H_2O$	5.15
Na_2SO_4	1.51
$Mg Cl_2$	0.47
KCl	1.49
$K_3C_6H_5O_7H_2O$	1.79
Iron and ammonium citrate (17 per cent Fe)	.07

Having experienced some administrative difficulties in its use on a large scale, it was replaced at the end of about one month by two mixtures which were suggested and prepared for us by Dr. Elias Elvove, of the division of chemistry of the Hygienic Laboratory. Together these furnished, qualitatively and quantitatively, the same inorganic elements as had the first mixture, but each could be separately dissolved in water and thus conveniently mixed with the food.

The composition of each of these is as follows (for one individual per day):

Mixture A

		Grams
$Ca(C_2H_3O_2)_2$ H_2O		4.187
$CaCl_2$		0.685
$Mg\ Cl_2$		0.470
KCl		0.495
NaCl		0.054
$FeCl_3$		0.007

Mixture B

$Na_2\ SO_4$	1.510
KH_2PO_4	4.079

Mixture B, in aqueous solution, was stirred up with the breakfast cereal and hash and A with the food at the mid-day meal. In order to make sure of a liberal supply of iodine, we began, at about the time the change to the two mixtures (A and B) was made, the daily addition to the evening meal of two drops of the sirup of the iodid of iron (U. S. P.). Incidentally, this increased somewhat the allowance of iron, an element in which the ash of milk is poor.

The amount of each of the nine mineral elements believed to be essential in mammalian nutrition which these daily supplements yielded is shown in Table 59, which has been prepared to permit also of a comparison with the elements yielded by the salt mixtures extensively used in their studies by Osborne and Mendel (1919) and by McCollum (1917) and associates, respectively.

It will be noted that while there are some differences among these three mixtures, there is a quite marked general similarity in the quantity of the elements yielded. On the basis of an identical yield of calcium the quantity of K, Na, P, and Cl supplied by our minerals is seen to be intermediate between that furnished by the mixture of Osborne and Mendel on the one hand and that of McCollum on the other. Our supplements differed perhaps most markedly from either of the other mixtures in the much lower yield by ours of iron.

At this juncture it may be noted that the bulk of the institution diet—the diet of the inmates whose attacks of pellagra we are about to consider—consisted of the cereals maize, wheat, and rice, some dried legumes, and a little beef. The mineral element supplied by such diet is, according to McCollum (1919), too low in the elements sodium, chlorine, and calcium.

Recalling that in the preparation of the various dishes constituting the diet, table salt is always freely used, there could here, therefore, quite independently of the mineral supplements, at no time be a question of an inadequate supply of the elements sodium and chlorine. According to Sherman (1918) the standard allowance of calcium in a man of 70 kilograms, with an energy requirement of 3,000 calories, should be 0.69 gram. Accepting this, it follows that our mineral supplement afforded a very liberal supply of this element, and there can thus be no question of a calcium deficiency in the diet so supplemented even when this was not entirely consumed.

In spite of the undoubted improvement in the institution diet thus brought about, a number of cases of pellagra occurred in individuals consuming it. Following is a brief summary of the significant points in the history of five cases in individuals known to have consumed during considerable periods practically their entire allowance of minerals.

Case 1. C–O: White female, age 32, weight 44.5 kilograms, had pellagra in 1913, 1914, and again in October, 1920. Began taking the mineral supplement on December 10, at which time she presented no recognizable symptoms of pellagra. The sirup of the iodid of

TABLE 59—*Number of grams of the specified elements yielded by the daily supplement of minerals and a comparison with quantities which would be yielded by salt mixtures extensively used by Osborne and Mendel and by McCollum, respectively, if supplied to yield the same amount of Ca.*

	Ca.	Mg.	K.	Na.	P.	Cl.	S.	Fe.	I.
Mixtures A and B, with 2 drops of sirup of iodid of iron (U.S.P.)........	1.20	0.12	1.43	0.51	0.98	1.06	0.34	0.0034	0.005
Mixture of Osborne and Mendel..................	1.20	.16	.87	.30	.72	1.12	.07	.023	.0003[*]
Mixture No. 185, of McCollum...............	1.20	.24	1.83	.55	1.66	.46	.31	.83	Trace.[+]

[*]Besides the elements shown in the table, this mixture includes traces of fluorine and aluminum.
[+]Supplied in the drinking water.

iron was begun on January 25. On the following June 7 this patient developed a pellagrous dermatitis, notwithstanding that during this period of at least 4½ months she consumed practically 100 per cent of the minerals furnished.

Case 2. H–L. L: White female, age 44, weight 35.8 kilograms, had pellagra 1912, 1914, and 1918. Began taking the mineral supplement December 10, and the sirup of the iodid of iron on January 25. On the following June 17 this patient developed the distinctive dermatitis, although it is estimated that she consumed during the interval fully 95 per cent of the minerals furnished.

Case 3. K–S: White female, age 54, weight 62.5 kilograms, had pellagra 1915, 1918, and again in September, 1920. Began taking the mineral supplement on December 10, at which time she was free from recognizable symptoms of pellagra. Administration of the sirup of the iodid of iron was begun January 25. On May 4 she developed the dermatitis of pellagra, although her record of food consumption during the interval indicated an intake of fully 95 per cent of the minerals furnished.

Case 4. S–E: Colored female, age 55, weight 39.2 kilograms, had pellagra in 1915, 1918, and again in August, 1920. Began taking the mineral supplement on December 16, by which time she was free of recognizable symptoms of pellagra. The sirup of the iodid of iron was begun on January 26. On the following May 30 she developed the dermatitis of pellagra, although she is recorded as having taken during the interval fully 95 per cent of the minerals.

Case 5. W–M: Colored female, age 55, weight 41 kilograms, had pellagra in 1917, 1918, 1919, in April, and a second dermal attack early in November, 1920. Like "S–E" she began taking the mineral supplement on December 16, by which time recognizable symptoms of pellagra had disappeared. The sirup of the iodid of iron was begun on January 26. On April 4 this patient developed the dermatitis of pellagra, although in the interval she consumed, we estimate, fully 95 per cent of the minerals furnished.

II. *Vitamins with supplement of minerals.*—Although, as will presently be indicated, there is reason to believe that the institution diet includes, in general, sufficient of the vitamin-containing foods to provide at least the minimum requirement of the known vitamins, the supply of these, particularly of vitamins C and A, is quite irregular and fluctuates widely, depending as it here does practically exclusively on the supply of fresh vegetables, a supply that is markedly influenced by season and other factors affecting availability. The supply of vitamin B fluctuates less and is more regular than that of

C and A, since such sources of this vitamin as unbolted maize (Mc-Collum, Simmonds, and Pitz, 1916) meal in form of corn bread is daily, and legumes (McCollum, Simmonds, and Pitz, 1917) (lima beans, navy beans, or cowpeas) are frequently (though irregularly) served at the midday meal. Accordingly, with the object of further improving the diet by correcting the possible faults arising from these causes, we replaced, on and after May 24, the fluctuating and irregular supply of fresh vegetables in the diet of those receiving the supplement of minerals, with a regular daily supply of 3 ounces of the juice expressed from canned tomatoes, and one-half ounce of cod-liver oil, and, on June 19, the variable and irregular supply of legumes with a regular daily ration of at least one-half ounce of cowpeas.

In this connection it may be observed that canned tomato juice has been shown to be an excellent antiscorbutic.[6] In comparison with lemon and orange juice, its antiscorbutic power would seem to be somewhat inferior. According to Hess, 4 cc. daily of strained canned tomato juice are sufficient to protect the guinea pig, whereas of either orange or lemon juice only about 3 cc. daily are required (1920)—a ratio of about 4 to 3.

Recalling that the experience of the British Navy and of Arctic expeditions has amply demonstrated that not over 1 ounce of lemon juice fully protects the sailor and the Arctic explorer against scurvy (Budd, 1839; Smith, 1918), it would follow, on the basis of this ratio, that about 1⅓ ounces of canned tomato juice should serve the same purpose. Our allowance of 3 ounces daily for these small, inactive inmates would therefore seem to be a very liberal one.

Tomato juice has also been found to be quite rich in the water-soluble and the fat-soluble vitamin. Its antineuritic potency is indicated by the fact that Hess and Unger (1919) have found that pigeons suffering from polyneuritis could be cured by giving them 5 cc. of this foodstuff daily. Presumably a smaller quantity would suffice to prevent the development of the polyneuritis in this highly susceptible animal. As a source of fat-soluble vitamin, tomato juice is far inferior to cod-liver oil.

This oil, of all foods so far studied, would seem to be the richest in vitamin A. Some samples quantitatively tested have been found 250 times as potent as butter (Zilva and Miura, 1921; Zilva and Drummond, 1921). Allowing for variations in potency of different samples and assuming that the sample used by us had only 10 per

6 Hess and Unger, 1918; 1919; 1919; Osborne and Mendel, 1919.

cent of this value, the daily administration of half an ounce of the oil would, on this extremely conservative basis, be equivalent to a daily consumption of the vitamin in some 12 ounces of butter. So far as can be judged, this quantity of butter would supply more than enough vitamin A for any human need. It would appear reasonably certain, therefore, that our cod-liver oil supplement alone furnished a more than ample quota of this food essential.

Besides its exceptional richness in the anti-xerophthalmic essential, cod-liver oil, it may be noted, seems also to carry an abundance of an as yet not fully defined antirachitic factor (McCollum *et al.*, 1920–21, Steenbock and Happert, 1921).

Notwithstanding these advantageous additions and modifications, three cases of pellagra developed in individuals known to have taken all of the cod-liver oil and tomato juice and to have consumed practically all of the cowpeas and minerals furnished. The following is a summary of the significant points in the history of these cases.

Case 6. J–F: Colored female, age 45, weight 54 kilograms; had pellagra in 1914 and again in April, 1920. Began taking the mineral supplement December 14, 1920, at which time she was free of active symptoms of pellagra. Beginning January 26, she was given 2 drops of the sirup of the iodid of iron daily. On May 24, began taking cod-liver oil (one-half ounce) and canned tomato juice (3 ounces) daily. Between June 3 and August 13 consumed daily, among other things, an average of approximately 1 ounce of dry cowpeas (boiled) and about 2 ounces of unbolted maize meal (as corn bread). After August 13 the daily consumption of cowpeas averaged approximately one-half ounce and of whole maize meal 3½–4 ounces. Throughout she took practically all of the mineral addition. Notwithstanding all this, however, this patient developed the beginning of a pellagrous dermatitis on August 24.

Case 7. S–M. L.: Colored female, age 37, weight 43.6 kilograms. Had pellagra in October, 1920. Began taking the mineral supplement on December 14, at which time she was free from active symptoms of pellagra. On January 26 she began receiving 2 drops of the sirup of iodid of iron daily. On May 24 began taking cod-liver oil (one-half ounce) and tomato juice (3 ounces) daily. Between June 3 and August 13 consumed daily, among other things, an average of approximately 1 ounce of dry cowpeas (boiled) and about 2 ounces of unbolted maize meal (as corn bread). After August 13 the daily consumption of cowpeas averaged approximately one-half ounce and of maize meal approximately 3½–4 ounces. Throughout she consumed practically all the mineral supplements. In spite of all this, however, this patient developed a mild but classical pellagrous dermatitis on September 16, 1921.

Case 8. T–E: Colored female; age 28, weight 40.2 kilograms. Had pellagra in October, 1916, and again in June, 1920. On December 14, at which time she was free of active symptoms of pellagra, began taking the mineral supplement. On January 26 she began receiving 2 drops of the sirup of iodid of iron daily with her supper. On May 24 she began taking cod-liver oil (one-half ounce) and tomato juice (3 ounces) daily. Between June 3 and August 13 she consumed daily, among other things, an average of approximately 1 ounce of dry cowpeas and 1½–2 ounces of unbolted maize meal (as corn bread). After August 13 the daily consumption of cowpeas averaged approximately one-half ounce and of maize meal 3½–4 ounces.

On September 19 this patient developed the beginning of a pellagrous dermatitis in spite of having consumed practically all of the minerals and vitamins furnished during a period of at least four months.

In addition to the foregoing we observed two cases in individuals who, because of capricious appetites, had not so regularly consumed the entire mineral supplement nor quite all the cowpeas, but who, by reason of the separate administration of the tomato juice and cod-liver oil, were known to have consumed all of their allowance of these foodstuffs. The significant points in the histories of these two cases are as follows.

Case 9. P–A: Colored female, age 45, weight 40.2 kilograms. Had pellagra in 1917, 1918, and 1919, and October, 1920. She was free from active symptoms of pellagra on December 14, 1920, when she began taking the mineral supplement. On January 26 she began receiving 2 drops of the sirup of iodid of iron daily. On May 24 began taking and thereafter took regularly fully one-half ounce of cod-liver oil and 3 ounces of tomato juice daily. Between June 3 and August 13 she consumed regularly as part of her diet practically all of a daily allowance of fully 1 ounce of cowpeas and of approximately 2 ounces of unbolted maize meal (as corn bread). Between August 13 and October 9 the consumption of cowpeas was reduced to a little under one-half ounce (approximately 10 or 11 grams) daily, but that of maize meal was increased to between 3 and 4 ounces a day.

During the period June 3 to October 9, 1921, the daily consumption of the mineral supplement was not complete, but is estimated to have equaled fully 80 per cent of that offered.

So far as can be judged, the shifts in food consumption noted would hardly seem to have effected any change in the quantity of vitamin B intake, the reduced consumption of cowpeas being probably fully compensated for by the increased consumption of maize meal. The reduced mineral intake would still, we should judge, furnish plenty of the elements sodium, chlorine, and calcium. In spite of all this, however, a pellagrous dermatitis made its appearance about October 10, 1921.

Case 10. N–M: Colored female, age 41, weight 41 kilograms. So far as known had her first attack of pellagra in July, 1920. She was free from active symptoms of pellagra on December 14, when she began taking the mineral supplement. Like Case 9, on January 26, she began receiving two drops of the sirup of the iodid of iron, and on May 24, one-half ounce of cod-liver oil and 3 ounces of tomato juice daily.

Between June 3 and August 13 she consumed daily as part of her diet an average of a little short of 1 ounce of cowpeas (about 25 grams) and upward of 1½ ounces of unbolted maize meal (as corn bread). After August 13 and up to September 20 the consumption of cowpeas was reduced to a daily average of slightly under one-half ounce (about 12 grams), but that of maize meal was increased to a daily average of between 3 and 4 ounces.

Between June 3 and September 20 her food consumption was such that her intake of calcium is estimated to have been fully 90 per cent of that offered.

It would appear that in this as in Case 9, the variation in appetite did not materially affect the intake of vitamin B and, since the cod-liver oil and tomato juice were regularly administered apart from the other food and always completely ingested, the intake of the other vitamins was not at all affected. With respect to the mineral elements of special interest (calcium, sodium, and chlorine), the slight reduction of intake, considering the liberal supply may, we judge, be regarded as negligible. Notwithstanding all this, however, a classical pellagrous dermatitis began its development on September 22.

Significance of Observations in Present Study

It will doubtless have been noted that in all the cases cited the individuals attacked had had one or more previous attacks of the disease. This was not an accidental circumstance. In selecting individuals for observation and study, we purposely chose those who had had previous attacks, in the belief that in a group so chosen there would be a greater chance of the development of cases than in a group of individuals not previously attacked, and therefore the failure of such development would be all the more significant of the value of the preventive measures being tested. For, although a pellagra recurrence must be regarded as etiologically fundamentally identical with an initial attack (Goldberger, 1916), there are nevertheless certain intrinsic factors which, exposure being equal, may conceivably operate to make more probable that a pellagrin will suffer a recurrence than that a nonpellagrin will develop an initial attack. Of these factors, three may be cited in the present connection.

There is, first of all, the possibility that some of those who have suffered an attack of the disease have not, by reason perhaps of inadequate treatment, fully recovered their normal nutritional status. For such, it may be assumed that the minimum supply of essential food factors must be greater than for the average normal individual since, conceivably, there is not only the need for taking care of current requirements, but also for the repair or correction of residual morbid processes or changes and, perhaps, also to satisfy a residual shortage of some essential nutritional elements.

There is next the probability that some, if not all, such individuals have suffered some (possibly permanent) damage to the digestive organs and glands which may conceivably lead to a lowering of efficiency or to an unfavorable modification of the digestive processes and thus to an inferior utilization of some of the ingested nutrients. It is known, in fact, that gastric anacidity is a frequent sequel of the disease and this, as both Murlin (1920) and Wilson (1921) suggest, probably explains the tendency in convalescents for intestinal putrefaction to take place high up in the intestines (Myers and Fine, 1913; Sullivan and Dawson, 1921) with the production of waste products, manifested by the appearance of an excess of hippuric acid and of indican in the urine. While this disturbed digestion may, as Wilson further points out, lead to serious loss of protein and, possibly of a little fat, it should perhaps be observed that it is not known that any other food factors are materially affected nor that the processes of absorption are appreciably interfered with.

Finally we have the possibility if not the probability that the pellagrin may be an individual whose minimum physiological requirements are normally somewhat above the average.

The circumstance, therefore, that our observations were in individuals with histories of one or several previous attacks and thus probably with requirements for a supply of nutrient factors in some measure above the normal average, makes it more than ordinarily important that in evaluating the significance of these observations due consideration be given to the question of the adequacy of supply of the dietary factors the rôle of which in pellagra prevention we are seeking to determine.

Mineral supplement.—It has already been pointed out that by reason of the nature of the shortcomings, with respect to the mineral element, of the type of diet provided the asylum inmates, the mineral supplement furnished by us coupled with the table salt used in the preparation of the several dishes, would, with reasonable certainty, not only correct such possible shortcomings but also provide a large margin of safety. So far as existing knowledge permits one to judge, both the total quantity and the composition of the mineral consumed may properly be regarded as having been fully adequate for the needs of the individuals concerned. Therefore the failure of our mineral addition to prevent the occurrence of the disease in the cases cited would seem quite clearly to indicate that a mineral deficiency is not an essential factor in the production of the disease. This interpretation is materially strengthened by the fact that lean meat, known to be poor in ash, is a valuable preventive of the disease. Indeed our experience leads us to believe that on the basis of protein, fresh lean beef is, gram for gram, at least as efficient a prophylactic as is milk, a food exceptionally rich in minerals.

Vitamins with minerals.—The failure of our attempt to prevent pellagra by supplementing the institution diet with mineral elements which, it seems safe to assume, made good the shortcomings of the ash constituents of the diet, is significant, however, not only in relation to the mineral factor itself but also as relates to a combination of this with the known vitamins.

In the large section of the asylum (colored females) under our observation, we have found symptoms of scurvy and of beriberi of such very exceptional occurrence as to leave no room for doubt that the institution diet provides at least the minimum requirement of the essential antiscorbutic and antineuritic vitamins. Similarly, although inflammatory conditions of the eye occur from time to time among the asylum inmates, we have at no time observed among them any condition which did not respond quite readily to mild local antisepsis, a response which, it is believed, would not have occurred in cases of ophthalmia the result of a vitamin-A deficiency. Therefore, if this form of ophthalmia has occurred among the inmates under our observation such cases must, we feel, have been both rare and very mild, for, although on the alert, we have recognized none. This suggests that the asylum diet contains, in general, sufficient vitamin A to prevent the development of this specific eye disease.

In the light of these considerations it would seem to follow that cases 1–5, cited above, developed in spite, not only of what, we believe, may properly be regarded as a liberal mineral intake (supplement of minerals plus minerals in institution diet), but also in spite of an intake at the same time of each of the three known vitamins included in the institution diet, an intake which, if not liberal, would seem, in general, to be at least adequate to prevent recognizable symptoms of a specific deficiency.

Recalling what has already been said of the richness in vitamins A, B, and C of canned tomato juice, and in vitamin A and the antirachitic factor of cod-liver oil, and taking into account also the fact that both dry cowpeas and unbolted maize meal are good sources of vitamin B (McCollum, Simmonds, and Pitz, 1916; idem, 1917), it would seem that the modifications of the institution diet, already referred to, as the result of which these vitamin-bearing foods were regularly included in the daily ration, very greatly improved it in all these respects. If, as we believe, the institution diet, in general, supplies at least the minimum needs of each of the three known vitamins, the diet modified and supplemented, as described, may reasonably, we believe, be regarded as supplying them in fully adequate quantities even for individuals of the type with which we were dealing.

Therefore, the development of recurrences in five individuals (Cases, no. 6, 7, 8, 9, and 10), each of whom had, as already detailed, consumed daily for periods of at least two and one-half months before the appearance of the eruption not only what we believe to have been an adequate mineral supplement but also what we judge to have been an abundance of all known vitamins, would seem to indicate that a deficiency of these dietary factors, individually and collectively, is not essential in the causation of the disease.

The development during the past few years in our knowledge of nutrition seems to warrant the belief that besides an adequate energy supply the following dietary factors are essential for normal physiological well-being: An adequate quota of protein of good biological quality; a suitable mineral supply; a sufficient supply of vitamins, A, B, and C, and, possibly, of an as yet not definitely identified antirachitic factor.

With regard to energy supply we estimate that the food actually consumed yielded an average of approximately 1,800 calories daily.[7] Considering the mild climate, the small size and inactive habit of the

7 In computing the caloric value the factor 4 was applied to protein and carbohydrate, and the factor 9 to fat. This therefore represents the available, not the gross, energy.

patients concerned, this should have fully supplied their energy needs. The cases of pellagra under consideration would seem to have occurred therefore in spite not only of a liberal intake of essential minerals and vitamins but also of an adequate energy supply.

Thus, by a process of exclusion we are led to conclude that of the known dietary essentials the protein factor alone was concerned in our failure to prevent the development of the cases herein cited. And if our interpretations are, as we believe, sound (and if all dietary factors essential in human nutrition are known) the further conclusion may properly be drawn, namely, that the dominating rôle of diet in the prevention and causation of pellagra must be referred primarily to the character of the protein supply.

The distinctive clinical physiognomy of the disease precludes the assumption of any but a specific etiology; it must be assumed, therefore, that the essential etiological dietary factor is a specific defect in the protein mixture or, since protein is but a complex of amino-acids, different for different proteins, that it is a specific defect in the amino-acid supply either in the nature of an improper balance or more probably of a deficiency of some one or of some combination or combinations of amino-acids. This does not mean and we do not wish to be understood as suggesting that the diet associated with the production of pellagra is always complete with respect to all but the specific amino-acid factor. On the contrary, there is reason to believe that such diets may, and probably frequently, have other more or less serious shortcomings which may operate as accessory etiological factors and thus perhaps account for some of the "Protean" clinical manifestations of the disease.

In 1918 Goldberger and Wheeler (Goldberger, Wheeler, and Sydenstricker, 1918) gave expression to the opinion that as conventionally defined pellagra not improbably includes at least two commonly associated but etiologically distinct though fundamentally closely related syndromes, namely, (1) the syndrome comprehended by the phrase "pellagra sine pellagra," and (2) the dermal complex or pellagra without or with only slight subjective manifestations. While according to this idea, both syndromes are dependent primarily on a faulty diet, the first is to be regarded as the expression of a nutritive or metabolic failure, not in all respects peculiar to pellagra, whereas the second is to be considered as a reaction to a toxic substance or substances of a fairly specific type. Furthermore the initial appearance of the eruption on the genitalia in each of the cases with eruption occurring in their feeding experiment in convicts (Goldberger and Wheeler, 1920) suggested to Goldberger and Wheeler that the initial site of the eruption must be looked upon as a specific reaction, direct or indirect, to some special factor or combination of factors in the diet.

Our experience at this asylum lends support to the distinctions suggested by Goldberger and Wheeler. We have seen cases in female inmates in which, clinically, there was nothing appreciable but a well-marked dermatitis. Indeed, in one such instance there was, during the period immediately preceding the appearance of the erythema, a slight but steady gain in weight. Our observations here have also strongly impressed us with the idea that there is, as Goldberger and Wheeler suggest, some correlation between the type of diet and the site of the initial localization of the eruption.

It is of interest to note that this differentiation into a constitutional and a dermal type gains some support also from the study of the metabolism by Sullivan, Stanton, and Dawson (1921), who found greater abnormality in the urinary findings in the systemic than in the dermal type of the disease.

With these considerations in mind we would suggest that with the conception of a specific amino-acid deficiency as the primary etiological factor should be coupled the idea that the character of the deficiency (the precise amino-acid combination) may vary within certain, probably narrow, limits. Hence it would seem permissible to conclude that the deficiency etiologically related to pellagra is probably some special combination or, within narrow limits, special combinations of amino-acids.

In this connection it should be pointed out that the possibility that some as yet unknown dietary essential, either alone or in combination with the protein factor, plays the dominating rôle in this disease, while perhaps very remote, is not excluded, and should, therefore, not be wholly disregarded.

In closing this section we should perhaps make clear that in dealing with the etiology of the disease we have intentionally centered our attention on those extrinsic factors which we believe to be essential to the production of the disease in the average normal individual. In doing so we have not been unmindful of the possibility that other, both extrinsic and intrinsic, factors may operate either to accelerate or to retard the development of the disease or of some of its distinctive manifestations. We have confined ourselves to a consideration of primary essential factors in the belief that progress in unraveling the complex problem of etiology could best be made by determining the fundamental essentials before dealing with accessory factors, however important these may be in certain individuals or special groups.

Discussion

It is of interest to note at the outset that the conclusion suggested by the observations herein reported, namely, that the primary etiological factor in pellagra is a specific defect in the amino-acid supply, probably of the nature of a deficiency, is in harmony with the other previously reported results of the series of studies of which the present is a part. These had in succession permitted the exclusion of one known vitamin after the other as an essential etiological factor (Goldberger, Wheeler, and Sydenstricker, 1920); but not until the present observations were made did it seem permissible to exclude not only each of them individually but all of them together and with them, also, the mineral element as essential factors.

Most, if not all of the older dietary theories (zeist and antizeist), some of them seemingly very discordant, can, we believe, be harmonized on the basis of an amino-acid deficiency.

Of the newer viewpoints, that first suggested by Funk gains no support from our work; although, as we have already indicated, it is quite possible that a low or inadequate intake of any or all of the known vitamins or other food factors may play a more or less important accessory rôle.

On the surface there may seem to be a lack of harmony in our results with those of Voegtlin, Neil, and Hunter (1920), who, as we noted in reviewing the literature, report observing very favorable therapeutic results following the administration of liver and thymus extracts containing both the antineuritic and the fat-soluble vitamin. Since these extracts are also reported to have contained unidentified amino-acids, the possibility is present that the beneficial effects noted are primarily attributable to these protein-building stones rather than to the contained vitamins. It should perhaps be recalled that these workers themselves did not attribute the favorable effects exclusively to the vitamins.

Our conclusions are in substantial agreement with those reached by Wilson. However, his use of Thomas' figures to appraise the biological value of a protein mixture, although in general, perhaps, very useful, seems to us to have the serious drawback, so far as pellagra is concerned, that a low biological protein value (so appraised) is not, in our view, necessarily indicative of a pellagra-producing defect. Since, as has already been pointed out, it must be assumed that the fault in the amino-acid complex related to pellagra is a specific one, it follows that individuals may conceivably subsist on diets faulty with respect to the protein mixture in other than this specific respect and not develop pellagra. Thus a pellagra-producing protein mixture may, according to Wilson's method of appraisal, always be of low biological value; but a protein of low biological value, so determined, may, we believe, not only not be pellagra-producing but actually be pellagra-preventing, so far, at least, as the distinctive dermatitis is concerned.

We think it important to keep this distinction in mind. It will aid in minimizing some of the perplexity and confusion of thought evidenced from time to time in discussions of the etiology of the disease. It may help to explain why the people of the Central Powers during the war and since, though living on presumably faulty, perhaps, starvation diets, and suffering severely from malnutrition, have remained practically free from pellagra.

Some of the perplexity and confusion will also be prevented if it is not forgotten that the biological quality of a protein and its adequacy in relation to pellagra may, and doubtless frequently do, depend on the plane of intake. In our experience, a supplement of not over 40 grams of milk or beef proteins will, for practically all normal individuals, adequately supplement a pellagra-producing mixture of proteins from maize, wheat, rice, and cowpeas, but 20 grams (representing somewhat over a pint of milk or a quarter of a pound of round steak) may not do so. Thus it does not suffice merely to include milk or meat in a diet to prevent pellagra; the quantity of either of these or of other like foods alone or as supplements must be considerable to be effective. This may help to explain some of the instances of pellagra in individuals (including some of those very rare ones in nursing infants) who are alleged to have had a "good" diet. They did not consume enough for their particular needs.

It is readily understandable that the necessary minimum of a protein or mixture of proteins will, so far as pellagra is concerned (other things being equal), depend on its amino-acid make up. Unfortunately our knowledge of the latter is so meager that judgment must, for the present, be very tentative. Wilson (1921), judging by the biological value of the protein as appraised on the basis of Thomas' figures—the amount available for assimilation, not the gross amount, being considered—suggests 40 as the minimum safe value for this factor. On the basis of practical experience, Goldberger (1920) has tentatively suggested that for preventive purposes the diet should include a minimum of approximately 40 grams of animal protein (milk, cheese, meat, eggs) per day. This is a higher figure than

Wilson's (if estimated by his method) and is higher than is needed by the average normal individual, but is not, we believe, too high when all types of individuals are considered.

For the purposes of treatment, the primary lesson to be drawn from this study is the need for emphasis on the protein factor. From the time of Casal, clinicians have repeatedly emphasized the importance of a "nutritious" diet, particularly one rich in animal foods, in the treatment of the disease. But notwithstanding Roussel's emphatic affirmation over half a century ago, that without diet all remedies fail, the full significance of a proper diet as the specific treatment is but just coming to be realized. Prevailing opinion, at least up to within three or four years ago, was probably accurately expressed by Dyer (1916) when he said: "We are emphatic in the belief that most cases of pellagra will get well under medication, irrespective of diet." In consequence, medicinal specifics were sought for, and arsenic, atoxyl, arsphenamine, quinine hydrobromate, etc., were, from time to time, proposed as having virtues but little short of those of a specific remedy. Nor could the full significance of diet be justly appreciated until Goldberger, Waring, and Willets, in 1915, for the first time convincingly showed that pellagra was completely preventable by diet without intervention of any other factor, hygienic or sanitary. This demonstration went far toward proving that diet is the primary controlling factor in the prevention and causation of the disease and thus pointed towards a proper diet as containing within itself the specific remedy for the disease.

With the search for the primary etiological factor narrowed down to a faulty amino-acid supply, we may expect, when the precise amino-acid defect is finally determined, that the specific remedy for the disease will at the same time have been found.

With this double end in view, we have made some tentative therapeutic tests with certain amino acids. These tests have not as yet been extensive enough to warrant any conclusions. We may say, however, that in two cases the dermal lesions seemed to show a markedly favorable response to cystine, and in a third the administration of a daily dose of one gram of cystine and two grams of tryptophan during a period of 31 days (the diet remaining unaltered), was accompanied by a weekly gain in weight and a slight improvement in diarrhea.

We hope to continue this line of study; but it seems wise to report these preliminary results, such as they are, in the hope that clinicians may be led to try cystine and tryptophan in the treatment of suitable cases, and thus aid in the determination of their value therapeutically and of their significance etiologically.

Summary

The more important part of the evidence proving diet to be the primary controlling factor in the prevention and causation of pellagra is briefly summarized.

Cases of pellagra are reported that were observed to occur in individuals who were known to have consumed daily, during periods of not less than two and one-half months immediately before the onset of the distinctive eruption, what is judged to have been a liberal supply of mineral elements and the known vitamins, which would indicate that a deficiency of these dietary factors is not essential in the causation of the disease.

These factors having thus been excluded, the dominating rôle of diet in the prevention and causation of pellagra must be referred primarily to the character of the protein (amino-acid) supply, this being the only other dietary factor at present known to be necessary to physiological well-being.

On the assumption that all the dietary factors essential in human nutrition are known, it may be concluded that the essential etiological dietary factor is a specific defect in the amino-acid supply, probably in the nature of a deficiency of some special combination or combinations of amino acids.

There is reason to believe that besides the specific amino-acid defect, pellagra-producing diets may and probably frequently have other more or less serious faults, including nonspecific amino-acid deficiencies which may operate as accessory etiological factors.

In some preliminary therapeutic trials with amino-acids the dermal lesions in each of two cases seemed to show a markedly favorable reaction to cystine; and in a third case a steady gain in weight, with some improvement in diarrhea, accompanied the administration of both cystine and tryptophan.

References

Bouchard, C. *Recherches Nouvelles sur la Pellagre* (Paris, 1862), p. 280.
Boyd, F. D., and Lelean, P. S. *Report of a Committee of Enquiry Regarding the Prevalence of Pellagra Among Turkish Prisoners of War* (Alexandria, 1919). Also *J. Roy. Army Med. Corps* (December, 1919, to March, 1920).
Budd, G. *Remarks on the Cause of Scurvy*, etc. (London, 1839).
Buniva. Cited by Roussel.

Calmarza, J. B. *Memoria Sobre la Pelagra* (Madrid, 1870).

Chick, H., and Hume, E. M. *Biochem. J.* (Cambridge), Vol. 14 (1920), p. 136.

Chittenden, R. H., and Underhill, F. P. *Am. J. Phys.*, Vol. 44 (1917), pp. 13–66.

Deeks, W. E. *Med. Record* (New York), Vol. 81 (1912), pp. 566–69.

De Rolandis. Cited by Roussel.

Dyer, I. *Am. J. Trop. Dis. and Prevent. Med.*, Vol. 3 (1916), p. 580.

Funk, C. *J. State Med.* (London), Vol. 20 (1912), pp. 341-68.

Goldberger, J. *Public Health Rep.* (Washington, D.C.), Vol. 29 (1914), pp. 1683–86.

——. *Public Health Rep.* (Washington, D.C.), Vol. 29 (September 11, 1914), p. 2353. *Ibid.*, Vol. 29 (October 23, 1914), p. 2821.

——. *J. Am. Med. Assn.*, Vol. 66 (1916), pp. 471–76.

——. *Public Health Rep.* (Washington, D.C., 1916), pp. 3159–73.

——. "Pellagra," *Practice of Medicine* (Tice), Vol. 9 (1920), p. 226.

——, and Tanner, W. F. Unpublished data.

Goldberger, J., Waring, C. H., and Willets, D. G. *Public Health Rep.* (Washington, D.C.), Vol. 30 (1915), pp. 3117–31.

Goldberger, J., and Wheeler, G. A. *Hyg. Lab. Bull.* (Washington, D.C.), No. 120 (1920).

——. *Arch. Int. Med.*, Vol. 25 (1920), pp. 451–71.

——, and Sydenstricker, E. *J. Am. Med. Assn.*, Vol. 71 (1918), pp. 944–49.

——. *Public Health Rep.* (Washington, D.C.), Vol. 35 (1920), pp. 648–713.

——, and King, W. I. Unpublished data.

Harris, W. A. *J. Am. Med. Assn.*, Vol. 60 (1913), pp. 1948–50.

Hart, E. B., Steenbock, H., and Happert, C. A. *J. Biol. Chem.*, Vol. 48 (1921), pp. 33–50.

Hess, A. F. *Scurvy, Past and Present* (New York, 1920), pp. 154 and 167.

——. *J. Am. Med. Assn.*, Vol. 76 (1921), footnote p. 700.

——, and Unger, L. *J. Proc. Soc. Exp. Biol. and Med.*, Vol. 16 (1918), pp. 1–2.

——. *Am. J. Dis. Children*, Vol. 17 (1919), pp. 221–40.

——. *J. Biol. Chem.*, Vol. 38 (1919), pp. 293–303.

La Pellagra in Italia (Roma, 1880), pp. 344, 345, 351.

Lavinder, C. H. *Public Health Rep.* (Washington, D.C.), Vol. 26 (1911), pp. 1459–68.

——, Francis, E., *et al. J. Am. Med. Assn.*, Vol. 63 (1914), pp. 1093–94.

Lussana, F., and Frua, C. *Su la Pellagra* (Milano, 1856).

McCafferty, E. L. *Gulf States Journal of Med. and Surg.* and *Mobile Med. and Surg. J.* (1909), pp. 228–36.

McCarrison, R. *Studies in deficiency diseases* (London, 1921).

McCollum, E. V. *J. Am. Med. Assn.*, Vol. 68 (1917), pp. 1379–86.

——. *The newer knowledge of nutrition* (New York, 1919).

——, Simmonds, N., and Parsons, H. T. *J. Biol. Chem.*, Vol. 33 (1918), p. 421.

————. *Ibid.*, Vol. 38 (1919), p. 125.

————, and Pitz, W. *J. Biol. Chem.*, Vol. 28 (1916), pp. 153–65.

————. *Ibid.*, Vol. 29 (1917), pp. 521–36.

McCollum, E. V., Simmonds, N., Shipley, P. G., and Park, E. A. *Proc. Soc. Exper. Biol. and Med.* (New York), Vol. 18 (1920–21), pp. 275–77.

Murlin, J. R. *Hyg. Lab. Bull.* (Washington, D.C.), No. 116 (1920).

Myers, V. C., and Fine, M. S. *Am. J. Med. Sc.*, Vol. 144 (1913), p. 720.

Nesbitt, C. T. *J. Am. Med. Assn.*, Vol. 64 (1916), p. 647.

Nightingale, P. A. *Brit. Med. Jour.*, Vol. 1 (1914), pp. 300–302.

Osborne, T. B., and Mendel, L. B. *J. Biol. Chem.*, Vol. 37 (1919), p. 572.

————. *J. Biol. Chem.*, Vol. 39 (1919), pp. 29–34. *Ibid.*, Vol. 41 (1921), pp. 549–63.

Petrof, T. *Rev. d'Hyg. et de Police Sanitaire* (Paris), Vol. 29 (1907), pp. 301–33.

Roussel, T. *Traité de la pellagre et des pseudo-pellagres* (Paris, 1866).

Sambon, L. W. *Reports on pellagra in the West Indies* (London, 1917), p. 39.

Sandwith, F. M. *Trans. National Assoc. for the Study of Pellagra* (1914), pp. 97–100; *Trans. Soc. Trop. Med. and Hyg.*, Vol. 6 (1913), pp. 143–48.

Sherman, H. C. *Chemistry of food and nutrition* (New York, 1918).

Smith, A. H. *Lancet* (London), Vol. 2 (1918), p. 737.

Stannus, H. S. *Trans. Roy. Soc. Trop. Med. and Hyg.* (London), Vol. 14 (1920), pp. 16–17.

Steenbock, H., and Happert, C. A. *J. Biol. Chem.*, Vol. 48 (1921), pp. 33–50.

Strambio, G. *Abhandlungen über das Pellagra* (Leipzig, 1796), pp. 65, 100.

Sullivan, M. X., and Dawson, P. R. *Arch. Int. Med.*, Vol. 28 (1921), p. 72.

————, Stratton, R. E. *Arch. Int. Med.*, Vol. 27 (1921), pp. 387–405.

Takaki. *Sei I Kwai* (Tokyo, 1885), Vol. 4, pp. 29–37.

Voegtlin, C. *J. Am. Med. Assn.*, Vol. 63 (1914), pp. 1094–96.

————. *Public Health Rep.* (Washington, D.C.), Vol. 35 (1920), pp. 1435–52.

————, Neil, M. H., and Hunter, A. *Hyg. Lab. Bull.* (Washington, D.C.), No. 116 (1920).

White, R. G. *Report on an Outbreak of Pellagra Amongst Armenian Refugees at Port Said, 1916–17* (Cairo, 1919).

Wilson, W. H. *Appendix I*, to R. G. White's *Report on an Outbreak of Pellagra Amongst Armenian Refugees at Port Said, 1916–17* (Cairo, 1919), pp. 44–46.

————. *J. Hyg.*, Vol. 20 (1921), pp. 1–59.

Wood, E. J. *Edinburgh Med. J.* (1920), p. 373.

Zilva, S. S., and Drummond, J. C. *Lancet* (London), Vol. 1 (1921), p. 753.

————, and Miura, M. *Lancet* (London), Vol. 1 (1921), p. 323.

15. A Study of the Pellagra-Preventive Action of Dried Beans, Casein, Dried Milk, and Brewers' Yeast, with a Consideration of the Essential Preventive Factors Involved[1]

JOSEPH GOLDBERGER
W. F. TANNER

The results of the general study of the prevention of pellagra begun in the early fall of 1914, though clearly demonstrating the preventability of the disease by means of an appropriate diet (Goldberger, Waring, and Willets, 1915; Goldberger, Waring, and Tanner, 1923), did not show what foods or food factors were the essential ones. The modified diet employed in that study, while satisfactorily serving its particular purpose, was relatively expensive and, it was suspected, in excess of minimal requirements. These considerations, it was felt, would stand in the way of its ready adoption by households and institutions of restricted incomes. It was extremely desirable, therefore, to attempt to devise a diet that was adequate to prevent pellagra and at the same time inexpensive. For this further investigation was of course necessary. Accordingly, as the clinical opportunities at the Georgia State Sanitarium seemed very favorable and as the trustees and officers were keenly interested in the problem and were ready and willing to cooperate, new studies were started at that institution on January 1, 1918, and have been carried on ever since. Some of the results, more particularly such as seemed to have a significant bearing on the essential dietary factors concerned in the prevention and causation of pellagra, have already been published.[2] In the following we record some additional results bearing on this fundamental question together with the results of the study primarily designed to afford a solution of the practical question which appealed to us at the outset.

Dried Beans

Soon after beginning the field study of pellagra, one of us (J. G.) encountered evidence strongly suggestive of the value of beans and

1 *Public Health Rep.*, Vol. 40, No. 2 (January 9, 1925), 54–80.
2 Goldberger and Tanner, 1922; 1922; 1924.

322

peas in the prevention of the disease. Influenced by this, the legumes were recommended in the treatment and prevention of the disease and were included in generous quantities in the diets used in the test of the preventability of pellagra at the orphanages and at the Georgia State Sanitarium (Goldberger, Waring, and Willets, 1915; Goldberger, Waring, and Tanner, 1923). The very favorable outcome of this test tended, of course, to support the earlier indications of the value of the legumes and thus suggested that a study of individual foods might well begin with one of this class.

Soy beans.—The unusually high food value, cheapness and ready availability of the soy bean led us to begin our study with this bean, which was furnished as an addition to the general diet of the inmates of the section of the Georgia State Sanitarium for colored women. The study began January 1, 1918.

The quantity of soy beans supplied averaged fully 2½ ounces per head per day during the first month, and this was increased on February 4, and thereafter maintained at a daily average of fully 3 ounces per person.

During the first month of the study all of the beans were boiled (in a steam-jacketed kettle). Thereafter, in order to favor as large a consumption as possible, the proportion of the beans so prepared was from time to time reduced, a correspondingly increased proportion, after being ground into a coarse meal, was incorporated in the corn bread and in the boiled grits of the diet. During February (February 4 to March 8) the boiled beans constituted 80 per cent of the total served. On March 8 this proportion was reduced to 75 per cent and so maintained until June 4. During the period of June 4 to July 4 the proportion was held at approximately 60 per cent and after July 4 at 50 per cent.

Despite this supplement several cases of pellagra developed among the inmates receiving it. An abstract of illustrative cases in individuals who were known to have consumed their fully daily ration of soy beans follows (unless otherwise indicated, the date of onset in the cases represents the date of the first appearance of the distinctive dermatitis):

Case 1.—A colored woman, 61 years old, weighing 42.6 kilos, began taking the supplement of soy beans January 1, 1918, at which time she was without symptoms of pellagra. Ate all her soy-bean ration; she nevertheless developed pellagra June 19, 1918.

Case 2.—A colored woman, 37 years old, weighing 50 kilos, began taking the supplement of soy beans January 1, 1918, at which time she was without symptoms of pellagra. Regularly ate all her soy-bean ration, but, nevertheless, developed pellagra June 25, 1918.

Case 3.—A colored woman, 20 years old, weighing 48.4 kilos, began taking soy beans January 1, 1918, at which time she was without symptoms of pellagra. She regularly ate all her ration of soy beans, but developed pellagra October 14, 1918.

Case 4.—A colored woman, 25 years old, weighing 59.8 kilos, began taking soy beans January 1, 1918, at which time she was without symptoms of pellagra. She regularly ate slightly more than the average allowance of the beans; nevertheless she developed pellagra September 18, 1918.

Case 5.—A colored woman, 43 years old, weighing 49 kilos, began taking the soy-bean supplement January 1, 1918, at which time she was without symptoms of pellagra. Regularly ate at least the average allowance of soy beans, but she nevertheless developed pellagra September 18, 1918.

Case 6.—A colored woman, 25 years old, weighing 42.8 kilos, began taking the soy beans January 1, 1918, at which time she presented some slight symptoms of a receding attack of pellagra, which were no longer perceptible two days later. She regularly ate all her allowance of the beans, but developed a recurrent attack on October 22, 1918.

Case 7.—A colored woman, 15 years old, weighing 43 kilos, began taking the soy beans on admission, January 10, 1918, at which time she had some symptoms of active pellagra. These symptoms cleared up between January 22 and 29. No further symptoms were noted until September 4, which date marked the onset of a recurrence. Throughout she had eaten her full allowance of the beans.

Case 8.—A colored woman, 56 years old, weighing 58 kilos, began taking the soy beans on admission, February 23, 1918, at which time she presented no symptoms of pellagra. She ate at least all of her allowance of the soy beans, but nevertheless developed the beginning of an attack of pellagra on September 17, 1918.

As has already been stated, the soy beans issued as an addition to the institution diet averaged fully 2½ ounces per head per day between January 1 and February 3. On February 4 the quantity furnished was increased and thereafter, to the end of the study, maintained at an average of fully 3 ounces per patient per day. In estimating the amount actually consumed some deduction should be made for unavoidable loss in handling in the kitchen and in distribution in the dining rooms; a small allowance should also be made for table waste, even in instances such as we have cited in which the individuals left "clean plates," consuming all of their portions. We believe that a deduction of one-half ounce probably more than covers all possible losses and that it is conservative to estimate that in each of the cases cited the individual ingested an average of fully 2½ ounces of soy beans daily during a period varying between four-and-one-half and eight-and-one-half months before developing the attack of pellagra.

It thus appears that the daily consumption of fully 2½ ounces of soy beans as here described was inadequate to prevent the development of the disease.

Discussion.—The failure of the soy bean supplemented diet would seem to indicate that this legume in spite of its relatively high food value lacked, or, in the quantities and form in which it was used, supplied too little of the essential preventive factor or factors to serve as an adequate pellagra-preventive supplement. While it is conceivable that a larger quantity might have been effective, this consideration is not of much importance practically, since for the average individual the practicable day-to-day limit of consumption had, we believe, about been reached in the test. In this connection, however, some consideration must be given to, and allowance, perhaps, made for, the degree of digestibility of the food in question. This is particularly pertinent in the present connection, since we have found that as served after boiling, this bean still retained a rather firm consistency, requiring relatively considerable pressure to mash it, and thus suggesting that unless well masticated digestion might be interfered with, with consequent serious loss of nutrients. Holmes (1920), discussing the results of a study of the digestibility of this bean, makes a very similar observation, remarking that "the digestibility of the protein supplied by steam-cooked soy beans is apparently less than that of soy-bean flour, owing to the fact that the thin unbroken skin that surrounds the cooked soy bean is impervious to the action of the digestive juices." Now it is well known that among the insane the "good eaters" are very frequently those who bolt their food with little or no mastication. The possibility is therefore present that in our patients a more than ordinarily large proportion of the boiled portion of the bean ration was subjected to very imperfect mastication before exposure to the digestive juices. How much, if at all, this actually contributed to the result under consideration we are unable to state, but we are inclined to assume that a deduction of one-third from the quantity of the soy beans ingested in the boiled form would perhaps quite fully cover the possible loss from this cause. Now since several of the above-cited cases of pellagra developed after periods of upward of two or three months, during which the boiled beans formed only about one-half of the daily bean ration, it would appear on the basis of this assumption that the disease developed in some instances in spite of a daily ingestion of the equivalent of approximately 2 ounces of soy beans of average (normal) digestibility (Table 60). But even this reduced quantity would seem to be a fairly liberal day-to-day intake of this legume, so that its failure as a preventive food, while not conclusive as to its absolute deficiency in preventive power, is, nevertheless, rather strongly suggestive of at least a practical inadequacy in this respect.

Soy-bean purée.—With the idea in mind that the failure of the soy-bean supplement might have been due to an inadequate quantity

TABLE 60—*Estimated average composition of soy-bean-supplemented institution diet furnished the colored female inmates of the Georgia State Sanitarium, 1918.*

(Calories, 2,263)

Diet	Nutrients			
Articles of diet	Quantity (grams)	Protein (grams)	Fat (grams)	Carbo-hydrate (grams)
Wheat flour............................	100	11.4	1.0	75.1
Corn meal*	140	11.8	6.6	103.6
Corn grits............................	60	5.5	1.1	45.7
Rice.................................	28	2.2	.1	22.1
Cowpeas⁺	14	3.0	.2	8.5
Meatⱦ	56	13.0	1.4	....
Fat..................................	42	....	42.0	....
Sugar"	50	....	.....	50.0
Sweet potatoes**	120	2.1	.8	32.9
Soy beans⁺⁺	56	20.0	9.8	17.2
Total nutrients........................		69.0	63.0	355.1
Nutrients per 1,000 calories....................		30.5	27.8	157.1

*A whole meal, sifted in the kitchen, used in making corn bread, for which a small amount of buttermilk was frequently used.
⁺The cowpeas were from time to time replaced by Lima beans or navy beans.
ⱦThe "meat" was principally beef and most commonly thoroughly "roasted" in a steam-jacketed cooker. Some of the beef so prepared was ground up, baked in an oven, and mixed with grits or grits and potatoes to make a "hash." The quantity stated is an estimate of the total served in terms of lean muscle.
"Includes sugar for coffee and cane sirup served at supper.
**This represents the fresh vegetable component, which actually varied considerably as to kind and quantity and was markedly seasonal. Irish potatoes, turnips, cabbage, collards, or turnip greens, singly or in various combinations, were the most common substitutes.
⁺⁺Quantity ingested, after deducting waste and allowing for reduced digestibility.

and a relatively (unusually) low digestibility of the beans, a further test of their preventive power was undertaken, beginning January 25, 1919. In this test the soy bean after being boiled was rubbed up into a purée. The composition of the daily ration of this purée during the period January 25 to February 8, 1919, was as follows: Dry soy beans, 228 grams; sucrose, 228 grams; pork fat, 28 grams; table salt, 4 grams; fresh lemon juice, 4 grams; and water enough to make approximately 2 liters. In order to insure an abundance of vitamin A, the daily ration of purée was modified so that after February 9 it had the following composition: Dry soy beans, 114 grams; creamery butter, 56 grams; sucrose, 228 grams; cornstarch, 85 grams; table salt, 4 grams; fresh lemon juice, 4 grams; and water enough to make 2 liters. The pureé was offered to a small group of pellagrins. It was very well taken during the first six or eight weeks, after which there was a more or less rapidly progressive decline in appetite with some nausea and vomiting, necessitating a change to another type of diet. In 3 of about 12 pellagrins in whom this treatment was tried, there was noted, either just before or very shortly after the change to another diet was made, the development of symptoms either very suggestive of, or quite definitely those of, a recurrence of pellagra or of *pellagra sine pellagra.*

Thus the daily intake of at least 114 grams (4 ounces) of soy beans in the form of a purée during a period of not less than seven to eight weeks appeared insufficient to prevent the recurrence of pellagra and tended to confirm the indications of inadequacy afforded by the result of the experience with the soy-bean supplemented diet of 1918.

Cowpeas.—The cowpea is one of the most highly esteemed legumes among the people of our southern states. While not possessed of quite so high a food value as the soy bean, it has an important practical advantage over the latter in that it requires much less cooking to prepare it for the table. These considerations, coupled with the fact that our previous field observations and experience were largely concerned with this legume, made it seem desirable to study it more closely. Using the variety known as the California blackeye pea, a test was begun in a small group of pellagrins (nine in all) on February 4, 1919, and carried on concurrently with the study of the value of the soy bean.

To insure as high a degree of digestibility as possible, the cowpeas were prepared as a purée. The composition of the daily ration was as follows: Dry cowpeas (California blackeye) 200 grams; creamery butter, 85 grams; sucrose, 170 grams; cornstarch, 28 grams; table salt, 4 grams; fresh lemon juice, 4 grams; and water enough to make approximately 2 liters.

This soup was quite well taken during at least the first three or four months. Then, as in the case of the soy-bean purée, the appetite of the patients more or less rapidly fell off, with the development of some vomiting, eventually leading to a change of diet in all cases. In two of the pellagrins of this group, mild but definite symptoms of a recurrence of pellagra developed, in one at the end of about four, and in the other at the end of about five, months of the cowpea soup feeding.

The indication of a failure to protect in these two patients suggests that the dry cowpea has little, if any, pellagra-preventive value (we have not yet studied the preventive value of the fresh green or string bean), and thus fails to support certain of the seemingly favorable indications afforded by the earlier clinical and epidemiological observations.

Summary and conclusion.—The pellagra-preventive value of the dry soy bean as an addition to the general diet of the colored female inmates of the Georgia State Sanitarium was studied during 1918. The daily issue was 3 ounces but, allowing for various possible losses, it is estimated that those who ate well ingested the equivalent of approximately 2 ounces (56 grams) of soy beans of normal digestibility. In spite of this, however, several cases of pellagra developed.

Concurrently with the soy-bean soup study a trial was made of the preventive value of a daily ration of approximately 200 grams of dry California blackeye peas, also in the form of a soup, with results indicating that this, too, was inadequate fully to prevent recurrence of pellagra.

The dry soy bean and the California blackeye pea would appear to possess little, if any, pellagra-preventive value.

Casein

The disappointing indications afforded by the study of the soy bean and the cowpea led us to turn to a study of milk, another one of the foods that had been included in the diet used in the successful test of pellagra prevention (Goldberger, Waring, and Willets, 1915; Goldberger, Waring, and Tanner, 1923). Some of the results of this and of related studies have already been published.[3] These showed that while milk (in the form of buttermilk) was capable of preventing pellagra, certain of the components of milk, namely, fresh butter

3 *Ibid.*

(that tested was, like the buttermilk, produced in the vicinity of the Georgia State Sanitarium) and the inorganic minerals (in the form of an artificial mineral mixture resembling in composition that of the ash of milk) appeared to be devoid of this action. Since certain other evidence incidentally adduced appeared to indicate that none of the known vitamins were essential factors in the prevention of the disease, there remained for consideration in attempting to explain the pellagra-preventive action of milk only (*a*) the quality of its protein, (*b*) some as yet unrecognized or unappreciated dietary factor, or (*c*) a combination of these. Since, as between the protein and an as yet unrecognized factor, the probabilities seemed to us to favor the former, it appeared reasonable to expect that the prevention of pellagra might be accomplished by improving the quality of the protein of the diet with a sufficient supplement of a good protein. For this purpose we chose casein and (hopeful of accomplishing our aim) began a study of its therapeutic and preventive value late in the summer of 1922. The study was carried on until late in February, 1924.

The casein principally used was a grain curd casein specially prepared for us by the Grove City Creamery, Grove City, Pa. Its preparation was under the supervision of Mr. A. C. Weimar, dairy manufacturing specialist of the Bureau of Animal Industry, United States Department of Agriculture, who advised us that the mode of preparation was essentially as follows: The casein was precipitated from sweet skim milk with hydrochloric acid of the pH of casein. After drawing off the whey, the curd was pressed and immediately ground fine in the moist state. Then for five days this casein was washed with tap water acidulated with acetic acid to the pH of casein, the acidulated water being changed daily. At the end of this period the casein was washed in distilled water to remove the acid and then dried and stored in sealed lacquered tin containers.[4] Desiring as highly purified a preparation (so far as vitamins were concerned) as practicable, a considerable part of this casein was subjected to further treatment before being used in our study. This additional treatment (a modification of a method of purification kindly recommended by Prof. E. V. McCollum) consisted first of a washing in three or four changes of scalding hot tap water on the

4 Young rats fed a diet which derived all its vitamin A from 18 per cent of this casein developed xerophthalmia after about eight weeks, showing a deficiency of vitamin A. When the same casein formed the sole source of vitamin B, the growth of young rats promptly ceased, followed at once by a rapid decline in weight, showing absence of factor B.

first day, then of a leaching in acidulated water (acetic acid 0.2 per cent in tap water) for six days with a daily change of the acidulated water. The acid was then removed by washing in three or four quick changes of tap water, after which the water was drained off and the casein dried in a current of air at about 80° C.

During two short periods, the first of 10 days at the very outset of the study and the second of 9 days near its close, a commercial vitamin A free casein (Harris laboratories, Tuckahoe, N. Y.) was used.

In all, some 34 pellagrins were offered the casein treatment. Of these six took it for periods (seven days to three and one-half months) too brief to serve as a sound basis for judging its value.[5] The remaining 28 took it for the more significant periods of from 5 to 13½ months.

The study included 9 pellagrins who, when treatment was begun, presented active symptoms of the disease, and 19 who were free of evidence of active pellagra when they came under observation. In the former, the casein supplement was nearly always begun at 85 or 90 grams a day and so maintained for at least 8 to 10 weeks and then reduced to 46 grams (after June 21 to 69 grams), the allowance made those pellagrins who when taken under treatment no longer presented any symptoms of the active disease.

In deciding on the allowance of casein to be made in the latter class of cases, that is, for the purpose of purely preventive treatment, we were guided by our experience with buttermilk, 1,200 grams of which (approximately 36 grams protein) was at that time proving itself adequate for preventive purposes. We began with approximately 46 grams (approximately 40 grams protein) per patient per day, in order to supply somewhat more protein than that furnished by the buttermilk, thus allowing, in some measure, for the inferiority of the casein protein as compared with the mixed proteins of milk. After some months—as will presently be explained—a suspicion arising that 46 grams of casein might not be quite sufficient in all cases, the supplement of casein was increased by 50 per cent to 69 grams a day. Toward the close of the study this was further increased to 85 grams.

Condensed clinical notes of 10 representative cases that received casein treatment follow:

5   The normal tendency for the clinical manifestations of pellagra to fluctuate in intensity, at times within the widest limits, may mislead the observer in appraising the effect (particularly the seemingly favorable effect) of treatment if the period of observation is brief.

Case 9.—A colored woman 34 years old, admitted to the Georgia State Sanitarium August 30, 1922, with dermal and mental manifestations of pellagra. Came under our observation September 2, 1922, presenting marked dry dermal lesions having the distinctive characters of the pellagrous dermatitis involving the back of the hands, fingers, lower third of the forearms, elbows, and the back of the neck and feet. There was present also some seborrhoea about the nose and some incrustation about the angles of the mouth. The bowels were constipated. She was confused and disoriented. With the idea in mind that gelatin might improve the protein mixture of the diet and thus prove beneficial, she was given a daily supplement of 85 grams of this protein. Stirred into her food, she took it well for some 10 or 11 days. Having lost somewhat in weight and strength during this period and the bowels having become somewhat overactive, the gelatin was replaced by an equal amount of casein on September 14. (From September 14 to September 24 the casein was the Harris "vitamin A free" casein; after September 24 it was our purified grain curd casein.) The daily allowance of 85 grams was maintained until January 3, 1923, when it was reduced to 46 grams, at which it was maintained until June 22, when it was increased to 69 grams (Table 61).

A few days after the change from gelatin to casein her appetite returned and she ate well. Weighing 38.5 kilos on September 18, 1922, her weight rose, attaining 54.5 kilos on June 4 and 56.5 kilos on October 29, 1923. The dermatitis and seborrhoea slowly improved and she gained in strength so that by November 6, 1922, she felt strong enough to be up and about. By December 4 all dermal lesions had cleared up, leaving but a residual pigmentation; mentally, however, she was still somewhat confused.

Early in January, 1923, and again early in June she suffered from some menorrhagia. In June also there was noted some tachycardia. From June 24 to August 8 she received a daily dose of 15 grams of Seidell's "activated solid" with the idea that it might have a beneficial effect on the tachycardia. No notable effect on the pulse rate having been accomplished, it was discontinued on the latter date. Except for a tendency to an accelerated pulse rate she continued in good condition until September 11, 1923, at which time there was noted a slight fissuring at the angles of the mouth with dryness and scaling of the vermilion border of the lower lip. At this time, too, her bowels were constipated.

By October 4 the vermilion border of the upper lip had also become dry and scaly. This condition of the lips persisted without significant change and on October 25 there was noted a slight roughening of a patch of skin of the upper lip just under the nasal septum. At this time she was again suffering from a somewhat prolonged though scanty menstrual flow. Meantime her mental condition had improved so that she seemed about at her normal.

On November 15, 1923, she was noted to be in good general condition except for the dryness and scaling of the lips with slight fissuring of the lower one, and as she desired to go home the casein supplemented diet was discontinued. Without further change in condition she left the institution on December 20, 1923.

Summary.—A case of dermal and mental pellagra in which treatment with casein was accompanied by gain in weight and strength and a clearing up of the marked dermal and mild mental manifesta-

TABLE 61—*Approximate composition of the casein-supplemented diet offered daily to each of a group of colored female pellagrins during 1922.*

(Calories, 2,356)

Diet		Nutrients		
Articles of Diet	Quantity (grams)	Protein (grams)	Fat (grams)	Carbo- hydrate (grams)
Basic:				
Corn meal*	130	10.9	6.1	96.2
Corn grits	66	6.1	1.3	49.8
Wheat flour	100	11.4	1.0	75.1
Rice	28	2.2	.1	22.1
Cow peas+	14	3.0	.2	8.5
Lard	56	.....	56.0	.....
Sirup	90	.....	.....	63.9
Supplemental:				
Casein#	69	60.5	.....	.....
Cod-liver oil"	15	.....	15.0	.....
Tomato juice	130	.....	.....	.....
Dilute hydrochloric acid (U.S.P.), 90 drops**	....	.....	....	.....
Calcium carbonate++	3	.....	....	.....
Sirup iodid iron (U.S.P.), 2 drops++				
Total nutrients		94.1	79.7	315.6
Nutrients per 1,000 calories		39.9	33.8	133.7

* Whole maize meal, sifted in the kitchen.
+ Served in place of the dry legume ration of the institution diet.
# This was 46 grams up to June 22.
" From canned tomatoes. Served in place of the variable institution ration of fresh vegetables.
**Given with a view of correcting a possible gastric anacidity so very common in pellagrins.
++Given to improve mineral composition of the diet.

tions without definite evidence of relapse of the dermatitis or mental disturbance during a period of approximately 14 months. The development during the latter part of this period of dryness and scaliness of the vermilion border of the lips with slight fissuring of the lower lip and at the angles of the mouth and of a tendency to constipation and to tachycardia, is regarded, however, as suggestive of an incomplete recovery or of a relapse of a larval *pellagra sine pellagra*.

Case 10.—A colored woman, 24 years old, admitted to the Georgia State Sanitarium in 1919. Developed an attack of *pellagra sine pellagra* (a well-marked stomatitis with slight looseness of the bowels and seborrhœa of the chin) in October, 1922.

Treatment with a supplement of 85 grams of our purified grain curd casein was begun October 28, 1922. This daily allowance of casein was continued until January 3, 1923, when it was reduced to 46 grams. On June 22, 1923, it was increased to 69 grams and so continued to October 22, when treatment with casein was discontinued.

For about a week after beginning the casein the appetite was poor. It then improved and she ate well until after the middle of September, 1923. Her strength improved and she gained in weight. (During the period January 1 to July 16, 1923, her weight rose from 58.5 to 67 kilos.)

By December 28, 1922, evidence of the attack had almost completely cleared up, after which she continued in good condition until about September 11, 1923. At this time there were noted erosions of the skin at the angles of the mouth with a moist soggy appearance of the vermilion border of the lower lip and a diminution of food taking. Gradually the condition of the lower lip changed so that by October 4 it had become dry and crusty and a little reddened with fissuring at the angles. In the course of the succeeding two weeks scattered, irregular, ill-defined patches of dark somewhat dry sebum developed over the forehead, nose, cheeks, and malar prominences. This washed off readily with soap and water, leaving a smooth skin, but within two or three days the condition re-formed. By October 25 there was present a definite though mild stomatitis, increased salivary flow, and a tendency to nausea. The food taking having gradually declined, a change in diet was made on October 22, 1923.

Summary.—A case of *pellagra sine pellagra* in which the inauguration of the casein supplemented diet was followed by physical improvement and a clearing up of the evidence of *pellagra sine pellagra.* At the end of a period of about 11 months of the casein treatment symptoms of a recurrence began to develop and in the course of a month had progressed so that a diagnosis of *pellagra sine pellagra* was made.

Case *11.*—A colored woman, 18 years old, admitted to Georgia State Sanitarium November 25, 1921. On October 2, 1922, she was found to have a stomatitis suspected of being pellagrous. She came under our observation on October 5, presenting a tongue with beefy red tip and margins, increase in saliva, reddened mucosa of lower lip, and constipation. A diagnosis of *pellagra sine pellagra* was made. On the same day treatment was begun with a liquid diet which included approximately 600 grams of milk, 15 grams of cod-liver oil, and 100 grams of butter. She took this well, and her symptoms subsided, so that at the end of three weeks there was nothing notable except some overactivity of the bowels. In the course of another two weeks, however, there was a relapse of mouth symptoms—a mild stomatitis. On November 11 the liquid diet was abandoned and a solid diet, including approximately 140 grams of fresh butter, was begun. She ate this well, her appetite continuing excellent. There was, however, no consistent improvement in her condition, there being alternations of improvement and relapse in the stomatitis as also of constipation and overactivity of the bowels. Although, as has been mentioned, she ate well, there was no gain in weight nor in strength.

On December 7, 1922, her diet was changed to the casein diet which case 9 and case 10 were at this time taking. During the first two weeks following this change her appetite was poor and her food consumption was considerably reduced, but she took practically her entire daily allowance of 85 grams of casein. After this there was improvement in food taking and gradual improvement in her condition. On January 3, 1923, the casein supplement was reduced to 46 grams, and by the end of that month she was practically free of any evidence of pellagra. By April 1 she had gained approximately 6 kilos in weight.

She continued in good physical condition until near the end of June, when her appetite showed some falling off, her temperature was found to have risen, and, there being indications that she might be suffering from an acute miliary tuberculosis, she was transferred to another section of the institution on July 1, 1923, and passed from observation.

Summary.—A case of *pellagra sine pellagra.* During the period of two months (October 5 to December 6) immediately after coming under observation this patient continued in a state of mild *pellagra sine pellagra*, brief periods of improvement in symptoms alternating with periods of relapse, indicating inadequacy of the treatment with the high butter diets during this period.

On the casein supplemented diet she gained in weight and strength, her symptoms cleared up without any evidence of a relapse at any time to the close of the period of observation, which came after upward of seven and one-half months of the casein.

Case 12.—A colored woman, 42 years old, who was a pellagrin with a record of active attacks in 1913, 1915, and 1919. Taken under observation January 3, 1923, for the purpose of preventive treatment. At this time she was without recognizable evidence of active pellagra, so she began with a daily supplement of 46 grams of our purified grain curd casein. She ate well and gained slowly in weight (about 3 kilos) during the first five or six months.

On June 22, 1923, or, roughly, about five and one-half months after beginning the casein, a dermal lesion about 2 centimeters in diameter was found to be present on the back of the left hand over the proximal end of the second metacarpal. The lesion was slightly pigmented, dry, and just beginning to desquamate. In the course of the succeeding three or four days the lesion desquamated centrifugally, leaving a clean central area slightly over 1 centimeter in diameter encircled by a desquamating fringe. In appearance it resembled a pellagrous lesion. There was no other discoverable lesion. She was in good physical condition, was eating well, and presented no other symptoms. Suspecting, however, that this lesion might be pellagrous, and, if so, that the casein supplement might not be fully adequate, the daily allowance for this patient and all other patients receiving casein was at once increased to 69 grams.

Within 10 days after the discovery of the lesion on the left hand (and after the increase in the casein) practically all evidence of it had cleared up. At about the end of this period—that is, about July 2, 1923—the presence of an unusual increase or accumulation of a caseous material in the folds at the angles of the nose was observed. Removal of this caseous material exposed a slightly reddened linear surface. In two or three days, however, this lesion, which was new to us, had cleared up. She continued in good condition, eating well, and nothing further of interest was again noted until about the beginning of October, when a mild seborrhœa made its appearance over the lower part of the nose and alae nasi, and then gradually the skin of these parts became slightly rough and scaly. This condition persisted and about November 1 a small area (about 1 centimeter in diameter) of skin just below the left angle of the mouth became somewhat eroded in appearance. In the course of the succeeding two weeks—that is, by November 15—a similar lesion developed below the right angle of the mouth. At this time, too, there was noted the reappearance of the pasty, caseous accumulation in the fold or groove at the angles of the nose and in that beneath the nasal septum.

In the course of the next two or three weeks all these lesions cleared up completely, so that by December 3, 1923, there was nothing notable in her condition.

About January 7, 1924, however, it was noted that the vermilion border of her lower lip was dry, glazed (somewhat parchment-like) in appearance. The allowance of casein was now increased to 85 grams.

Toward the end of January the patient began to complain of pain in her feet, particularly at night, and it was found that the patella reflex was much diminished. During February the pain seemed gradually to subside, but some stiffness and uncertainty in gait developed. The vermilion border of the upper lip became glazed and some fissuring at the angles of the mouth appeared.

On February 27 the treatment of the patient was radically modified, so that this marks the end of the casein preventive treatment, which had thus lasted upward of 13 months.

Summary.—A pellagrin without active manifestations when treatment was begun. At the end of about five months of the preventive casein treatment (46 grams a day) this patient developed a very suspicious but slight and evanescent dermatitis on one hand which did not reappear during a subsequent further period of observation of about eight months on an increased casein allowance. During this second period (of increased casein) other manifestations in part familiar (seborrhœa and roughening of skin of nose, erosions of skin at, and fissuring of, oral commissures, glazing of vermilion border of lips, pain in the feet suggesting *pellagra sine pellagra*) and in part (pasty accumulation overlying a reddened linear surface in the fold at angle of nose and beneath nasal septum) new to us made their appearance.

Case 13.—A colored woman 39 years old; a pellagrin with a record of an attack of the disease in 1920 and in 1921. She was taken under observation for preventive treatment with casein on January 3, 1923, at which time she was without evidence of active pellagra so, as in case 12, she began with a daily supplement of 46 grams of our purified grain curd casein. Because of suspicious development in case 12 the dose of casein in this, as in all other patients receiving the treatment, was increased to 69 grams on June 22.

Her appetite was good and she ate the casein supplemented diet (Table 61) well until about the middle of September, when there began a falling off in food consumption. Up to this time, that is, during a period of about eight months, she had gained 10 kilos in weight. About the time (or a little before) her appetite began to fail, the vermilion border of the lower lip became dry and scaly and in the course of the following week the mucosa of the lower lip became reddened; some fissuring at the angles of the mouth developed and there seemed to be some increase in salivary secretion.

During the last week of September a definite though mild stomatitis developed and a slight seborrhœa at the angles of the nose made its appearance.

Early in October a slight conjunctivitis developed with a secretion that tended to dry and accumulate on the margin of the lids at the inner canthus. The stomatitis persisting with a more marked diminution in appetite and a tendency to flurries of looseness of the bowels, the casein supplemented diet was discontinued on October 7 and a liquid nourishment offered instead.

Summary.—A pellagrin without active symptoms when preventive treatment was begun. During a period of seven to eight months following the inauguration of the preventive casein supplemented diet this patient gained in weight and appeared in good physical condition. At about the end of this period there began a falling off in food taking, with the gradual development of a stomatitis, a tendency to looseness of the bowels and a mild conjunctivitis, constituting a *pellagra sine pellagra*.

Case 14.—A colored woman 21 years old; admitted to the sanitarium April 29, 1922, with pellagra. Taken under observation for preventive treatment January 23, 1923, at which time she no longer presented evidence of active pellagra. The casein supplement offered daily was 46 grams until June 22, when, by reason of developments noted in case 12, an increase to 69 grams was made. At the outset and until about the middle of July, that is, during about six months, her appetite was good and she gained about 5 kilos in weight.

About the middle of July food taking began to lessen, and about a month later a mild conjunctivitis affecting the right eye made its appearance. Under boric acid solution irrigation the condition of the eye cleared up in the course of about a week. About a week later, that is, about August 30, erosions of the skin at the angles of the mouth appeared and in the course of the succeeding three or four days the symptoms (reddening of the mucosa of the lips, cheeks, and soft palate) of a mild but definite stomatitis developed. In the course of another three or four days the vermilion border of the lips became dry and began to exfoliate. At the same time there appeared along about the inner third of the cutaneous aspect of the margin of the eyelids what seemed to be a dark adherent film of ocular secretion. The bowels were constipated. Meanwhile the appetite had become so much diminished that a change to another type of diet was deemed desirable and was made on September 14, 1923, or toward the close of a period of approximately eight months.

Summary.—A pellagrin without active symptoms when preventive treatment was started. After about six months of the casein preventive treatment, the appetite began to diminish; then after about six weeks more a mild but definite stomatitis developed (accompanied by a peculiar, unfamiliar condition of the eyes) suggesting *pellagra sine pellagra.*

Case 15.—A colored woman 35 years old with history of pellagra in 1915, 1920, and 1921. Taken under observation for preventive treatment January 3, 1923, at which time she was free from recognizable evidence of active pellagra. The casein supplement was 46 grams daily until June 22, when it was increased to 69 grams. The diet so supplemented was well taken until early in May, when a slight diminution in food taking developed. At about this time or shortly thereafter the bowels became markedly constipated. She maintained her initial weight and physical condition until about August 7, when a further reduction in appetite developed, slight erosions appeared at the angles of the lips, the lower lip appeared somewhat reddened, and the tip and upper surface of the tongue became slightly eroded. In the course of another week the condition of the lips and tongue returned virtually to normal, but the erosions at the angles of the mouth reappeared a few days later. About September 11 it was noted that slight fissuring had developed at the oral commissures and that there was present in the fold at the angles of the nose and below the septum a somewhat linear lesion consisting of a pasty, caseous accumulation over a reddened surface. The lesion at the oral commissures persisted but fluctuated in degree at irregular intervals but the linear lesion at the angles of the nose and below the septum faded out before the end of September, only to reappear early in October. By November 12 the symptoms of a mild stomatitis developed and, as the appetite had been capricious since May and food taking had since early in August become increasingly unsatisfactory, a change to another type of diet was made on November 18, or after a period of about ten months of the casein preventive treatment.

Summary.—A pellagrin without evidence of active pellagra when preventive treatment was started. The appetite declined and became capricious after about four months of the casein treatment. After a further period of about three or four months, erosions and fissures developed at the oral commissures and a peculiar, unfamiliar dermal lesion, linear in form, appeared in the fold at the angles of the nose and below the nasal septum. Finally at the end of about 10 months there developed a definite stomatitis suggesting a *pellagra sine pellagra.*

Case 16.—A colored woman 27 years old with a record of an attack of pellagra in 1921. Was taken under observation for preventive treatment January 3, 1923, beginning with a casein supplement of 46 grams. At this time she was without evidence of active pellagra. Her appetite was good and remained good throughout the year, that is, until January, 1924, when food taking began gradually to decline. There was a gradual and steady though slight gain in weight during the year, so that by the middle of November (1923) she had gained approximately 6½ kilos. With the falling off in appetite beginning with January, 1924, there was a decline in weight.

There was nothing notable in her condition until about the beginning of October, when the lower lip was observed to be somewhat reddened and the oral commissures slightly fissured. By October 22 there had developed a mild but definite stomatitis. The stomatitis faded out in the course of three or four days, but the reddening of the lower lip and fissuring of the angle of the mouth persisted. About November 1 it was noted that a crusty accumulation of secretion had formed about the inner canthus of each eye. About the middle of November the signs of a stomatitis reappeared. During the last week of the month all signs previously noted, except the reddening of the lower lip, cleared up. For about three weeks there was again little notable in her condition. Then, during the last week of December, the vermilion border of the lower lip became scabby and fissured.

About January 8, 1924, the casein supplement was increased to 85 grams, but the slightly reddened mucosa and the scabby and fissured condition of the vermilion border of the lower lip persisted, though with some fluctuations, to the end of the period of observation, February 27, 1924, when a radical modification in her diet was made.

Summary.—A pellagrin without active symptoms when preventive treatment was begun. Signs of a mild but definite stomatitis (*pellagra sine pellagra*) appeared after about nine months.

Case 17.—A colored woman 30 years old, admitted to the sanitarium on April 3, 1923, at which time she presented an extensive pellagrous dermatitis, seborrhœa of the face, slightly reddened tongue, normal bowels, and mental confusion. At this time she was offered the infirmary diet with supplementary milk. The appetite was poor at first, but slowly improved.

On April 23 she came under our observation, and treatment with a casein supplement of 90 grams was begun. She ate this well. On June 15 the casein allowance was reduced to 46 grams, but because of the suspicious developments mentioned in case 12 the casein allowance was increased to 69 grams on June 22. By the end of May 11 evidence of active pellagra had cleared up but there was still present a slight mental retardation. The food taking continued excellent and her weight rose gradually. Weighing 48 kilos on April 23, when the casein treatment was begun, she attained a weight of 54 kilos on July 9 and maintained substantially this weight to the end of the period of treatment.

About September 27, that is, at the end of a period of five months of casein, she developed a somewhat comma-shaped patch of erythema, about 2 to 3 centimeters in length, extending downward and outward from the inner palpebral angle of each eye. At this time she was in fair touch with surroundings but still, apparently, somewhat nervous. Within three or four days after its appearance the erythema gave place to pigmentation. At this point (September 30, 1923) she was furloughed and left the institution. She was seen by one of us about a week later, at which time the pigmented patch had faded, leaving a hardly perceptible trace, nor did she present any other recognizable indications of a recurrence of the disease.

Summary.—A case of pellagra with an extensive dry dermatitis and mild mental symptoms when patient came under observation. Signs cleared up and patient gained in weight and strength on the casein-supplemented diet but at the close of a period of treatment of about five months very slight dermal lesions, suspected to be pellagrous, made their appearance but quickly faded out.

Case 18.—A colored woman, 31 years old, taken under observation for treatment with casein June 9, 1923. At this time she presented a pellagrous dermatitis over the lower third of the radial aspect of the forearms and of the back of the left hand, a seborrhœa of the face, and a reddened mucosa of the lower lip with a dry and fissured vermilion border. The bowels were normal. Her appetite was good, and by about the middle of July she had gained about 3 kilos in weight. The evidence of pellagra rapidly cleared up, so that by July 9 she was apparently free of active pellagra. She so continued until early in September when the vermilion border of the lower lip was observed to have become abnormally dry and a pasty caseous accumulation overlying a reddened surface, linear in form, along the fold at the angles of the nose had formed. This persisted thereafter without notable variation. About September 24 a little dried secretion was noted to have gathered on the lids of the left eye at the inner canthus. At about the same time the appetite began to diminish. Early in October it was noted that the angles of the mouth had become fissured and eroded. By October 11 a mild but definite stomatitis was present and dried secretion had gathered on the lids at the inner canthus of the right eye, so that both eyes were now affected. Early in November the stomatitis subsided markedly, but the lips continued dry and had become crusty and a pasty, caseous accumulation on a linear reddened surface formed in the transverse groove just below the nasal septum. The condition of the eyelids remained unchanged, but gradually the evidence of a conjunctivitis became pronounced, so that by November 22 it was quite marked. There was at this time some photophobia, particularly of the right eye, which presented an ulceration apparently about 1 millimeter in diameter in the lower inner quadrant of the cornea. The secretion from the eyes seemingly overflowed and dried on the lower lids along the palpebral border. That portion of the lower lid of the right eye over the tarsal cartilage presented, in addition, a slightly reddened erythematous appearance. Food taking having meanwhile fallen off quite markedly, a change in diet was made at this time. The therapeutic preventive period of treatment extended in this case from June 9 to November 22, 1923, somewhat over five months.

Summary.—A case of dermal pellagra when treatment was started. On the casein the distinctive pellagrous dermatitis and the other signs of pellagra cleared up rapidly. The dermatitis did not relapse during the five months of observation, but at about the end of four months there developed evidence of a mild stomatitis (*pellagra sine pellagra*) and a conjunctivitis later accompanied by a mild ulceration of the cornea.

Results.—Summarizing our experience, it may be stated that following upon the inauguration of the casein-supplemented diet the general physical condition (weight and strength) improved in all but one or two patients and the symptoms of active pellagra (including *pellagra sine pellagra*) if such were present at the beginning of treatment, cleared up in all but three or four. In all cases presenting the distinctive dermatitis on beginning treatment this cleared up. In a few instances (illustrated by case 11) the improvement and freedom from symptoms persisted to the end of the period of observation. In all the others in which improvement apparently had taken place, this improvement was followed after varying periods by the relapse or recurrence of unfavorable signs and symptoms. Very commonly, though not invariably, there was some falling off in food taking and generally this was the first unfavorable sign to appear. Accompanying or independently of any diminution in appetite there developed some one or more of the signs or symptoms illustrated by the cases above cited, namely, a dry, glazed, vermilion border of one (usually the lower) or both lips with or without scaling or exfoliation; erosions of the skin at the angles of the mouth with or without fissuring of the commissures; perlèche; reddening of one or both lips, alone or associated with stomatitis; slight seborrhœa about the nose and, in two or three instances, reduction in or loss of the patella reflex and some disturbance (spasticity) in gait accompanied in one by pain in the feet. All of these signs and symptoms have been observed in or associated with pellagra. In addition there appeared in several of the patients a peculiar, to us unfamiliar and heretofore undescribed, lesion (a more or less marked accumulation of a pasty, caseous material on a linear reddening of the skin) in the groove at the angles of the nose and in the transverse groove below the nasal septum; in some there developed a conjunctivitis with a secretion that tended to accumulate and dry at the inner canthus of the eyes or on the lids along the palpebral margin. The linear lesion at the angles and below the septum of the nose and the conjunctivitis were entirely new in our experience with pellagra. That they were of dietary origin was rather strongly suggested by their very prompt response to a change in diet (dried yeast).

With three exceptions at the most, none of our patients showed any evidence of a relapse or of a recurrence of the distinctive dermatitis. The exceptions included cases 12 and 17 above cited and a case in a patient in whom there developed after about nine months of the casein supplemented diet a dry, scaly condition of the skin across the bridge of the nose subsequently extending slightly to the cheeks. This was quite suggestive of the butterfly lesion of pellagra. In none of these three cases did the suspicious lesion develop sufficiently to permit of its confident recognition as pellagrous. In other words, while nearly all of our patients sooner or later developed some symptoms either suggestive of or definitely of *pellagra sine pellagra*, with only three possible exceptions none had a relapse or recurrence of the distinctive dermatitis of pellagra. This is all the more striking since ordinarily we would expect fully 40 or 50 per cent of such patients to develop the characteristically marked eruption.

Conclusion.—It would appear, then, that the casein supplement had had a beneficial effect on the general nutrition of our patients and in considerable measure prevented or, at least, notably delayed the development of the distinctive dermatitis. It did not prevent, though it may have delayed, the relapse or recurrence of some of the other symptoms and signs of the disease (*pellagra sine pellagra*).

Dried Milk

Our very favorable experience with buttermilk (Goldberger and Tanner, 1924) during 1922 naturally emphasized the desirability of improving the availability of milk as a measure looking to the eradication of the disease from institutions and localities affected by it. Climatic and economic considerations suggested that this purpose might most satisfactorily be served by dry skim milk. While in the light of our previous experience with milk it seemed entirely permissible to assume that dry skim milk would be effective in pellagra prevention, it nevertheless seemed worth while to demonstrate by trial that such was actually the case. With this in view we began a trial of dry skim milk as a pellagra preventive in July, 1923, and carried on the study until September, 1924.

In order to make the study at least roughly comparable to that of buttermilk, the daily allowance of the milk was fixed at 105 grams in order to supply approximately the same amount of protein (approximately 36 grams) as was supplied by the supplement of 1,200 grams of buttermilk. During the first three months it was stirred into the food, but after that it was found more convenient to dissolve it in water and give this in equal portions at each of the three meals (Table 62).

Of some 22 pellagrins taking this milk supplemented diet, one developed mild but definite symptoms of a recurrence including a superficial but distinctively marked dermatitis, one a mild, intermittently relapsing dermatitis and two others some dermal lesions very suggestive, but not certainly those of pellagra. None of the others, 12 of whom were under observation for fully one year, showed any recognizable indications of the disease unless some loss in weight in a few instances is to be so regarded.

It would appear indicated, therefore, that the dry skim milk, in the quantity offered, had some, but not fully adequate, pellagra-

preventive action, and since the quantity of dried milk consumed
was approximately equal (on the basis of protein content) to that
of the buttermilk offered during the study of the latter and found
fully adequate for all of a group of 25 patients, we would seem to
have here a suggestive indication of a difference in pellagra-preventive power in favor of the fresh buttermilk. In this connection it may
be noted that, as compared with casein, the dried milk may, perhaps,
have been less efficient in preventing the recurrence or relapse of the
distinctive dermatitis but more efficient in preventing the other
symptoms and signs of the disease. The difference as relates to the
dermatitis was slight, probably too slight and based on too small
a number of observations to be significant. As relates to the symptoms other than the dermatitis, the difference was very marked and
unmistakable.

TABLE 62—*Approximate composition of dried skim-milk-supplemented
diet offered daily to each of a group of white female pellagrins during
1923–24.*

(Calories, 2,121)

Diet		Nutrients		
Articles of diet	Quantity (grams)	Protein (grams)	Fat (grams)	Carbo- hydrate (grams)
Basic:				
Corn meal*	130	10.9	6.1	96.2
Corn grits	40	....	....	.....
Wheat flour	80	9.1	.8	60.0
Rice	14	.7	.0	11.1
Cowpeas+	28	6.0	.4	17.0
Lard	20	....	20.0	....
Vegetable cooking oil	30	....	30.0	....
Sirup	90	....	....	63.9
Supplemental:				
Dried skim milk	105	36.6	.3	55.5
Tomato juice#	130	....	....	.....
Cod-liver oil	15	....	15.0	.....
Dilute hydrochloric acid (U.S.P.), 90 drops"	......	......	......	.....
Total nutrients		63.3	72.6	303.7
Nutrients per 1,000 calories		29.8	34.2	143.2

*Whole maize meal, sifted in the kitchen.
+Served in place of the variable dry legume ration of the institution.
#From canned tomatoes. Served in place of variable institution ration of fresh
vegetables.
"Given with a view of correcting possible gastric anacidity so very common in
pellagrins.

The results of this study would seem to warrant the conclusion that dried skim milk may have some pellagra-preventive action.

Brewers' Yeast

Certain observations in connection with an experimental study of black tongue in dogs having afforded highly suggestive indications that yeast possessed valuable therapeutic and preventive action in this condition (Goldberger and Wheeler, n.d.), and being impressed with the possibility that this canine disease might be the analogue of pellagra in man (Wheeler, Goldberger, and Blackstock, 1922; Goldberger, Tanner, and Saye, 1923) it seemed desirable to try yeast in the treatment and prevention of the human disease.

A beginning was made on May 26, 1923, with two patients. The effect of the yeast in these appeared so favorable that gradually more and more patients were taken under treatment, so that by May 10, 1924, 26 in all had come under observation. The results of this study up to December, 1924, are summarized in the following:

The study of yeast has been carried on along the same lines as was that of casein, of which, indeed, the former may be regarded as a continuation.

The yeast employed has throughout been a commercial preparation of brewers' yeast (Harris laboratories, Tuckahoe, N.Y.) in the form of a dry powder.

The therapeutic dose was arbitrarily fixed at approximately 1 gram per kilo of body weight. As the majority of our patients weighed in the neighborhood of 50 kilos, we found it convenient to adopt 50 grams as the daily dose of yeast to be given all patients with marked active symptoms. As soon as convalescence appeared established, a matter of 1 or 2 to 3 or 4 weeks, depending on the severity of the case, the dose was reduced to 15 grams. This smaller allowance was also that given the milder active cases and those without active symptoms. On February 27, 1924, the daily allowance was raised to 30 grams (Table 63). This increase was made because of a suspicion that 15 grams might not be a fully adequate allowance in all cases, since two or three patients who had been eating well for periods of four to six months had for some weeks before that date shown some diminution of appetite. Although no very significant effect on the appetite of these patients followed this increase, the dose was not again reduced.

The yeast was given in the food in equal portions at each of the three meals until December 1, 1923. After this date it was found

TABLE 63—*Approximate composition of dried yeast-supplemented diet offered daily to each of a group of colored female pellagrins during 1923–24.* (Calories, 2,224)

Diet		Nutrients		
Articles of diet	Quantity (grams)	Protein (grams)	Fat (grams)	Carbo-hydrate (grams)
Basic:				
Corn meal*	140	11.8	6.3	103.6
Grits..............................	48	4.4	.9	36.2
Wheat flour........................	70	8.0	.7	52.5
Rice...............................	28	2.2	.1	22.1
Cowpeas+	14	3.0	.2	8.5
Lard..............................	56	....	56.0	.....
Vegetable cooking oil.............	15	....	15.0	.....
Sirup.............................	90	....	.....	63.9
Supplemental:				
Dried brewers' yeast..............	30	12.5	.5	14.2
Cod-liver oil.....................	15	.....	15.0	......
Tomato juice#	130	.....	.....	......
Dilute hydrochloric acid (U.S.P.), 90 drops"	....	.....	.....	......
Calcium carbonate**	3	.....	.....	......
Sirup iodid of iron (U.S.P.), 2 drops**....		.....	.....	......
Total nutrients.............................		41.9	94.7	301.0
Nutrients per 1,000 calories....................		18.9	42.7	130.6

* Whole maize meal sifted in the kitchen.
+ Served in place of the variable dry legume ration of the institution.
# From canned tomatoes: Served in place of the variable institution ration of fresh vegetables.
" Given with a view of correcting a possible gastric anacidity so very common in pellagrins.
**Given to improve the mineral composition of the diet.

convenient to give the daily dose at one time, generally in the cane sirup served at the supper meal.

As has been already mentioned, 26 patients in all were taken under treatment with yeast between May 26, 1923, and May 10, 1924. Nearly all presented more or less pronounced symptoms of pellagra or *pellagra sine pellagra*. The majority were patients with mild recurrent attacks that had developed, as already described, while taking the casein-supplemented diet. With one exception all made prompt recoveries from the immediate attack. The exception was a case in a recently admitted patient with symptoms of central neuritis who died within 96 hours after admission and within 72 hours after coming under our observation.

The patients remained under observation on the yeast for varying periods. In one, this was for barely one month, at the end of which time she went home on furlough. In another, a complicating condition arose at the end of about four months, necessitating a transfer to another ward and withdrawal from yeast for about eight weeks, at the end of which time she returned and resumed the yeast supplemented diet. In the third, the development of active pulmonary tuberculosis made permanent withdrawal necessary by reason of transfer to another section of the institution. Two others went home on furlough in good physical condition at the end of five and six months, respectively. Of the remaining 20 patients, 1 has been under observation for about 7, and 19 for from 12 to 18 months. None has shown any recognizable evidence of a relapse or recurrence of the disease.

Since experience has convinced us that without the yeast supplement fully 40 or 50 per cent of our patients would have developed a relapse or recurrence of pellagra (with the distinctive dermatitis) within the period of observation, this result would appear very clearly to indicate that the brewers' yeast supplied an essential or the essential preventive factor or factors.

Preventive Factors

Having presented the results of our studies, we may now consider the significance of their indications with respect to the dietary essentials concerned in the prevention and, incidentally, in the causation of pellagra.

The results of previously published studies (Goldberger and Tanner, 1924) have indicated that vitamin A, vitamin B, vitamin C, the antirachitic factor, and the mineral mixture could, with a very high degree of probability, be excluded from consideration in relation to the prevention of the disease. We need not at this time, therefore, concern ourselves further with these, but may pass on to a consideration of the other dietary essentials at present recognized, namely, the antisterility factor X of Evans and Bishop and the protein or, more specifically, the biological quality of the protein, since previous studies have already indicated that the quantity of protein is not necessarily involved.

With respect to the factor X, it may be said that since fresh green leaves and whole cereals are reported by Evans and Bishop (1923) to be rich in this factor, our experience would tend to warrant its elimination from the relationship under present consideration, for the occurrence of the disease has been repeatedly observed by us in association with diets containing sifted whole cornmeal and such leafy vegetables as cabbage, collards, and turnip greens. (See, for example, diet shown in Table 60.) That factor X may be excluded would seem even more strongly indicated by the results of our study with yeast. Reported by Evans and Bishop (1923) to be devoid of their antisterility factor, dried yeast has in our experience clearly shown itself to possess pronounced pellagra-preventive action.

Turning to the protein factor, we may consider in relation thereto the significance, first of all, of the preventive failure of the soy-bean-supplemented diet (Table 60). From the best estimate that we have been able to make, it appears that the basic institution diet of 1918 probably furnished our patients with not over about 50 grams of protein. If to this is added the protein of the soy-bean supplement, estimated at approximately 20 grams (soy beans 56 grams × 36.5 per cent protein), the total gross protein supply of this diet amounted to some 70 grams. Of this protein mixture, very nearly one-half was a combination from meat and soy beans. Since there is reason to believe that both of these (when taken in sufficient quantity) yield protein of adequate quality, it is possible that the protein mixture of this diet was adequate for the nutritive needs of our patients, and thus it is possible that the preventive failure of the diet under consideration was not due to an amino-acid defect but to some heretofore unrecognized complex. Whether this protein mixture was actually nutritively adequate cannot be decided on the basis of available data, so that the result of the soy-bean study does not in itself afford a sound basis for judging of the preventive rôle of the protein factor.

Passing next to the outcome of the casein study, we find that a supplement of 69 grams appeared in considerable measure to prevent or notably to delay the distinctive dermatitis, but failed to prevent, though it may have delayed, the relapse or recurrence of some of the other symptoms of the disease. Since the quality (and quantity) of the protein mixture resulting from the large casein addition may reasonably be assumed to have been adequate for normal nutrition in our patients, it would seem permissible to conclude that the protein of the diet, if it be concerned in the prevention (or causation) of pellagra, is not the sole preventive (or causative) factor, and thus that some other heretofore unrecognized or unappreciated dietary complex also plays an essential part.

This interpretation would appear to receive support from the results of the dried-milk study. As has already been stated, the dried skim milk appeared decidedly more efficient than the casein in the prevention of symptoms other than the distinctive dermatitis. This would tend to suggest that the milk supplied something other than protein having this beneficial action of which the casein supplied little or none at all. This suggestion gains some weight from the indication of inferior preventive potency of dried skim milk as compared (on the basis of protein content) with fresh buttermilk. It gains very much more weight, however, from the evidence of a pronounced pellagra-preventive action of dried yeast. In a daily dose of between 15 and 30 grams, representing less than 15 grams of protein, this has, as we have already seen, shown itself very efficient in preventing the disease. In view of the failure of the casein to prevent the *pellagra sine pellagra* syndrome, it is difficult to attribute the very favorable action of the yeast to its protein content, which, at best, was not over one-fourth that supplied by the casein. It seems warranted to conclude, therefore, that in the prevention of pellagra there is concerned a heretofore unrecognized or unappreciated dietary factor that was contained abundantly in our dried yeast, slightly in our dried skim milk, and inappreciably in our casein.

Considering the relatively small amount of protein furnished by the effective dose of yeast, it would seem as if the heretofore unrecognized pellagra-preventive factor, to which we shall hereafter refer as factor P–P, were capable of preventing the disease with little if any cooperation from the protein factor of the diet. On the other hand, in the light of the outcome of our casein study, it would seem as if a liberal supply of a presumably good protein mixture may in itself be capable of modifying the clinical picture of the disease by notably delaying or preventing the appearance of the distinctive dermatitis. This, it may here be recalled, is in harmony with Goldberger and Wheeler's suggestion (Goldberger, Wheeler, and Sydenstricker, 1918) that pellagra, clinically, possibly includes at least two commonly associated but etiologically essentially distinct though closely related syndromes, namely, (*a*) the syndrome that is comprehended by the phrase "*pellagra sine pellagra*," and (*b*) the dermatitis or pellagra without or with only slight subjective manifestations. But since the action of the protein mixture of the diet in the casein study may conceivably have been due not to the protein *per se* but to factor P–P carried as an impurity in the casein or since this action, on the more reasonable assumption that it was due entirely to the protein, may be conceived to have been of an indirect or sparing nature, it is possible that factor P–P plays the sole essential rôle in the prevention (and thus in the causation) of pellagra.

The foregoing discussion and the results presented would seem to warrant the following conclusions:

(*a*) A liberal supply of protein presumably of good biological quality does not completely prevent, though it may modify, the clinical picture of pellagra by notably delaying or preventing the development of the distinctive dermatitis. This modifying action may be of an indirect, sparing nature.

(*b*) In the prevention (and presumably causation) of pellagra there is concerned a heretofore unrecognized or unappreciated dietary factor which we designate as factor P–P. This may be effective with but little, possibly without any, cooperation from the protein factor.

(*c*) Factor P–P may possibly play the sole essential rôle in the prevention (and causation) of pellagra.

(*d*) Factor P–P is present in brewers' yeast, in milk and (on the basis of our experience with fresh meat) in lean beef; it is very low or lacking in dry soy beans, dry cowpeas, butter, cod-liver oil, and canned tomatoes. (See diet Table 61.)

References

Evans, H. M., and Bishop, K. S. *J. Am. Med. Assn.*, Vol. 81 (September 15, 1923), pp. 889–92.

Goldberger, J., and Tanner, W. F. *Public Health Rep.*, Vol. 37 (1922), p. 462.

———. *J. Am. Med. Assn.*, Vol. 79 (1922), p. 2132.

———. *Public Health Rep.*, Vol. 39 (1924), p. 87.

———, and Saye, E. B. *Public Health Rep.*, Vol. 38 (1923), p. 2711.

Goldberger, J., Waring, C. H., and Tanner, W. F. *Public Health Rep.*, Vol. 38 (1923), p. 2361.

Goldberger, J., Waring, C. H., and Willets, D. G. *Public Health Rep.*, Vol. 30 (1915), p. 3117.

Goldberger, J., and Wheeler, G. A. Unpublished Data.

———, and Sydenstricker, E. *J. Am. Med. Assn.*, Vol. 71 (1918), pp. 944–49.

Holmes, A. D. *J. Am. Med. Assn*, Vol. 74 (1920), p. 798.

Osborne, T. B., and Wakeman, A. J. *J. Biol. Chem.*, Vol. 40 (1919), p. 383.

Wheeler, G. A., Goldberger, J., and Blackstock, M. R. *Public Health Rep.*, Vol. 37 (1922), p. 1066.

16. A Further Study of Butter, Fresh Beef, and Yeast as Pellagra Preventives, with Consideration of the Relation of Factor P–P of Pellagra (and Black Tongue of Dogs) to Vitamin B[1]

JOSEPH GOLDBERGER   G. A. WHEELER
R. D. LILLIE   L. M. ROGERS

A pellagra-preventive feeding experiment begun in 1914 by Gold-berger, Waring, and Willets and carried on for a period of three years resulted in demonstrating the complete preventability of pel-lagra by diet alone (Goldberger, Waring, and Willets, 1915). This experiment was of such a character, however, that it did not in itself reveal just what food or foods were to be credited with the preven-tive action. It could be considered as suggesting, at most, that the fresh meat and milk of the diet were concerned in bringing about the protective effect. The probability that both meat and milk con-tained the factor or factors which operated to prevent the develop-ment of the disease gained strength from the results of a study of the relation of diet to pellagra incidence among households of certain South Carolina cotton-mill villages carried out during 1916 by Goldberger, Wheeler, and Sydenstricker (1920). In that study it was found not only that pellagra occurred less frequently or not at all in households having a daily minimum average supply of approxi-mately a pint of milk or 30 grams of fresh meat per adult unit, but also that an increasing supply of each of these foods independently of the other was definitely associated with a decreasing pellagra incidence.

The soundness of the inference drawn from these studies, together with the inference from such epidemiological observations as the well-known rarity of the disease in nursing infants, that milk when a generous element in the diet operates to prevent pellagra was, in 1922, demonstrated by Goldberger and Tanner (1924) by direct test. In that test it was found that a daily supplement of approximately 1,200 grams (40 fluid ounces) of fresh buttermilk prevented the devel-opment of recognizable evidence of the disease in all of a group of

1 *Public Health Rep.*, Vol. 41, No. 8 (February 19, 1926), 297–318.

25 insane patients during a period of observation of one year when, in the absence of the buttermilk or other equivalent preventive, upward of 40 or 50 per cent of the group would, judging by previous experience, have developed the disease within a period of three to seven or eight months. A test of dry skim milk (a Merrel-Soule product) carried out by the same workers (Goldberger and Tanner, 1925) during the period July, 1923–September, 1924, resulted in showing that when taken in a daily quantity (105 grams) approximately equivalent (on the basis of protein content) to that of the fresh buttermilk, the dry skim milk was not fully adequate as a pellagra-preventive, and thus distinctly inferior to fresh buttermilk, since of some 22 pellagrins taking the dry skim milk, four developed either definite or very suggestive evidence of a recurrence of the dermal lesions of pellagra. The inferior potency of dried skim milk was recently further impressed on us by observing the occurrence of two recurrent attacks in a patient on a liquid diet containing 125 grams of such milk. As this observation has a number of interesting bearings, mention of the more significant details may here be made:

A white, insane, female pellagrin, thirty-five years old and weighing 47 kilos, came under observation May 14, 1924, with mild dermal pellagra. The dermal lesions persisting, though with remissions, and the patient being so poor an eater as to make tube feeding from time to time necessary, she was changed on July 19, 1924, from the general ward diet to the following liquid diet: Dry skim milk (Merrel-Soule), 125 grams; cod-liver oil, 28 grams; cottonseed oil, 70 grams; sucrose, 200 grams; tomato juice (from canned tomatoes), 170 grams; table salt, 5 grams in water. The dermal condition now cleared up, but a stomatitis gradually developed, and on September 29, 1924, that is, about two months after beginning this milk diet, the distinctive dermatitis reappeared. On October 10 she began taking a supplement of "Yeast Vitamin-Harris Powder," 25 grams daily. Eight days later this was reduced to 10 grams. Gradually the dermatitis and stomatitis cleared up. On January 15, 1925, the patient appearing in excellent condition, the "yeast vitamin" supplement was discontinued. She continued seemingly in good condition, taking all the milk ration until April 29, 1925, when lesions that proved to be those of a pellagrous dermatitis began to appear on her hands. Thus, this patient had a relapse of her attack of pellagra at the end of a period of about two months, during which she daily consumed 125 grams of dry skim milk (representing about 44 grams of milk proteins), and a recurrence of the disease at the end of a further period of about seven months of this diet, or about three and a half months after discontinuing the supplement of a commercial yeast concentrate.

Butter

The evidence that milk had preventive action in pellagra naturally suggested an inquiry as to whether butter had similar properties. In a previous communication (Goldberger and Tanner, 1924) mention was made of the very disappointing results of such an inquiry. The butter to which this had reference was from the general supply of the Georgia State Sanitarium and was produced in batches of a few pounds each by farmers in the general vicinity of this institution in central Georgia and sold by them to the sanitarium. The study was made at a season when the cows yielding the butter were and had for some time been largely pasture fed. Although tried repeatedly and in increasing quantities (in several instances the patients were known to have consumed an average of approximately 135 to 145 grams daily during a period of from three to upward of five months), this butter practically invariably failed to prevent recurrence of the disease.

The favorable results in the treatment and prevention of the Chittenden-Underhill (1917) pellagralike disease of dogs (black tongue (Wheeler, Goldberger, and Blackstock, 1922)), reported by Underhill and Mendel (1925), with butter from a northern locality suggested, in view of the possibility, if not probability, that this canine disease may be the analogue of human pellagra, the desirability of trying butter from a similar locality in the human disease. And this all the more as it seemed possible that butter from a northern dairying locality, presumably affording superior pasture at certain seasons, might be more potent in the factor preventing black tongue (and, possibly, pellagra) than that from the nondairying region of central Georgia. Accordingly, a supply of such butter laid down in Vermont early in July, 1924, was secured. It was kept in cold storage at New Haven, Conn., until the fall of the year (October), after which time express shipments in quantities as needed were made to us at the Georgia State Sanitarium, where the study was carried out. At the sanitarium it was kept in the sanitarium refrigerator room and issued daily in the required amounts. The approximate composition of the butter-supplemented diet is shown in Table 64.

The results of trials in pellagra prevention made with this butter were no more favorable than those made with butter locally pro-

TABLE 64—*Approximate composition of butter-supplemented diet offered daily to certain pellagrins during the fall, winter, and spring of 1924–25.* (Total calories: 2,301)

Diet		Nutrients		
Articles of diet	Quan-tity	Protein	Fat	Carbo-hydrate
Basic:	Grams	Grams	Grams	Grams
Corn meal*	185	15.5	8.7	136.9
Wheat flour	85	9.7	.9	63.8
Rice	14	1.1	.0	11.1
Cowpeas (Vigna sinensis)+	28	6.0	.4	17.0
Lard	4	....	4.0	.....
Tomato juice#	130	....	....	.....
Supplemental:				
Creamery butter (Vermont)"	147	1.5	125.0	.....
Calcium carbonate**	1.5	....	....	.....
Dilute hydrochloric acid (U.S.P.) (90 drops)++	....	....	....	.....
Sirup iodid iron (U.S.P.) (2 drops)**	....	....	....	......
Total nutrients		33.8	139.0	228.8
Nutrients per 1,000 calories		14.7	60.4	99.5

* Whole maize meal, sifted in the kitchen and made into corn bread and mush.
+ Served in place of the variable dry legume ration of the institution.
# From canned tomatoes, pressed through a cloth.
" A portion served at each meal; thoroughly stirred into the hot mush or mush, rice, and peas.
** Given to improve the mineral composition of the diet.
++ Given with a view of correcting a possible gastric anacidity so common in pellagrins.

duced. Recurrence of the disease was observed in some patients (weighing between 40 and 50 kilos) in spite of a daily consumption of approximately 147 grams (about 5 ounces) of the Vermont butter during periods ranging from two to seven months.

It is possible that these periods were in most instances somewhat longer, that is, that the recurrence of the eruption was somewhat later, than would have been the case had the butter been absolutely devoid of preventive action. In this respect the Vermont butter did not differ appreciably from that locally produced. Our study was not on a sufficient scale to permit of sound judgment on this point; the indications afforded by our preliminary trials were so decidedly unsatisfactory as not to justify their continuation. Recalling, however, that fresh buttermilk was found to have pellagra-preventive action (Goldberger and Tanner, 1924) it would seem reasonable to expect that butter may carry at least a trace of the special pellagra-preventive essential (factor P–P). Considering the very large quantity of butter daily consumed by some of our patients, its definite failure to prevent in these a recurrence of the disease seems to us, however, to indicate that if the butter with which we worked (both the Vermont and the Georgia product) contained this factor it contained it in a practically negligible quantity.

Assuming, as seems reasonable in view of Underhill and Mendel's report, that the Vermont butter contained the black-tongue-preventive substance, then it would seem as if this substance and factor P–P were not identical or that it had undergone deterioration during the time before the butter was used. The latter possibility would seem all the more plausible, as Underhill and Mendel (1925) report that butter of known origin and rich in the black-tongue-protective substance gradually loses its effectiveness when kept in cold storage for a period of approximately one year or less. In considering this possibility it must be noted that our Vermont butter began to be served to our patients about the middle of October, 1924, or about three months after it was laid down, and the first recurrence of pellagra in patients taking it developed during the latter half of February, 1925,[2] or not over about 7½ months after the butter was made. If our disappointing experience with Vermont butter was due to loss of potency, then it would seem as if the P–P factor (in butter) undergoes deterioration surprisingly quickly.[3] Since our Georgia butter was always relatively quite fresh, loss of potency incident to long storage can hardly enter into consideration in relation to the failure of this product, so that it would seem as if this must have been poor or lacking in the P–P factor from the outset. Considering our experience with butter as a whole and in the light of the fact that our study of fresh buttermilk produced near the sanitarium showed this to contain the P–P factor, it would seem more probable that, like our Georgia butter, the Vermont product was poor or lacking in the P–P factor in the first place rather than that this had undergone deterioration and therefore that this factor and the black-tongue-preventive substance are not identical. So far as the above recorded experience with butter goes, these factors may, indeed, be distinct;

2 In a patient who had come under observation and had begun taking the full allowance of this butter at about the middle of December, 1924.
3 A test of the vitamin A potency of this butter made during December, 1925, when it was about 17 months old, showed it to be quite efficient in curing xerophthalmia in a dose of 100 mgm. of the fat daily. A smaller dose was not tested.

but we should here perhaps state that our own experience with butter in experimental black tongue is in harmony with that in pellagra. In our own study, butter has failed us in the treatment and prevention of experimental black tongue just about as it has failed us in the treatment and prevention of pellagra. We have no explanation to suggest of the difference in our results with butter in black tongue from those reported by Underhill and Mendel, except the possibility that the black-tongue-preventive factor entered into their basal diet from some unsuspected source. It was just such occurrence in our own work that led to the discovery of the black-tongue-preventive potency of yeast.

Beef

The belief that fresh meat contains the pellagra-preventive factor or factors was, up to 1924, based on indirect evidence of the character cited in a preceding section of this report. In that year Goldberger and Tanner (1924) added to that evidence by reporting very favorable results of treatment in eight well-marked though not very severe (mainly dermal) cases, with fresh beef as the only known therapeutic element in the diet. Though carried out with all possible care it was realized that a therapeutic test on so restricted a scale could at best hardly be more than strongly suggestive; and while it was in harmony with and strengthened previous indications that fresh beef contains the pellagra-preventive factor or factors, it was, nevertheless, felt that a preventive feeding test would be needed to prove this conclusively. We have carried out such a test as a detail of the study of pellagra prevention that has been in progress at the Georgia State Sanitarium since 1914, the pertinent facts in relation to which are as follows:

In this test we used fresh beef drawn from the sanitarium supply. The muscle meat was trimmed free of tendon, gristle, and visible fat, run through a meat chopper and a weighed amount, at the rate of seven ounces (200 grams) per patient per day, was stirred into a little water, seasoned with salt, and quickly brought to a boil. This daily ration was served and well taken in equal portions at breakfast and at the midday meal.

The determination of the daily allowance was largely arbitrary. Since our purpose was, if possible, to show that the disease could be prevented completely by a liberal though not excessive quantity of this food, we decided on the allowance (200 grams) that had served us very satisfactorily in the treatment of active cases (Goldberger and Tanner, 1924), judging that this would be very likely to fulfill the, presumably, somewhat less exacting requirements of prevention. The approximate composition of the diet thus supplemented is shown in Table 65. The test was begun December 17, 1924, and carried on for one year to December 31, 1925. During this period 26 pellagrins were taken under observation for preventive treatment with the beef-supplemented diet. Of this number, two were under observation for periods so brief as to have no significance, three were under observation for fully ten months, and the remaining 21 for fully one year. In none of these patients was there observed any recognizable evi-

TABLE 65—*Approximate composition of fresh beef-supplemented diet offered daily to each of a group of colored female pellagrins during the period December 17, 1924–June 22, 1925.**

(Total calories: 2,080)

Diet		Nutrients		
Articles of diet	Quan-tity	Protein	Fat	Carbo-hydrate
Basic:	Grams	Grams	Grams	Grams
Cornmeal[+]	140	11.8	6.3	103.6
Corn grits..................	48	4.4	.9	36.2
Wheat flour.................	70	8.0	.7	52.5
Rice.......................	28	2.2	.1	22.1
Cowpeas (Vigna sinensis)[#]	14	3.0	.2	8.5
Sirup......................	90	....	....	63.9
Lard.......................	42	....	42.0	.....
Tomato juice"	130	....	....	.....
Supplemental:				
Fresh beef**	200	44.8	5.8	.....
Cod liver oil[++]	15	....	15.0	.....
Calcium carbonate[##]	3	....	....	.....
Dilute hydrochloric acid (U.S.P.) (90 drops)	....	....	....	.....
Sirup iodid of iron (U.S.P.), (2 drops)[###]	....	....	....	.....
Total nutrients...........................		74.2	71.0	286.8
Nutrients per 1,000 calories...............		35.7	34.1	137.9

*Tabulation for the period June 26, 1925-December 31, 1925 deleted. ED.
[+]Whole maize meal sifted in the kitchen and made into corn bread and mush.
[#]Served in place of the variable dry legume ration of the institution.
"From canned tomatoes, pressed through a cloth.
**Lean muscle free of visible fat.
[++]Given in place of the variable butter or margarine ration of the institution.
[##]Given to improve the mineral composition of the diet.
[###]Given with a view of correcting a possible gastric anacidity so common in pellagrins.

dence of a recurrence of pellagra, although in the light of repeated experience with this class of patients (five of the 21 who were under observation a full year had had at least two previous attacks of the disease) it is safe to state that in the absence of the beef or other equivalent preventive food upward of 40 or 50 per cent of them would have suffered a return of the disease within a period of from three to seven or eight months. The complete absence of any indication of a recurrence in any of this group of pellagrins—twenty-one of whom, as stated, were under observation for a year—would therefore seem to be conclusive evidence of the preventive action of the fresh lean beef.

Although no recurrence of pellagra was observed in any of these patients it is of much interest to note that mild evidence of beriberi developed in five of them. The most striking and constant indication of beriberi was a slight and variable edema of the legs beginning over the shins, in the feet, or in both these parts, and was noted in the first case of this group of patients about June 11, 1925, or nearly six months after the patient had begun the beef diet. Following an increase in the whole maize meal and the cowpeas at the expense of the grits and rice, designed to increase the vitamin B (antineuritic) content of the diet, the edema began to subside and before the close of the period of observation this and such other symptoms as may have been present (tachycardia, pain and tenderness of the legs) had cleared up completely. Evidently the beef diet, while adequate to prevent pellagra, was, during about the first six months of this study, slightly deficient in the beriberi vitamin. [Tabulation of composition of revised diet deleted. ED.]

Yeast

Some very favorable indications afforded by therapeutic and preventive tests of yeast in experimental black tongue of dogs (Goldberger and Wheeler, n.d.) led to a study of the action of this preparation in pellagra. The results of that study were published a year ago (Goldberger and Tanner, 1925); they indicated that dried yeast was an efficient pellagra-preventive. Toward the close of the study its favorable progress, particularly in view of the failure of casein, suggested the desirability of studying in a similar way the protein-free yeast fraction of Osborne and Wakeman (1919), and this all the more as a commercial preparation of what we understood was this fraction was available on the market. This has been done with results as follows:

We have worked with the commercial preparation marketed under the name of "Yeast Vitamin-Harris Powder" of the Harris Laboratories, Tuckahoe, N.Y. This preparation appears to have come into use in a number of laboratories as a convenient supposedly protein-free concentrate of vitamin B and is commonly but, we find, erroneously assumed to be the Osborne and Wakeman yeast fraction II (1919). It is possible that when first marketed it may have been this yeast fraction; we are advised, however, by Dr. I. F. Harris, director of the Harris Laboratories, and, with his permission, state that now this preparation is simply the dried watery (acidulated) extract of yeast prepared according to a somewhat modified Osborne and Wakeman (1919) technique. This is claimed by Doctor Harris to be but negligibly, if at all, inferior in vitamin B potency to fraction II of Osborne and Wakeman (1919).

The dose of this preparation decided on for administration to our patients was one-half of that used in the study of dried yeast, that is, 15 grams a day. (It may well be that considerably less than this may suffice as a preventive.) In a few instances and for brief periods this was increased for therapeutic purposes to 30 grams. It was given dissolved in a little tap water in equal portions at each meal during the first three months of the study. After this period it was all given at one time at the supper meal.

The basic diet given the patients receiving this vitamin powder supplement was essentially identical with that given the patients receiving beef, and is shown in Table 66.

The study was begun May 26, 1924, with the treatment of a case in a recently admitted patient with a sharp attack (dermal and mental). Since then 22 patients in all have come under this treatment. Of these, 12 presented more or less pronounced active symptoms, including the dermatitis, and 3 the stomatitis, etc. of a *pellagra sine pellagra*. Seven came under observation for purely preventive treatment, being without active symptoms of the disease at the time.

Of these 22 patients, 1 has been under observation for 16 months, 1 for 14 months, 1 for 13 months, 5 for 12 months, 2 for 8 months, 2 for 7 months, and the others for various shorter periods.

Under the treatment, the active symptoms of the disease, in those presenting such, cleared up and, what is of much greater significance, in no case while taking the yeast extract has there been any recognizable evidence of a recurrence.

Recalling that our expectation, based on long experience with this class of patients, was that some 40 or 50 per cent of them would have developed evidence of a recurrence within some three to seven or eight months in the absence of the vitamin powder or equivalent

TABLE 66—*Approximate composition of "yeast vitamin"-supplemented diet offered daily to each of a group of colored pellagrins during the period up to June 22, 1925.*[*]
(Total calories: 2,104)

Diet		Nutrients		
Articles of diet	Quan-tity	Protein	Fat	Carbo-hydrate
Basic:	Grams	Grams	Grams	Grams
Corn meal[+]	140	11.8	6.3	103.6
Corn grits...................	48	4.4	.9	36.2
Wheat flour..................	70	8.0	.7	52.5
Rice.........................	28	2.2	.1	22.1
Cowpeas (Vigna sinepsis)[#] ...	14	3.0	.2	8.5
Sirup........................	90	....	....	63.9
Lard.........................	42	....	42.0	.....
Vegetable cooking oil........	28	....	28.0	.....
Tomato juice"	130	....	....	.....
Supplemental:				
Yeast vitamine (Harris) powder[**]	15	....	....	.....
Cod liver oil[++]	15	....	15.0	.....
Calcium carbonate[##]	3	....	....	....
Dilute hydrochloric acid (U.S.P.) (90 drops)[""]	....	....	....	....
Sirup iodid of iron (U.S.P.) (2 drops)[##]	....	....	....	....
Total nutrients..................		29.4	93.2	286.8
Nutrients per 1,000 calories................		14.0	44.4	136.6

[*] Tabulation for the period June 26, 1925-December 31, 1925 deleted. ED.
[+] Whole maize meal sifted in the kitchen and made into corn bread and mush.
[#] Served in place of the variable dry legume ration of the institution.
[""] From canned tomatoes, pressed through a cloth.
[**] A commercial preparation.
[++] Given in place of the variable butter or margarine ration of the institution.
[##] Given to improve the mineral composition of the diet.
Given with a view of correcting a possible gastric anacidity so common in pellagrins.

preventive, the absence of any recurrence whatever in any of the patients, eight of whom were under observation for at least one year, is, in our judgment, conclusive evidence of the pellagra-preventive action of this yeast extract.

Here we wish to record that, as in the case of the beef study, a number of the patients taking the yeast extract developed evidence of beriberi.[4] In these, six in all, as in the five mentioned in con-

4 Having been led to believe from the literature that this preparation was exceptionally rich in vitamin B (antineuritic), this occurrence both surprised and perplexed us at first, but the development of the same syndrome in some of the patients in the beef study, together with the clearing up of

nection with the study of beef, the most striking and constant indication was a slight edema of the feet or feet and legs. This appeared first about May 24, 1925, in a patient of this group who began taking the yeast vitamin preparation on November 21, 1924, or about six months after beginning this treatment.

The changes in diet looking to an increase in the beriberi vitamin, mentioned in connection with the cases observed in the patients taking beef, were made between June 22 and June 26, 1925, and also affected the patients taking the "yeast vitamin" powder. By this date, however, three of the patients had already completed an observation period of a year, one of fully 11 months, one of 9½ months, and one of 7 months. Following the indicated modifications in the basic diet the evidence of beriberi gradually subsided and disappeared. [Tabulation of composition of revised diet deleted. ED.]

Thus the yeast extract-supplemented diet, like the beef-supplemented diet, was adequate to prevent pellagra, but, until certain modifications were made (which for certain patients were not in effect until after 7 to 12 months after beginning the "yeast vitamin" treatment), was slightly deficient in the beriberi vitamin.

Discussion

The results of previously published studies[5] have been interpreted as indicating that in the prevention and, presumably, causation of pellagra there is concerned a previously unrecognized or unappreciated dietary essential (designated as factor P–P) which may be effective with but little, possibly without any, cooperation from the protein factor. The results of the studies presented above serve, we believe, to strengthen this interpretation and to increase the probability that factor P–P plays the sole essential rôle in the prevention of the disease.

It seems well established that the muscle of beef is relatively poor in all the commonly recognized dietary essentials except protein. So that, at first thought, it might plausibly be suggested that the preventive action of fresh beef is due to this constituent. When it is recalled, however, that, in a study carried out by Goldberger and Tanner (1925), a daily supplement of 69 grams of casein (approximately 60 grams of protein) failed fully to prevent the disease, it is

---

the symptoms following upon the changes in diet designed to increase the antineuritic vitamin, convinces us that the 15 grams of "yeast vitamin" powder supplied little if any more antineuritic than did the 200 grams of fresh beef.

5　Goldberger and Tanner, 1924; 1925.

difficult to attribute the marked potency of the beef supplement to its 45 grams of protein, or, at least, to this protein alone. This difficulty is enhanced and the presence of another factor in the beef more strongly suggested when we recall the distinctly inferior pellagra-preventive potency (on the basis of protein content) of dried skim milk as compared with fresh buttermilk already referred to in the introductory section of this report.

The evidence of pellagra-preventive activity of the supplement of 15 grams of the yeast extract appears to us to point still more strongly to the existence of a special pellagra-preventive essential (factor P–P), and to the probability that this may be effective without any cooperation from the protein. This preparation is believed to be low in or lacking appreciable amounts of protein, and while it has a fairly high nitrogen content[6] it seems reasonably certain that only part of this is in a form conceivably capable of supplementing the protein of the diet. Assuming, however, that all of its nitrogen is in the form of protein, the 15 grams of the dried extract would, on this assumption, contribute at most about 7.5 grams of protein. To attribute to this small addition the preventive potency of this preparation would imply that its nitrogen is in a form possessing supplementing properties notably superior to those of not less than about 36 grams of milk proteins (dried skim milk) and to those of 60 grams of casein protein. While this may conceivably be the case it seems so highly improbable as to warrant the conclusion that the preventive action of the yeast extract is due primarily to a special pellagra-preventive substance (factor P–P).

It would appear then, that, unlike butter, fresh lean beef and yeast contain a factor (factor P–P) which probably plays the primary rôle in the prevention and the causation of pellagra.

Relation of Factor P–P to Vitamin B

If the foregoing interpretation is, as we believe, sound, it follows that the "yeast vitamin" powder with which we have worked is not, as it has generally been considered, a concentrate of vitamin B alone, but contains also and, apparently, in considerable concentration, the pellagra-preventive factor P–P. (So far as the above recorded experience with this preparation goes, it would suggest that this preparation may be richer in factor P–P than in vitamin B.)

It seems necessary at this juncture to anticipate the publication

---

6 One sample analyzed in the Division of Chemistry of the Hygienic Laboratory was found to contain 7.59 and another 7.14 per cent nitrogen.

of the results of our experimental study of black tongue of dogs. This study, begun over four years ago, is still in progress, but we may now state that we have experimentally induced this canine disease by feeding dogs certain diets previously found associated with the occurrence of pellagra, including the Rankin prison farm experimental diet (Goldberger and Wheeler, 1920). Some modifications of certain of these diets have resulted in giving us our standard experimental black-tongue-producing diet. This is shown in Table 67. In this study, white and yellow maize meal, casein, cod-liver oil, and butter have been found very poor, or lacking, in the black-tongue-preventive factor. Milk has been found to possess inferior preventive activity. A test of fresh lean beef, although not yet completed (it has three more months to run to complete a period of one year, our usual period in such cases), is sufficiently far advanced to warrant the statement that this possesses considerable black-tongue-preventive potency. [Tabulation of data deleted. ED.] Dried yeast and the commercial yeast extract referred to above have been found very efficient preventives of black tongue. Seidell's activated solid (1922) in a daily dose at the rate of 2 grams per kilo of body weight as a supplement to basic diet 123, shown in Table 67, has black-tongue-preventive action. Thus the black-tongue-preventive factor is present in lean beef muscle, in yeast, and in the commercial dried watery extract of yeast, and it is adsorbed from a watery extract of yeast by English fuller's earth. Our data appear to indicate that this factor is a dietary essential, heretofore either not recognized or not appreciated as such, necessary for the nutrition of the dog.

From the foregoing it appears that the substances that have been found to possess black-tongue-preventive potency have, when tried in pellagra, been found efficient preventives of the human disease; those that had failed in pellagra or were of low pellagra-preventive potency (milk) when tried in black tongue have failed or were feeble as preventives of the canine syndrome. In view of this striking similarity, if not identity, of behavior we feel justified in adopting, and are planning our studies of pellagra on, the working hypothesis that black tongue of dogs is the analogue of pellagra in man. Accordingly, it may tentatively be assumed that factor P–P is the dietary essential primarily concerned in the prevention and causation of both black tongue and pellagra. The assumption of this identity seems all the more reasonable as otherwise it would (and it still may) be necessary to conclude that the "yeast vitamin" powder contains in addition to the pellagra-preventive essential, also a special black-tongue-preventive factor. Thus assuming that we are

364

The Pellagra-Preventive Factor

TABLE 67—*Composition of experimental black tongue-producing diet No. 123.* On this diet recognizable signs of black tongue begin to appear in from one to three or four months. When adequately supplemented with "yeast vitamin" powder, Seidell's activated solid, autoclaved yeast, etc., black tongue does not develop.†*

(Total calories: 2,400)

Diet		Nutrients		
Articles of diet	Quan-tity	Protein	Fat	Carbo-hydrate
	Grams	Grams	Grams	Grams
Cornmeal[#]............,,......	400	33.6	18.8	296.0
Cowpeas (Vigna sinensis)"	50	10.7	.7	30.4
Casein[**] (purified)............	60	52.0	....	......
Sucrose.....................	32	.....	....	32.0
Cottonseed oil...............	30	.....	30.0	......
Cod-liver oil.................	15	.....	15.0	......
Sodium chlorid[++] ,,,..........	10	.....	.....	......
Calcium carbonate[++]	3	.....	.....	......
Total nutrients.......................		96.3	64.5	358.4
Nutrients per 1,000 calories.................		40.3	26.9	149.3

* The cornmeal, cowpeas, and salt are stirred into water and cooked one and one-half hours. Then the other ingredients are well stirred in, the total weight being brought to 2,400 grams with water (so that one gram equals one calorie) and this finished mixture is served to the dog ad libitum.
+ Tabulation of data for similar diet deleted. ED.
# This is whole maize meal sifted as for human consumption.
" The variety known as the California black-eye pea.
**Leached for a week in daily changes of acidulated water, after McCollum.
++The salt and calcium carbonate may be replaced by 22 grams of the well-known Osborne and Mendel salt mixture.

dealing with one factor (P–P) let us consider its relation to "water soluble B."

Although this water-soluble vitamin has quite generally been considered as representing a single dietary factor having both antineuritic and growth-promoting properties, a number of investigators[7] have dissented from this view and have advanced reasons for believing that it includes at least two distinct dietary essentials—one the antineuritic or beriberi vitamin (vitamin B *sensu stricto* according to Funk [1922]) and the other a "growth-promoting" factor which some workers (Funk and Dubin, 1921; Heaton, 1922) believe iden-

7 Osborne and Mendel, 1919; Mitchell, 1919; Emmett and McKim, 1917; Emmett and Luros, 1920; Sherman and Smith, 1922; Eijkman, 1922; Heller, 1923; Levene and Muhlfeld, 1923.

tical with Wildiers' bios. Thus with the possibility before us that vitamin B may include at least two distinct dietary essentials, it becomes necessary to consider the relation of factor P–P to these two at least.

In previous publications (Goldberger and Tanner, 1924; 1925) evidence was adduced that was interpreted as excluding vitamin B from consideration as essential in relation to the prevention and causation of pellagra. This had reference to vitamin B in the generally accepted sense of the antineuritic or antiberiberi vitamin. That vitamin B in this sense, that is, as the antiberiberi essential, and factor P–P are distinct and may perform their physiological functions independently, is also, and we believe quite conclusively, shown by the fact of the rare association of the two diseases beriberi and pellagra. An interesting example of this independence of action is the observation, mentioned in a preceding section, of the occurrence of beriberi in some of the patients taking the beef and in others taking the yeast extract-supplemented diets. The fact that very exceptionally the two diseases may occur together in the same patient[8] emphasizes the significance of the rarity of such association. In other words, while the diet may at the same time be deficient in both the beriberi- and the pellagra-preventive essentials, ordinarily, in endemic localities of these diseases, the diet concerned is deficient in one and not (or but inappreciably) in the other factor.

With respect to the relation of factor P–P to the second, the so-called growth-promoting essential, possibly included in the designation "water soluble B," the studies presented in the foregoing afford no basis for judgment. It may be stated in this connection, however (again anticipating the publication of certain of the results of the experimental study of black tongue), that the discovery of the black tongue- (and pellagra-) preventive potency of yeast has led to a study designed to elucidate the characters of factor P–P and thus, perhaps, aid in the determination of its identity. This study has revealed that factor P–P is adsorbed from an acidulated watery extract[9] of yeast by English fuller's earth (Seidell's activated solid); that yeast heated to charring no longer possesses appreciable black-tongue-preventive activity. After heating in the steam autoclave at 15 pounds for two and one-half hours, the yeast retains, our tests in dogs show, much, if not all, of its activity in the prevention of black tongue; but when

---

8 Schüffner and Kuenen, 1912; Saunders, 1914; Mendelson, 1923.
9 We have gained the impression that factor P–P is relatively much more soluble in acidulated water than in 85 per cent (by volume) alcohol, whereas the antineuritic is relatively readily soluble in both.

young rats are fed a diet in which the sole source of "water soluble B" is derived from as much as 30 or 40 per cent of this autoclaved yeast, and which is otherwise complete for growth, their growth is quickly arrested, their weight then declines, and they die with or without symptoms of polyneuritis. [Tabulation of composition of rat diets and graphic representation of weight changes deleted. ED.] The unheated yeast,[10] it may be noted, when fed young rats in diets at an 8 or 10 per cent level, provides sufficient "water soluble B" for good, though not for optimal, growth. Thus, according to current ideas, the heating for two and one-half hours inactivates the water-soluble vitamin (as it exists in dried yeast; it does not appreciably affect it as it exists in Seidell's activated solid), but obviously does not notably affect the P–P factor. Evidently, too, factor P–P is not of itself growth promoting. Furthermore, if the so-called growth-promoting water-soluble vitamin of the yeast is distinct from the antineuritic and from the P–P factor, then either the heating has inactivated it or, like factor P–P, it is not a special "growth" factor.

But that factor P–P or some associated (and, in yeast, relatively thermostable) factor, distinct from the antineuritic, is essential for growth (of the rat at least) would appear from the following: (1) When young rats are fed a diet complete for growth except as to "water soluble B" and containing as the sole source of this vitamin as much as 30 or 40 per cent of yeast[11] previously heated in the autoclave at 15 pounds for two and one-half hours (and from tests in dogs shown to contain P–P), they quickly decline in weight after a slight initial rise and die with or without signs of polyneuritis (antineuritic deficient). (2) When young rats are fed a diet complete for growth except as to the "water soluble B," but containing as the sole source of this vitamin as much as 40 per cent of a preparation of an alcohol extract[12] of corn meal that can alleviate or cure polyneuritis in the rat, the weight of such animals, after slight initial

10   Fleischmann's wort-grown, low temperature dried yeast was used.
11   Fleischmann's wort-grown, low temperature dried yeast was used.
12   This extract is prepared by intermittent percolation of whole white corn-meal at room temperature with alcohol of 85 per cent by volume strength, until about 6.5 liters are obtained from 5 kg. corn-meal. The percolate is put into a distilling flask and concentrated to about one-fifth to one-fourth its volume. This is then poured into a pan on a water bath and corn starch stirred into it at the rate of 125 gm. of starch to 5 kg. of corn-meal used. The remaining alcoholic liquid is driven off by fanning. The damp residue is then transferred to glass dishes and further dried in a current of warm air, after which it is ground into a powder. For each 18 to 18.5 gm. of corn-meal 1 gm. of this product is thus obtained.

growth, is arrested and then declines. (3) If, however, young rats are fed a diet, as before, complete for growth except as to the "water soluble B," but containing as sources of this vitamin as little as 8 or 10 per cent of the autoclaved yeast and as little as 5 per cent of our extract of maize meal, the animals grow.

Again, when young rats are fed a diet complete for growth except as to the "water soluble B" and containing 20 per cent of dried fresh lean beef (which, judging by experience with pellagra and black tongue, contains factor P–P) as the sole source of this vitamin, such animals, as is well known, after slight initial growth, decline in weight and die with or without polyneuritis (antineuritic deficient). [Graphic representation of growth changes deleted. ED.] If, however, when signs of polyneuritis begin to appear, there be included in such diet as little as 5 per cent of our alcoholic corn extract (40 per cent of which as the sole source of water-soluble vitamin in a diet does not enable the rat to grow), the animals, if not too far gone, recover from polyneuritis and resume growth. Evidently our alcoholic extract of maize contains an essential that cures polyneuritis in the rat, and while not growth promoting (relatively, not absolutely so) of itself, permits or promotes growth when combined in a diet otherwise complete for growth except for "water soluble B" with a suitable proportion of a P–P-containing substance such as autoclaved yeast or beef (which itself, within certain limits, neither prevents polyneuritis nor permits growth).

Thus, autoclaved yeast and beef muscle contain a factor distinct from the polyneuritis-preventing vitamin which in combination with the antineuritic is essential for the growth of the rat. From the facts presented, it seems probable that this is the same as factor P–P, and some of the work in the very confusing literature relating to the identity of the "growth-promoting" complex of "water soluble B" with bios appears to us to be in harmony with this interpretation. Further investigation will, however, be required to determine this.

In any event investigators using the rat-growth test must hereafter recognize and take due account of at least two essentials (B *sensu stricto* and P–P) where heretofore only one was considered. This is, perhaps, of special importance to those heretofore occupied in the chemical isolation of the beriberi vitamin. It may well be suspected that the highly "active" concentrates, supposedly of vitamin B (*sensu stricto*) that some of these workers have succeeded in preparing, in proportion as they enable the rat to grow in the absence of any other source of the "water soluble B" in the diet are concentrates of at least two factors. The rat-growth test may continue to be used as a test of the purity of a concentrate, but must be interpreted in a sense opposite to that heretofore current. The pure concentrate will be seemingly inert. The complete test of such a concentrate (or a food substance) will necessitate combining it alternately with an adequate proportion of a proved preparation of the antineuritic and of the P–P factor, respectively, and, perhaps, of both, and this or some equivalent test will have to be made before an apparently inactive preparation (or food) can be adjudged as really inert. It is, at least, possible that in the past, workers in discarding "inactive" fractions have unwittingly been throwing away the very thing they were laboriously seeking. This may perhaps explain, at least in part, the somewhat unaccountable losses of vitamin in the process of fractionation of "active" preparations.

In closing it may be permitted to suggest that investigators interested in the isolation of vitamin B may find maize a better source of this factor than yeast, since maize is much poorer in the associated thermostable factor or factors than is yeast.

Summary and Conclusions

1. Previous trials of butter in a daily quantity of about 140 grams (5 ounces) using a Georgia product had practically invariably failed to prevent recurrence of pellagra. Further trials with a Vermont product proved no more favorable than those with the Georgia butter.

Butter would seem to be poor, or lacking, in the pellagra-preventive factor or factors.

2. The pellagra-preventive action of a daily allowance of 200 grams (7 ounces) of fresh meat in the form of lean beef was tested and found capable of completely preventing the disease, thus proving that fresh beef contains the pellagra-preventive factor or factors.

The beef-supplemented diet, though adequate for pellagra prevention, was, during about half of the period of study, slightly deficient in the beriberi vitamin.

3. The pellagra-preventive action of a dried yeast extract was tested in a daily quantity of 15 grams (half an ounce) and found efficient in preventing the disease.

The yeast-extract-supplemented diet was adequate to prevent pellagra, but, during a part of the period of observation, was slightly deficient in the beriberi vitamin.

4. The results of the studies presented are believed to strengthen the interpretation of those previously reported, namely, that in the prevention and presumably causation of pellagra there is concerned

a heretofore unrecognized or not fully appreciated dietary essential (factor P–P), and to indicate the probability that this may play the sole essential rôle in relation to the disease.

5. A statement of a preliminary character is made of some of the results of an experimental study of black tongue, and it is briefly pointed out that the substances that have been found to possess black-tongue-preventive potency have, when tried in pellagra, been found efficient preventives of the human disease and that those that had failed in pellagra, or were of low pellagra-preventive potency, when tried in black tongue have failed, or were feeble, as preventives of the canine disease. The working hypothesis has therefore been adopted that black tongue of dogs is the analogue of pellagra in man, and thus that factor P–P is concerned in the prevention and causation of both black tongue and pellagra.

6. The relation of the factor P–P to "water soluble B" is considered and evidence is cited showing: First, that the antineuritic factor (vitamin B *sensu stricto*) is distinct from the factor P–P and does not in itself suffice for the growth of the rat; second, that if the term "water soluble B" includes, as some investigators have suggested, in addition to the antineuritic factor a so-called growth-promoting essential (possibly identical with Wildiers' bios), this, like the antineuritic factor, is either inactivated by autoclaving, or does not suffice by itself for the growth of the rat; third, that factor P–P or some associated, and, in yeast, like P–P, thermostable factor (possibly the so-called growth-promoting factor) distinct from the antineuritic vitamin, though not sufficing in itself for the growth of the rat, is, in combination with the antineuritic, essential for growth in rats.

7. Whether factor P–P is, as at present seems most probable, identical with the so-called growth-promoting essential heretofore included (with the antineuritic) in the term "water soluble vitamin B," or whether these are distinct, further investigation must determine.

References

Annual Report of the Surgeon General of the Public Health Service of the United States for the Fiscal Year 1924 (Washington, D.C., 1924), p. 22.
Chittenden, R. H., and Underhill, F. P. *Am. J. Physiol.* (Baltimore), Vol. 44 (1917), pp. 13–66.
Eijkman, C., *et al. J. Biol. Chem.*, Vol. 50 (1922), p. 311.
Emmett, A. D., and Luros, G. O. *J. Biol. Chem.*, Vol. 43 (1920), p. 265.
Emmett, A. D., and McKim, L. H. *J. Biol. Chem.*, Vol. 32 (1917), p. 409.

Funk, C. *The Vitamines* (Baltimore, 1922), p. 39.
———, and Dubin. *J. Biol. Chem.*, Vol. 48 (1921), p. 437.
Goldberger, J., and Tanner, W. F. *Public Health Rep.* (Washington, D.C.), Vol. 39 (1924), pp. 87–107.
———. *Public Health Rep.* (Washington, D.C.), Vol. 40 (1925), pp. 54–80.
Goldberger, J., Waring, C. H., and Tanner, W. F. *Public Health Rep.* (Washington, D.C.), Vol. 38 (1923), pp. 2361–68.
Goldberger, J., Waring, C. H., and Willets, D. G. *Public Health Rep.* (Washington, D.C.), Vol. 30 (1915), pp. 3117–31.
Goldberger, J., and Wheeler, G. A. *Hyg. Lab. Bull.* (U.S. Public Health Service, No. 120), Washington, D.C., 1920.
———. Unpublished data.
———, and Sydenstricker, E. *Public Health Rep.* (Washington, D.C.), Vol. 35 (1920), pp. 648–713.
Heaton, T. B. *Biochem. J.*, Vol. 16 (1922), p. 800.
Heller, V. G. *J. Biol. Chem.*, Vol. 55 (1923), p. 394.
Levene, P. A., and Muhlfeld, M. *J. Biol. Chem.*, Vol. 57 (1923), p. 341.
Mendelson, R. W. *J. Trop. Med. and Hyg.*, Vol. 26 (1923), p. 6.
Mitchell, H. H. *J. Biol. Chem.*, Vol. 40 (1919), p. 399.
Osborne, T. B., and Mendel, L. B. *J. Biol. Chem.*, Vol. 37 (1919), p. 594.
Osborne, T. B., and Wakeman, A. J. *J. Biol. Chem.*, Vol. 40 (1919), p. 383.
Saunders, E. B. *Trans. Natl. Assn. for Study of Pellagra* (Columbia, S.C., 1914), p. 325.
Schüffner, W., and Kuenen, W. A. *Arch. f. Schiff u. Trop. Hyg.* (Leipzig), Vol. 16 (1912), pp. 277–304.
Seidell, A. *Public Health Rep.* (Washington, D.C.), Vol. 37 (1922), p. 801.
Sherman, H. C., and Smith, S. *The Vitamines* (1922), pp. 48–54.
Underhill, F. P., and Mendel, L. B. *Public Health Rep.* (Washington, D.C.), Vol. 40 (1925), pp. 1087–89.
Wheeler, G. A., Goldberger, J., and Blackstock, M. R. *Public Health Rep.* (Washington, D.C.), Vol. 37 (1922), pp. 1063–69.

PART FIVE

Summation

17. *Pellagra: Its Nature and Prevention*[1]

JOSEPH GOLDBERGER

In the following pages an attempt is made to answer as simply as possible some of the more important questions which the general public frequently asks in regard to pellagra.

Symptoms

Although the fully developed disease makes a picture which, when once seen, can hardly ever fail to be recognized even by one who is not a physician, the diagnosis of the disease is by no means always easy, because the fully developed cases form only a small proportion of the total. Difficulties may arise also in that other conditions at times present signs or symptoms which the untrained and inexperienced may mistake for those of pellagra.

The following sketch of the symptoms is presented, therefore, not with the idea that it will enable the untrained to recognize the disease, but rather to call attention to those symptoms or combinations of symptoms which should be looked upon as suspicious and as calling for the simple and effective measures of prevention to be outlined.

In a fairly well developed though not advanced case the disease shows itself by a variety of symptoms, of which an eruption, weakness, nervousness, and indigestion form the most distinctive combination.

Eruption.—The eruption is the most characteristic telltale of the disease and the main reliance in its recognition. When the eruption first shows itself it may look very much like, and frequently is mistaken for, a sunburn. The sunburned appearance soon changes and in many cases the reddened skin turns to a somewhat dirty brown and frequently acquires a parchmentlike appearance, then quickly becomes rough and scaly, or cracks and peels. In some instances, however, the beginning redness is not noticed or perhaps does not occur, the first and possibly the only thing observed being the dirty-looking scaly patch of skin appearing very much like and frequently thought to be no more than a simple weathering or chapping.

Among the most distinctive peculiarities of the eruption is its

1 *Public Health Rep.,* Vol. 42, No. 35 (September 2, 1927), 2193-2200.

preference for certain parts of the body surface. The backs of the
hands, forearms, and the backs of the feet are its favorite sites. Other
parts not infrequently attacked are the sides or front of the neck or
both, the face, arms, elbows, legs, and knees. Another marked
peculiarity of the eruption is its tendency to appear at about the
same time and to cover similar areas, both as to extent and peculiarities of outline, on both sides of the body. Thus it may be stated as
the rule that if the back of one hand or of one foot, one elbow, one
knee, one side of the neck, one cheek, or the lid of one eye is affected,
then the corresponding part on the other side of the body is, or soon
becomes, similarly affected, and affected to almost exactly the same
extent. This rule, however, is not without many exceptions. It must
not be hastily assumed, therefore, that the possibility of pellagra is
necessarily excluded because the back of one hand or of one foot
or of one side of the neck alone seems to be involved, or is involved
to so slight an extent as to be almost nothing in comparison with
the involvement of the other side.

Suspicious symptoms.—Although the main reliance in the recognition of the disease, the eruption of pellagra not infrequently is very
tardy in making its appearance. While it is ordinarily impossible to
determine the presence or absence of the disease with certainty until
the eruption appears, a shrewd suspicion may, nevertheless, be
formed from a careful consideration of the other symptoms. This
applies only to a limited extent to children, in most of whom the
manifestations of the disease, other than the eruption, are slight and
frequently difficult or impossible to make out. Notwithstanding this,
however, careful questioning of the mother, if she be observant, not
infrequently develops the fact that the child seems to her less active
than common; in some cases it is evidently listless or fretful, and the
mother may also recognize that it has fallen off in weight. In older
individuals a complaint of loss of strength with indigestion or nervousness, or both, coming on or made worse in the late winter or
spring and improving in the fall, are very frequently met with. The
patient may complain of being "worked out" or of having "blind
staggers" (dizziness, vertigo), of discomfort or pain in the pit of
the stomach, frequently of headache, sometimes of wakefulness, frequently also of sluggishness of the bowels requiring, possibly, the
habitual use of medicine to move them. Although, as has already
been said, these symptoms alone or even with the addition of such
symptoms as a burning or scalded feeling of the mouth, reddened
tongue, burning of the hands or feet, and loose bowels, are not
enough to distinguish pellagra from other conditions, they are ample

to justify a suspicion of the disease, especially if such individual is known to be finicky or a nibbler about food, or has been living on a diet made up largely of biscuits, corn bread, grits, gravy, and sirup, with little or no milk or lean meat and but a small amount of vegetables and fruit.

The suspicion of pellagra may with confidence be dismissed in one who is known to be, and to have been, a habitual milk drinker and meat eater. It is well to be warned, however, that it is very easy to be misled about what and, particularly, as to how much the individual actually eats. The question of quantity is of the utmost importance. It is not enough merely to nibble; one must consume a substantial quantity of these or other preventive foods to supply fully the body's needs.

Insanity.—In a small proportion of cases, fortunately much smaller than is commonly believed, the mind is affected to a degree requiring asylum care. Many of these cases get well under treatment. Recovery of the mind is not to be expected, however, when, as frequently happens, the pellagra occurs in a person whose mental disturbance is due to some other (incurable) cause.

Importance and Distribution

Under proper treatment and with careful nursing, only a small percentage of cases die; nevertheless, the actual number of deaths is deplorably large. As deplorable, if not even more so, is the great amount of sickness and debility, much of it vague and ill-defined and thus frequently unrecognized, which pellagra must be charged with causing. It is probable that in each year for every death attributed to the disease there are fully 20 persons with clearly recognizable attacks and probably as many more with debility from the same cause but not definitely marked as such.

In the United States the disease occurs most frequently in the area south of the Potomac and Ohio Rivers. Indeed, in many of the southern states pellagra still is one of the foremost causes of death. In other parts of the country the disease is very much less common. This difference is due mainly to the different dietary habits of the people in the northern and western part of the country and to the better conditions of food supply.

Relation to Living Cost

The disease may occur anywhere and in anyone, but it is the poor man who is the chief sufferer from it. This explains why hard times, especially when accompanied by rising food prices, are likely to be followed by an increase in the disease. This is well illustrated by the great increase that took place in 1915 following the hard times brought on by the outbreak of the war in Europe in the summer of 1914, and by the great decrease in 1916 following the improvement in conditions that developed during 1915. Unfortunately, the upward trend of living cost in the fall and winter of 1916 brought about an increase of pellagra in 1917 in many localities. Similarly, the postwar deflation of 1920 was followed by an increase of pellagra in many localities in 1921.

Cause

Pellagra not "catching."—Experimental tests and careful observations show that pellagra is not a communicable disease. No germ that can properly be considered its cause has ever been found. Attempts to give persons pellagra by inoculations of blood or saliva and of other body discharges from severe cases of pellagra have failed completely. On the other hand, when 11 convicts were fed on an unbalanced diet composed mainly of biscuit, corn bread, grits, rice, gravy, and sirup, with only a moderate amount of vegetables and no milk, meat, or fruit, at least six developed the disease. Furthermore, it was observed that in an asylum where many of the inmates developed pellagra year after year the nurses and helpers who lived with them never developed the disease. The only discoverable reason for the exemption of the nurses and helpers was a better diet. The nurses and helpers had a liberal allowance of lean meat and some milk, while the inmates had very little or none. When this observation was tested by giving the inmates a better diet—that is, by giving them more meat, milk, fruit, and vegetables—it was found that they stopped having pellagra. This test was also carried out at three orphanages where there had been many cases in the children every spring for several years, and always with the same result. After the diet was improved, although no other change was made, pellagra disappeared. Attempts to prevent pellagra by other means have succeeded only when a change in diet (whether intentional or not) was also made.

Unbalanced diet.—The foregoing facts, together with others which cannot be here set forth, show that pellagra is caused by subsisting on a special kind of faulty or unbalanced diet, and that people who consume a mixed, well-balanced, and varied diet—such, for example, as that furnished to our soldiers and sailors—do not have the disease. Stated more specifically, it may be said that pellagra results from a deficiency in the diet of a pellagra-preventing dietary essential **or** vitamin, which has been named vitamin P–P. This deficiency arises when the diet does not include *enough* of the foods which carry the vitamin P–P to supply the needs of the body for this food factor. This does not mean that the diet that leads to pellagra is entirely devoid of this essential vitamin. On the contrary, it is probable that what may be called a pellagra-producing diet always contains some but not *enough* for the nutritive needs of some or all of those living on it.

The main, or basic, portion of the diet of the rural population of the South is made up of the following foods: Cornmeal, hominy grits, white wheat flour, white-rice, dried beans, "white meat" (salt pork), sorghum or cane molasses, and collards, or "greens." Because of the three principal components, namely, meal, "meat," and molasses, to which this diet in hard times tends to be restricted, it is designated in common parlance as the "Three M's." This basic diet, when made up in conventional proportions, is pellagra-producing. It contains some vitamin P–P derived from the cornmeal, dried beans, and collards, but ordinarily this is much too little to prevent pellagra. A sufficient increase in the beans and collards, or, much better, the addition of some other food or foods containing this vitamin, would tend to diminish or altogether prevent the occurrence of the disease.

When the disease develops it may be taken as a certain indication that for some reason there has not been included in the diet *enough* of the foods containing vitamin P–P. This reason may be any one or some combination of the following:

1. Individual peculiarity or eccentricity of taste, particularly under circumstances affording but little variety of P–P rich foods from which to choose. This may be exemplified by some of those (including certain types of insane) who may have a dislike for milk, for eggs, for fowl, etc. In this connection may be mentioned also the improper dieting that may accompany a prolonged alcoholic debauch.

2. A short available supply of the P–P rich foods, resulting from (a) inaccessibility to market, (b) difficulties of transportation, particularly of the perishable foods, (c) an epizootic among some of the domestic animals (milch cows, poultry, swine), (d) fencing laws which may make it impracticable for many to keep milch cows, or (e) destructive storms or overflows which may lead directly or indirectly to a reduction in the number of domestic animals (milch cows, goats, poultry, or swine) and to a shortage of fresh vegetables from the loss of gardens, etc.

3. Insufficient cash or credit available for the purchase of such

food, resulting from unemployment, insufficient income from crops, extravagance with respect to expenditures for purposes (amusements, automobiles) other than for food, shiftlessness.

Prevention and Treatment

The pellagra-preventing vitamin is believed to be present in nearly, if not quite, all natural foods except the oils and fats, but in very greatly varying amounts. Thus, there is very little in corn meal, white flour, or rice; somewhat more in wheat middlings, and a great deal in lean meat and powdered yeast. Unfortunately, it is not yet known just how much each food contains nor how much the body must have for the maintenance of health. In considering prevention and treatment it is, therefore, necessary to proceed on general principles, guided by such knowledge of relative values as we already have.

Milk.—Although not rich in the pellagra-preventing vitamin, milk, whether as sweet milk or buttermilk, is one of the most valuable single foods for the prevention and cure of pellagra. But when lean meat, powdered yeast, vegetables, and fruits are not included in the diet or only infrequently, or in small amounts, it must be taken in liberal quantities—at least three or four glassfuls (about 2 pints) daily—in order to insure an adequate preventive effect.

Ownership of a good milch cow is a valuable means of insuring an adequate supply of milk for the family and thus of preventing pellagra, and should be encouraged to the utmost.

Lean meat (beef, mutton, pork, fish, fowl, etc.).—Lean beef has been found to be quite rich in the pellagra-preventing vitamin. The same is very probably true of such other lean animal flesh foods as those of mutton, pork (ham, shoulder, liver, kidneys), fresh or canned fish (as, for example, salmon), and poultry. For pellagra-preventive purposes, when it is the main reliance, an adult will need nearly half a pound of a lean meat a day.

Powdered yeast.—Dried pure yeast is the richest P–P containing food at present known. It is also very rich in protein and in the beriberi-preventing vitamin, so that it should rate high as a food. This yeast is a microscopic plant cell used in baking and brewing. For use as a food the yeast plant should preferably be dead. In the home it may readily be killed by stirring the dry powder into some water and then boiling for about one minute. In the adult, 1 ounce a day (or two teaspoonfuls three times a day) of the pure powdered yeast will of itself suffice to prevent pellagra. It may be taken in any way that is most convenient as, for example, in water, in milk, in tomato juice, in sirup or molasses, etc.

The valuable dietary properties of powdered yeast suggest the importance of its consideration for general inclusion in the dietary.

Eggs.—There is reason to believe that eggs contain the pellagra-preventing vitamin which is probably present exclusively in the yolk. As a preventive food, eggs are probably inferior to lean meat.

Vegetables and fruits.—There is reason to believe that all vegetables—potatoes, turnips, string beans, tomatoes, cabbage, collards, turnip greens, spinach—and the fruits contain the pellagra-preventing vitamin, but, probably like milk, in small amounts. Thus, it probably requires nearly 2 pounds of tomatoes (about 1 quart of canned tomato juice) to produce about the same preventive effect as a quart of buttermilk or as about half a pound of lean meat, or as 1 ounce of powdered yeast. Notwithstanding this, however, the vegetables are valuable foods for balancing the diet, but must be eaten in liberal amounts.

The cultivation of more and better gardens in the area of pellagra endemicity would be very helpful in the prevention and eradication of pellagra and should be encouraged in all possible ways.

The foods that have preventive action have, of course, also curative value; but in the face of an actual or impending attack of pellagra, it is manifestly advantageous to begin the treatment with foods that are rich in the P–P vitamin and that at the same time are within the digestive capacity of the patient. With these considerations in mind, powdered yeast, milk (sweet or buttermilk), lean meat (fresh meat juice, scraped beef), egg yolk, tomato juice (fresh or canned tomatoes) should be given preference.

The foods of first choice, in suitable quantities, should be given at regular intervals just as is done with medicine. Indeed, for the prevention and cure of pellagra the only medicine we have is food. There is no drug known that actually serves any useful purpose in this disease unless it is to mitigate or relieve painful or disturbing symptoms.

Care must be taken to see that the food prescribed is actually eaten. It is to be borne in mind that some individuals must be educated or re-educated to proper food habits. Unsatisfactory results from treatment are frequently attributable to a failure to bear this in mind and to take precautions accordingly.

Of the powdered yeast, 1 ounce a day will ordinarily be enough for an adult, or half of this for a child under 12 years of age. More may be given in cases of exceptional gravity. It may be advantageously administered (one or two teaspoonfuls three to six times a day) in milk, tomato juice, fruit juice, or sirup. Where yeast happens not to be available, and in cases where solid food cannot for any reason be taken, milk and tomato juice may be depended on. The juice pressed from fresh beef, or raw egg yolk, or both, may, and if practicable should, be given in addition to the milk and the tomato juice. A bean or pea soup (purée), with or without milk or meat juice, may be used as a palatable and valuable addition to the liquid diet.

As the ability to take solid food returns, scraped or finely minced beef or other lean meat may be included in the feeding. The diet should be increased as rapidly as the digestive ability of the patient permits. In the average case the patient, if carefully fed, will be fully convalescent in from six to twelve weeks.

Recurrence

Recovery from an attack does not mean, however, that thereafter the disease will not recur. It may or will return if one's diet again becomes faulty in the special way above described. To avoid having a return of the disease there is one and only one known way, and that is by a proper diet at all times and at all seasons. In order to assure this for those in the area of pellagra endemicity, every effort must be made by the individual and by persons in positions of influence to improve available food supplies by the promotion of diversified farming, the ownership of good milch cows, and the cultivation of more and better gardens.

Appendix

PUBLICATIONS ON PELLAGRA
BY GOLDBERGER AND HIS ASSOCIATES

*Items marked with asterisk
are those included in the text*

1914

*1. Goldberger, J. "The etiology of pellagra: the significance of certain epidemiological observations with respect thereto," *Public Health Reports,* 29 (June 26, 1914), 1683–86.

*2. ———. "The cause and prevention of pellagra," *Public Health Reports,* 29 (September 11, 1914), 2354–57.

3. Lorenz, W. F. "The treatment of pellagra: clinical notes on pellagrins receiving an excessive diet," *Public Health Reports,* 29 (September 11, 1914), 2357–60.

4. Goldberger, J., Waring, C. H., and Willets, D. G. "The treatment and prevention of pellagra," *Public Health Reports,* 29 (October 23, 1914), 2821–25.

1915

*5. ———, ———, and ———. "The prevention of pellagra: a test of diet among institutional inmates," *Public Health Reports,* 30 (October 22, 1915), 3117–31.

*6. Sydenstricker, E. "The prevalence of pellagra: its possible relation to the rise in the cost of food," *Public Health Reports,* 30 (October 22, 1915), 3132–48.

7. Goldberger, J., Waring, C. H., and Willets, D. G. "A test of diet in the prevention of pellagra," *Southern Medical Journal,* 8 (1915), 1043–44.

8. Willets, D. G. "The treatment of pellagra by diet," *Southern Medical Journal,* 8 (1915), 1044–47.

9. Goldberger, J., and Wheeler, G. A. "Experimental pellagra in the human subject brought about by a restricted diet," *Public Health Reports,* 30 (November 12, 1915), 3336–39.

1916

10. Goldberger, J. "Pellagra: causation and a method of prevention, a summary of some of the recent studies of the United

States Public Health Service," *Journal American Medical Association*, 66 (1916), 471–76.

11. ———, and Wheeler, G. A. "The alleged production of pellagra by an unbalanced diet—a reply," *Journal American Medical Association*, 66 (1916), 977.

*12. Goldberger, J. "The transmissibility of pellagra: experimental attempts at transmission to the human subject," *Public Health Reports*, 31 (November 17, 1916), 3159–73.

1917

13. ———. "The transmissibility of pellagra—experimental attempts at transmission to the human subject," *Southern Medical Journal*, 10 (1917), 277–86.

1918

14. ———, Wheeler, G. A., and Sydenstricker, E. "A study of the diet of nonpellagrous and of pellagrous households in textile mill communities in South Carolina in 1916," *Journal American Medical Association*, 71 (1918), 944–49.

15. Goldberger, J. "Pellagra: its nature and prevention," *Public Health Reports*, 33 (April 5, 1918), 481–88.

1920

*16. ———, and Wheeler, G. A. "The experimental production of pellagra in human subjects by means of diet," *Hygienic Laboratory Bulletin*, No. 120 (February, 1920), 7–116.

17. Sullivan, M. X., and Jones, K. K. "The chemical composition of the Rankin Farm pellagra-producing experimental diet," *Hygienic Laboratory Bulletin*, No. 120 (February, 1920), 117–26.

18. Sullivan, M. X. "A biological study of a diet resembling the Rankin Farm diet," *Hygienic Laboratory Bulletin*, No. 120 (February, 1920), 127–40.

19. ———. "Feeding experiments with the Rankin Farm pellagra-producing experimental diet," *Hygienic Laboratory Bulletin*, No. 120 (February, 1920), 141–56.

20. Goldberger, J., and Wheeler, G. A. "Experimental pellagra in white male convicts," *Archives Internal Medicine*, 25 (1920), 451–71.

*21. ———, ———, and Sydenstricker, E. "A study of the relation of diet to pellagra incidence in seven textile-mill communities of South Carolina in 1916," *Public Health Reports,* 35 (March 19, 1920), 648–713.

*22. ———, ———, and ———. "Pellagra incidence in relation to sex, age, season, occupation, and 'disabling sickness' in seven cotton-mill villages of South Carolina during 1916," *Public Health Reports,* 35 (July 9, 1920), 1650–64.

*23. ———, ———, ———, and Tarbett, R. E. "A study of the relation of factors of a sanitary character to pellagra incidence in seven cotton-mill villages of South Carolina in 1916," *Public Health Reports,* 35 (July 16, 1920), 1701–14.

*24. Goldberger, J., Wheeler, G. A., and Sydenstricker, E. "A study of the relation of family income and other economic factors to pellagra incidence in seven cotton-mill villages of South Carolina in 1916," *Public Health Reports,* 35 (November 12, 1920), 2673–2714.

25. Goldberger, J. "The pellagra outbreak in Egypt," *Lancet,* 2 (1920), 41–42.

26. ———. "Some commonly misapprehended points in the diagnosis of pellagra," *Military Surgeon,* 47 (1920), 94–99.

1922

27. ———. "The relation of diet to pellagra," *Journal American Medical Association,* 78 (1922), 1676–80.

28. ———. "A consideration of deficiency diseases: diseases resulting from faulty diets," *Virginia Medical Monthly,* 49 (1922), 489–94.

*29. ———, and Tanner, W. F. "Amino-acid deficiency probably the primary etiological factor in pellagra," *Public Health Reports,* 37 (March 3, 1922), 462–86.

30. ———, and ———. "An amino-acid deficiency as the primary etiologic factor in pellagra," *Journal American Medical Association,* 79 (1922), 2132–35.

31. Wheeler, G. A., Goldberger, J., and Blackstock, M. R. "On the probable identity of the Chittenden-Underhill pellagra-like syndrome in dogs and 'black-tongue,'" *Public Health Reports,* 37 (May 5, 1922), 1063–69.

1923

*32. Goldberger, J., Waring, C. H., and Tanner, W. F. "Pellagra prevention by diet among institutional inmates," *Public Health Reports,* 38 (October 12, 1923), 2361–68.

33. Goldberger, J., Tanner, W. F., and Saye, E. B. "A case of

black tongue, with post-mortem findings," *Public Health Reports,* 38 (November 16, 1923), 2711–15.

1924

34. Goldberger, J., and Tanner, W. F. "A study of the treatment and prevention of pellagra: experiments showing the value of fresh meat and of milk, the therapeutic failure of gelatin, and the preventive failure of butter and of cod-liver oil," *Public Health Reports,* 39 (January 18, 1924), 87–107.

1925

*35. ———, and ———. "A study of the pellagra-preventive action of dried beans, casein, dried milk, and brewers' yeast, with a consideration of the essential preventive factors involved," *Public Health Reports,* 40 (January 9, 1925), 54–80.

36. Goldberger, J., Wheeler, G. A., and Tanner, W. F. "Yeast in the treatment of pellagra and black tongue; a note on dosage and mode of administration," *Public Health Reports,* 40 (May 8, 1925), 927–28.

1926

*37. Goldberger, J., Wheeler, G. A., Lillie, R. D., and Rogers, L. M. "A further study of butter, fresh beef, and yeast as pellagra preventives, with consideration of the relation of factor P–P of pellagra (and black tongue of dogs) to vitamin B," *Public Health Reports,* 41 (February 19, 1926), 297–318.

38. Goldberger, J., and Lillie, R. D. "A note on an experimental pellagra-like condition in the albino rat," *Public Health Reports,* 41 (May 28, 1926), 1025–1029.

39. Goldberger, J. "The present status of our knowledge of the etiology of pellagra," *Medicine,* 5 (1926), 79–104.

1927

40. ———, and Wheeler, G. A. "A study of the pellagra-preventive action of the tomato, carrot, and rutabaga turnip," *Public Health Reports,* 42 (May 13, 1927), 1299–1306.

*41. Goldberger, J. "Pellagra: its nature and prevention," *Public Health Reports,* 42 (September 2, 1927), 2193–2200.

42. ———, and Wheeler, G. A. "A study of the pellagra-preventive action of the cowpea (vigna sinensis) and of com-

mercial wheat germ," *Public Health Reports,* 42 (September 30, 1927), 2383–91.

*43. Goldberger, J., and Sydenstricker, E. "Pellagra in the Mississippi flood area: report of an inquiry relating to the prevalence of pellagra in the area affected by the overflow of the Mississippi and its tributaries in Tennessee, Arkansas, Mississippi, and Louisiana in the spring of 1927," *Public Health Reports,* 42 (November 4, 1927), 2706–25.

44. Goldberger, J. "The present status of our knowledge of the etiology of pellagra," Johns Hopkins University School of Hygiene, *DeLamar Lectures, 1925–1926* (Baltimore, 1927), 128–53.

1928

45. ——, and Wheeler, G. A. "Experimental black tongue of dogs and its relation to pellagra," *Public Health Reports,* 43 (January 27, 1928), 172–217.

46. Goldberger, J., Wheeler, G. A., Lillie, R. D., and Rogers, L. M. "A further study of experimental blacktongue with special reference to the blacktongue preventive in yeast," *Public Health Reports,* 43 (March 23, 1928), 657–94.

47. ——, ——, ——, and ——. "A study of the blacktongue-preventive action of 16 foodstuffs, with special reference to the identity of blacktongue of dogs and pellagra of man," *Public Health Reports,* 43 (June 8, 1928), 1385–1454.

*48. Goldberger, J., Wheeler, G. A., Sydenstricker, E., and King, W. I. "A study of endemic pellagra in some cotton-mill villages of South Carolina: an abstract," *Public Health Reports,* 43 (October 12, 1928), 2645–47.

1929

49. ——, ——, ——, and ——. "A study of endemic pellagra in some cotton-mill villages of South Carolina," *Hygienic Laboratory Bulletin,* No. 153 (January, 1929), 1–85.

50. Goldberger, J., and Wheeler, G. A. "A study of the pellagra-preventive action of canned salmon," *Public Health Reports,* 44 (November 15, 1929), 2769–71.

51. Goldberger, J., "Pellagra," *Journal American Dietetic Association,* 4 (1929), 221–27.

1930

52. ——, Wheeler, G. A., Rogers, L. M., and Sebrell, W. H. "A study of the blacktongue preventive value of leached

commercial casein, together with a test of the blacktongue preventive action of a high protein diet," *Public Health Reports*, 45 (February 7, 1930), 273–82.

53. ———, ———, ———, and ———. "A study of the blacktongue preventive value of lard, salt pork, dried green peas, and canned haddock," *Public Health Reports*, 45 (June 6, 1930), 1297–1308.

54. Goldberger, J., and Sebrell, W. H. "The blacktongue preventive value of Minot's liver extract," *Public Health Reports*, 45 (December 12, 1930), 3064–70.

Index

387